D0913402

BETWEEN THEIR
WORLD AND OURS

BETWEEN THEIR
WORLD AND OURS

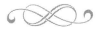

*Breakthroughs with
Autistic Children*

Karen Zelan

St. Martin's Press
New York

www.stmartins.com

ISBN 0-312-31375-6

First Edition: May 2003

10 9 8 7 6 5 4 3 2 1

To the children,
parents, and teachers
who inspired this book

To Kris, the guardian
of ideas

To Joe, the arbiter
of words

Contents

Note to the Reader

To protect their identities, I have given fictitious names to the young people whose stories comprise this book. The names of the teachers have also been changed. Throughout the book I use the personal pronoun appropriate to the subject of the narratives. If the ideas I advance were suggested by the progress of a young autistic girl, I use the pronoun *she*, even if I'm not describing a particular child.

Prologue

Michael, row the boat ashore,
Allaluyah . . .
Michael's boat is a music boat,
Allaluyah . . .
—CIVIL WAR FOLK SONG

Every author has a personally compelling reason for writing a book. Usually it embodies ideas one has been mulling over for years. One reason for my enduring interest in autistic children stems from my childhood. I couldn't have been more than four or five when I began to wish desperately that I had no feelings. These feverish desires no doubt stemmed from particular experiences when, like many a child, I felt buffeted about by an arbitrary world that often raised my hopes only to dash them. I'd seek comfort in music, running my fingers over the off-pitch keys of the piano my parents had just bought. The music seemed to envelop me in my sorrow, to purge my anger, to bathe me in euphoria as I caressed those piano keys and arranged them in a melodic jumble, in harmonic tiers.

Luck had it that the first autistic children I connected with often expressed themselves through music. They would communicate by singing, as if song were their special language. At other times, when they were isolated and wild, aloof and dreamy, they seemed to have accomplished what I tried out as a child. They would apparently turn off all sentiment as routinely as one flicks a light switch. One of my autistic charges, Marcia, could fade into nothingness, silently, unobtrusively, faster than the blink of an eye. I watched as her face quickly lost all feeling, as she began, then, to stare out at emptiness, blankly.

How does she *do* that? I asked myself, astonished. Why *would* she do it? Did she feel, as I had, frustrated by an arbitrary world?

I later realized that it was when Marcia felt surrounded by intrusive demands and noisy chaos that she vanished in this way; she simply was not there. Oh, how I had sometimes wished not to be anywhere when I was a child!

Eleven-year-old Marcia had fewer than a hundred words in her spoken vocabulary and scarcely any interest in using them. Yet she'd lapse into song frequently enough to reveal how she was feeling. Luckily, her singing vocabulary was larger than her speaking vocabulary! Once when she seemed comfortable in the company of the other children with whom she lived, she abruptly joined them to sing the folk song "Michael, Row the Boat Ashore." She sang expressively about coming ashore and even more so about coming ashore in a music boat. I was amazed at the mellifluous clarity of her song, how melodically she put her thoughts to music, whereas expressing anything in words seemed utter torture or completely beyond her. I thought Marcia, too, might "come ashore" to join with the others as she sang in her "music boat," to emerge from her solitude into the world of people, far from the lonely island she seemed to inhabit much of the time. Did she realize the implications of what she sang with us so lyrically?

I had begun to work at the University of Chicago's Orthogenic School, then directed by Bruno Bettelheim, some twelve years after psychiatrist Leo Kanner coined the term "early infantile autism." I spent eight years at the School, from 1956 to 1964. During my tenure there, I counseled fourteen girls in two groups of five to eight children. Some of the girls graduated during this time, one moved into another group, and I worked for the last five years with a stable group of eight girls. Marcia and another autistic child, Stacy, were with me for seven and six years, respectively. I also became acquainted with many students who were not in my group, including quite a few young autists. I found myself gravitating toward them on the way to the common dining room or on the playground.

Each dormitory group was staffed by two counselors. The children were in class with their teachers from nine to three, Monday through Friday, and in their dorms before and after class and on weekends. The students developed strong relationships with one or both counselors and with their teachers. The staff also spent individual time with their charges during shopping trips, during visits to the dentist or the doctor, and in psychotherapeutic sessions. I met with both Marcia and Stacy in individual sessions.

The School was also staffed by two psychiatric social workers who took the child's developmental history from the parents. Bettelheim interviewed the parents and the children upon their admission to the School. By design, the rest of the staff had no direct contact with the parents.

Bettelheim believed that to work effectively with a child, the staff must be free of the past's influence on the child, even that of the parents who, in many cases, had struggled valiantly to care for their wayward children. The children should be in a wholly new environment, one especially created for them, if they had failed to adjust to home and school and had failed to form friendships. Only a new and different setting, free of connotations from the past, would convince them that life could be different, that, ultimately, they could change their lives for the better.[1]

The staff wrote monthly reports for the parents. We described the gains made by the child and the work needed for a more complete recovery. We got glimpses of the parents from discussions with the children about the parents' letters to them, from conversations about their visits with their parents and their memories of home life before they entered the School. As I lived and worked with troubled children, including Marcia, who could evanesce into nothingness, and Stacy, who was wild and attacking, I learned how they agonized over their limitations, how they viewed themselves in their world and in ours.

Yet this was a time of personal upheaval for me, when my hopes, my dreams, my vision of the future broadened suddenly and propitiously. I was experiencing postadolescent optimism, sometimes unrealistic, I hope not foolhardy. I think my energy could not have escaped the notice of the sensitive, intelligent children I took care of, young autists among them. Because they would come up with inventive, surprising ideas that challenged the accepted and routine ways of thinking about things, I exulted in the work with these young people. Conversing with them was often rejuvenating, rarely tiresome. This was even true of the autistic youth. Once they had deigned to recognize me and had braved their insecurities to actually speak with me, I realized how interesting their ideas were, how thoughtful they could be. I firmly believed that any of the children in my care—the young autists, too—could achieve just about anything. This appeared to inspire my charges and encouraged them to take a good look at themselves as they lived and interacted with one another.

Soon I began to work intensively with autistic youngsters. I read Leo Kanner's seminal paper, published in the 1940s, wherein he described a young autistic boy, Donald, who, Kanner said, possessed good cognitive potential. "He appears to be always thinking and thinking," wrote Kanner, "and to get his attention almost requires one to break down a mental barrier between his inner consciousness and the outside world."[2]

Kanner asked five-year-old Donald to subtract four from ten. Instead of refusing to reply, young Donald responded elliptically, "I'll draw a hexagon." What an interesting response, I thought; how like the statements I'd heard from my autists—intriguing, intelligent, if not instantly comprehensible. Donald seemed to have cleverly, perhaps mischievously, analogized a six-sided figure to the number six.

Preparing *Between Their World and Ours* several decades later, I re-read Kanner's autism papers and the account of Donald. By then I had had conversations with more than forty young autists, time enough to convince me that I had sufficient insight into autism's mysteries to write about my efforts to reach these children, to detail my psychotherapeutic successes and the ways in which my attempts went awry. I remembered Kanner's description of the indifferent aloneness he sensed emanating from the dozens of afflicted children he studied. By "aloneness" he presumably meant the lack of human connectedness he felt was opposing his vigorous attempts to interact with and evaluate these self-contained youth. Like many of us who have since tried to get to know autistic young people, maybe Kanner felt his own sense of loneliness while being with his patients, who seemed to exist in an intolerable interpersonal vacuum. Perhaps they left him feeling suspended midair, effortlessly dangling him with the lack of an expected social response.

So was Donald's offer to draw Kanner a hexagon an attempt to breach the social chasm between him and his doctor yet remain true to his mathematical ideology? *I'll* (I will) draw a hexagon bespeaks purpose percolating in an otherwise unresponsive child. And willing something does not usually occur in a social void. Bowing to social expectation, perhaps this youngster simultaneously preserved his own aesthetic purpose. To him, thinking about hexagons might have been infinitely more compelling than subtracting numbers. If the topic had been hexagons, perhaps Donald would have talked more freely with his doctor.

Although Kanner began his work with autistic children long ago, we still have little clear idea and hardly a consensus about autism's causes and remedies. The latest professional word has it that the condition encompasses a range of behaviors and abilities—a "spectrum" of attributes—meaning individual differences obtain for autists just as they do for other people. For most experts, language development is key to differentiating between two components of the spectrum, "classical autism" and "Asperger's syndrome." Children with classical autism often do not speak or, in their infant years, lose what little speech they had developed. Children with Asperger's syndrome have little or no difficulty developing language and have fewer bothersome behaviors.

Another way of classifying children with autism is by their level of functioning. Language usage and level of intelligence determine whether a child is thought to be "high-functioning" or "low-functioning." High-functioning autistic youth have normal cognitive and learning abilities, but may have had difficulty acquiring language initially. Low-functioning autists are generally mute and less intelligent.[3]

There are other factors that may lead a parent to conclude that a child is "high" or "low" functioning—the range of the child's social behaviors, for example. Does the child abide by minimal standards of social conduct? Can he dress himself, adapt to family rules and routines, answer—at least minimally—when spoken to, initiate social contact in situations that are familiar or promising?

In the 1960s and 1970s, heated disputes erupted over the psychogenic versus the neurological theories of autism, over Bruno Bettelheim's view that young autists behave as though they have experienced an "extreme situation" versus Bernard Rimland's view that these children suffer from specific neurological dysfunctions. Autistic children do act "extremely," as if there is something disastrous about to happen to them. But this is due to the nature of their condition and not to anything their parents may have done to "cause" autism. Today, most experts agree that neurological and/or biochemical dysfunctions underlie much in autistic behavior. For example, investigators have found EEG abnormalities, atypical eye movements, and stereotypic body movements in some autistic children. A significant elevation of blood serotonin has been found in others. It is, however, important to remember that no physical marker unique to autism has yet been identified. In the words of researcher Sally Ozonoff and her colleagues, "[A]utism spectrum disorders have many faces, with some people being high functioning and others mentally retarded, some being highly verbal while others do not use language at all, some having severe problem behaviors . . . while others have no sign of such difficulties."[4,5]

Since my Orthogenic School days my view of the cause of autism has undergone a significant transformation. Though I sometimes did question the prevailing view that parents had, by misguided parenting, contributed to autism's onset, I had never met the parents of an autistic child and thus had little knowledge of their perspective. Marcia's mother did write newsy letters to her daughter, informing her of family events and expressing her best wishes for Marcia's recovery. But these glimpses into a parent's feeling for a child pale by comparison to the direct work with the parents of autistic kids that I have undertaken since 1968.

The parents I work with are remarkably responsive to my efforts with their young autists and to my attempts to help them meet their children's needs. Far from being the cause of autism, they are unusually sensitive to their children. As a group, they are forthcoming about their frustrations but also candid about their dreams and aspirations for their children. They are reliable and enthusiastic partners in a team effort to evoke discernible changes in their children's behavior, attitudes, and, especially, their feelings about *being autistic*.

It's actually healthy and productive for kids when their parents resonate to feelings—their own and those of their children. Natural human responses to even a wild or withdrawn child help him get to know the social world and to adapt to it. Through understanding their parents' emotions, autists are then able to tune in to the emotions of others.

Nationwide, parents of young autists are increasingly vocal in steering professional attention to autism's early identification and to remedies that work. They have spoken zealously of the need for medical science to originate new methods of treating their children.[6] Since doctors are now able to diagnose autism in children as young as two, the efforts of parents and schools to find ways to assist them have been on the rise.[7] I do not believe Bettelheim was correct when he wrote or implied that the parents of autistic children cause the condition by inattention to their kids, through neglect, or by misguided parenting.

Yet Bettelheim was, in many ways, right about the children themselves. His contribution lies in his empathy with the supersensitive child bent on maintaining sameness, as well as in his understanding of the predicaments the autistic child faces in getting along in a social world. Young autists soon learn that the best way to protect themselves from emotionally overloading excitants is to dodge human contact, to turn to an inner world.

But the tendency to avoid other humans has its costs. Some of the young autists I knew refused to eat in the company of others—the stimulation emanating from their mere presence was just too much to bear. Once Marcia could not eat because she had used her fingers to block her ears and her nostrils. She was intent on shielding herself from the hubbub of the common dining room and from the offensive smells that surrounded her. Her two forefingers pressed hard against her ears, and she covered her nose with her two little fingers. When encouraged by Bettelheim himself to try a new food, spaghetti, persnickety Marcia spoke in clear, ringing tones, "Broke my curtain!" Perhaps she meant to tell us that she visualized a curtain separating her from the intruding world. Protected by an imaginary barrier that controlled to some happy extent the stimuli that reached her sensitive sensoria, she could dispense with it as Bettelheim offered to free the fingers blocking her ears. To help her protect herself, he gently covered Marcia's ears with his own hands. Now, blocking only her nostrils with her forefingers, she began to eat the spaghetti, pushing it into her mouth with her little fingers one strand at a time. How inspiring! Maybe there was hope, I thought.

Memories of what seemed to work with autistic children at the Orthogenic School doubtless influence the way I approach them today. I had learned to view what young autists say as meaningful in some fashion. Now I like to settle into engrossing conversations with each and every one who can or will speak. I respond to their ideas about the world and themselves in it just as I do with the other children I talk to—respectfully, absorbedly, happily. For their part, these shy young people gradually adjust themselves to pleasing discourse.

I discovered anew how enormously gratifying it is to witness children who, against many odds, struggle to understand, to speak, to reciprocate. No matter how modest the social goal, no matter how small the actual gain, the young autists' mission to get to know us and to know themselves is always a noble one. Their gain is real, their labors honorable, their attitude earnest.

What, exactly, can be changed in the lives of young autists? To answer this question, I had to educate myself not just about their feelings but also about their minds. Though it is doubtless true that aspects of temperament and personality tend to remain stable across the life span, the perspectives and ideas of individuals do develop. I believe the same to be true of autists. What's more, the social context in which these children find themselves can make an enormous difference in how their perspectives and ideas unfold.

Between Their World and Ours begins with a discussion of the relevant issues in diagnosing young people as "autistic." I discuss the ways in which diagnosis can distort or prejudice our impression of these youth. I offer more complete and, I think, more humane ways of thinking about the quandaries inherent in the autistic condition.

Chapter 2 describes in detail the progress of an autistic child whom I knew when he was five and again when he was ten. His story illustrates many of the themes that are relevant to the upbringing and development of autistic children. In Chapter 3 I describe the remaining eight autists who are the subjects of this book. I depict their social and linguistic difficulties and the ways in which these young people overcame their troubles. To prepare the reader for the rest of the book, I briefly discuss how my friendship with them began and the themes around which we came to a meeting of minds.

The chapters that follow are arranged in roughly the order in which I undertook my psychological studies. My conjectures and conclusions are in large part based on conversations with autistic youth; many of these are presented in Chapters 4 and 5. Chapter 4 describes autists younger than ten; Chapter 5, older autists.

In speaking with young autists, I realized that their use of language opened a window to understanding their thinking processes. For at least two decades psychologists have studied theory of mind aspects— or their absence—in autistic children. These young people have been compared to other youth in the attempt to show that autists diverge significantly in their ability to conceptualize the *mind* concept, which refers to the belief that others have a mind capable of understanding things or events just as one's own mind does. The emphasis is on capability of understanding, not the particulars of understanding. For example, minds can disagree about whether the earth is flat. This is different from understanding that everyone has a thinking mind. It is the latter that has been called "theory of mind."

Since theory of mind is a necessary and often conspicuous human trait, its alleged absence in one human group is remarkable. As I speak with young autists, it does not appear to me that they lack an understanding of their own functioning minds nor do they seem to miss the fact that others possess this sense. The results of the *mind* studies are thus at variance with my own observations. In Chapter 6 I discuss the flaws in some of these studies and the evidence for a theory of mind sensibility in young autists. Many parents of autistic kids read anything they can get their hands on about the condition. It is important that they understand how to critique such scientific research.

While conversing with young autists, I wondered how their sense of self develops during their childhood. Could the talks I had with scores of autistic youngsters reveal how this sense had emerged? In Chapter 7 I argue that the autistic self develops through interacting with others in much the way a self develops in ordinary children. I do not believe, as Bruno Bettelheim did, that the autistic child passes through a self-development sequence different from that of other children. An autist's sense of self is compromised not, as Bettelheim would have it, by the child merging her identity with another person; nor is it impeded by an inability to reflect upon the self's qualities. It is rather limited by her social isolation. This denies her opportunities to consider qualities of the self in tandem with those of the other. It is my hope that this chapter will not only be helpful to psychotherapists of autistic children but also to their parents, who would benefit from knowing what to look for in a therapist treating their kids.

The social use of *mind* and an enhanced sense of self contribute to the young autist's ability and willingness to form and enjoy friendships. During my talks with autistic youth I would hear how their first friendships had originated, about the pitfalls and pleasures they experienced in relating to their friends and acquaintances, their dreams and fears of social contact. In Chapter 8 I discuss the complexities of autists' befriending attempts and the risks they must endure to initiate and sustain companionships.

I explored with young autists, their parents, and their teachers how they could be assisted at home and at school; about what could reasonably be expected of them as they endeavored to join or rejoin the family circle, to grasp learning assignments, and to meet social expectations in the classroom.

As I was writing *Between Their World and Ours*, I was invited to visit a public school that welcomed several young autists in its regular classrooms. The school's principal and I had many talks about how to encourage young autists in their struggles to learn and to socialize. These talks helped me enormously as I worked with my autistic kids and would hear from the principal how she and her teachers were doing with their autistic students. Chapter 9 is an account of the achievements of these youth. Their progress in school, sometimes startling, sometimes incomplete, reveals what can be accomplished in an ordinary classroom with motivated young autists and their dedicated teachers.

Chapter 10 gives specific recommendations to parents and teachers about what to do with the autistic youth with whom they live and work.

Finally, Chapter 11 discusses the attitudes and behaviors of parents, teachers, and specialists that are likely to increase young autists' chances of recovery and to kindle hopes for their future.

If we want to entice autistic children out of their private worlds, we ought to offer them something worthwhile. Offering them enticements is not likely to occur unless we are convinced that autistic youth will heed our attempts to help, unless we hope they will benefit from our overtures. Someone I once talked to about autism cautioned, "All one can do with these children is make their lives more bearable." Well, yes, in an important way. All we can do, which is quite a lot, is create a promising context in which their lives may become not only more bearable but actually enjoyable. And that is no small deal.

BETWEEN THEIR
WORLD AND OURS

CHAPTER ONE

The Diagnosis Is Not the Person

I love my family, truly, dearly, and profoundly, but from a
distance . . . A hyper-sensitive organism like mine can find
human contacts unendurable and deeply wounding,
even if the heart remains tender.
—HENRI MATISSE

Afflictions with unknown causes and cures educe in us a diverse array of
feeling. Autism, the uncanny tendency to turn one's focus inward and
away from others, resists and frustrates our most well-intentioned,
tender, and prodigious efforts to help. Parents of affected individuals and
professionals alike are glutted by lengthy, authoritative statements on
what autism is all about, what causes it, and what its likely course will be.
According to developmental psychologist Bryna Siegel, it is a "developmental disorder" that impacts the ways a child views the world.[1] Autism's principal quality, one that prevails across the entire spectrum and
the most upsetting to parents and teachers, is an indifference to or rejection of social contact. The autistic attitude seems almost "inhuman."
Though it is true that the condition influences how a child perceives the
world and learns about it, I emphasize how autism implicates social
learning and colors the youngster's view of the social world in particular.

The list of autistic behaviors is a mile long: difficulties conversing;
an evasion of human company; an inability to play freely; sensory
sensitivities, especially to human stimuli; a need for situations to remain the same; such repetitive, self-stimulating behavior as chin-

tapping, hand-flapping, or rocking; glassy-eyed staring and an avoidance of eye contact; a refusal, sometimes studied, to use the personal pronoun "I" or the word "yes." All this and more mystifies or appalls us. Self-injurious acts, such as biting, head-banging, or animal-like sniffing and attacking, are particularly hard to bear.

For this condition all sorts of nostrums have been ventured. Autistic children have been subjected to procedures intended to "bond" them with their parents. Some therapists have recommended that parents forcefully hold their wild or withdrawn children in order to convince them of the social benefits of being physically close. Young autists may be the subjects of structured behavioral regimes that ignore how autistic people feel. Medical aids may be recommended, including vitamin supplements, psychotropic medication, or auditory training. Psychologists may interview autists to show that they lack a "theory of mind" (ToM)—that is, they have little or no awareness of their own mentality or anyone else's.[2] Having a theory of mind means, simply, that you know you have a thinking mind and that others do, too. It means you know that minds function similarly even though people may arrive at different conclusions. Lacking this sense means that you're "mind-blind." Researchers agree that the child displays a sense of mindedness around four to five years.[3] The development of a theory of mind permits the child to engage in deceiving, storytelling, tricking, joking, analogizing, and symbolizing. In order to engage in these activities, the child must understand that other people are capable of recognizing his or her intent. Theory of mind activities are social activities *par excellence*.

Touting this or that theory of autism and treatment method, investigators often neglect to take seriously an important body of evidence, much of it from autistic individuals themselves, that cries out for a fundamentally different approach. Save the telling accounts of the autistic experience by autistic persons and by their parents, a deplorable sameness pervades what we are told: *they* are not like *us*. How ironic that we meet the autist's desire that situations remain the same with a misguided consistency of our own! However vexing the condition, autism calls for a humanistic approach, one that returns us to the whole child, notwithstanding his often withdrawn or wild behavior. *He has reasons for his actions and many a purpose behind them.*

When he found himself in unbearable family circumstances, Henri Matisse, who was obedient and passive as a child until his mother gave him a box of crayons, called attention to his hypersensitivity in the company of others and described human contact as distressing, even though his feelings remained affectionate. The "box of colours . . . was a tremendous attraction, a sort of Paradise Found in which I was completely free, alone, at peace."[4] Many young autists would understand this implicitly; quite often they experience an inner tenderness despite wishing to be alone with their pursuits and at peace.

What if we framed our views of the autistic dilemma in a radically different way? What if we perceived young autists as capable of shaping their lives in significant ways? What if we believed parents capable of helping them in this endeavor? What if we humanely presumed a commonality among *us* and *them?* By what moral or psychological tenets do we gloss over *their* agonizing struggles to relate to *us?*

A Recent Encounter

In my work as a psychologist to distressed young people, I've learned to take with a grain of salt what is reputed to be true of them. I like to visit their schools and even their homes to observe firsthand what is going on. On one such occasion, I am sitting cross-legged with some nursery-school children, listening to a child I work with talk to his teacher about the highlight of the day. The children will be creating a collage by dipping their hands in brightly colored paints and pressing them on a sheet.

Suddenly all eyes turn toward the door as a latecomer, a fragile-looking but pretty, slender girl, is quickly ushered by her mother into the art room, away from the other children. For her part, the girl is propelling herself as quickly as she can into the very room, as it will turn out, in which she'll excel. But what could be so wrong that the children's chatter must come to such an abrupt halt?

A while later I feel a quick tug on my shirtsleeve. I'm being pulled in the direction of the art room by the girl who came late. Staring intently in the general direction of my arm, she says urgently to the air, "No painting . . . no painting." I realize that I'm face-to-face with an autistic child.

"We think she's autistic," confirms her teacher. "She wears us out saying everything in opposites. If she wants to do something, like paint, she tells us she *doesn't* want to do it." (Why is the little girl stressing the "pain" in the word "painting," I wonder. It sounds like she's saying, "No *pain* . . . ting." Could she have been pained by being told "no" to painting so many times? Or maybe she knew *she* was a "pain" for asking to paint so many times.) Now her teacher exclaims, "She's driving me crazy!" And to the art teacher, "Isn't there room for her to paint *yet?*"

Later I peek into the art room, where I witness the little girl gazing blissfully at her fingernails as she carefully brushes them, one by one, with a deep cherry red. Remarkably her autism does not divert her from her artistic purpose. It's as obvious as any other child's as she paints her fingernails red. It shows determination, perhaps giftedness, does it not? Her contentment is unmistakable as she amuses herself tinting her nails, engrossed and attentive, revealing commendable fine-motor control. Doesn't it make a static diagnosis like "autism" un-necessarily binding? If another, undiagnosed child had concentrated so thoroughly, had created such beautifully colored fingernails, we might say, "How wonderful!" or ask, "Is she imitating the big girls painting her nails like that?"

"She does this kind of thing very well," says her teacher, noticing I am watching the little artist at work.

. . .

This episode stayed with me for weeks. It was the tug on my shirtsleeve from a seemingly spaced-out kid that did it. It got me thinking about my experience with autistic children decades before. I recalled how, while training to work with troubled youth, I'd been taken by the idea that our attempts to get to know a person in distress ought to be infused with the same kind of simpatico respect we pay to and expect from our closest, most trusted companions. I learned it wasn't disengaged professional distance, free from the muddying effects of human emotion, that helped my autistic charges. It was rather an attentive, gentle, caring approach that worked best. It wasn't "scientistic" diagnosis and preconceived notions of autistic infirmity that had helped them go beyond autism. Instead it was an open-minded attitude, a wondering whether young autists behave as they do for sound reasons, that got me beyond their autistic indifference.

And the little girl had chosen me, of all people, to advocate for her turn to paint. I felt a surge of elation, flattered to have been *the* one, much as I had felt overjoyed when years before my autistic protégées deigned to recognize my existence. True, our young autist seemed to use my arm as an instrument to get into the art room. If I hadn't known better, I might have felt dehumanized when she talked to the air while staring slightly off to the side of me or when later she looked right through me. I might have become steadfastly disinclined to attribute any reason at all to her odd behavior because she had the temerity to treat me the same way she would an object.

Knowing full well, though, the obstacles an autistic individual must surmount to reach out to another person, I could hardly contain my excitement at this unexpected opportunity to observe and reflect upon the autistic phenomenon once more. How I longed to take the little girl's hand and walk with her to the art room, countering, perhaps whispering, "Yes! Painting!" Who knew what this unusual child would do if I tried to interact with her in a different way? But, alas, I was only a visitor.

Parents and Children

Bruno Bettelheim, with whom I trained to be a psychotherapist at the University of Chicago's Orthogenic School, a residential treatment milieu for young people, thought troubled youth became so because they had always lived out an "extreme situation." Their acute anxieties and violence suggested to him that something in their experience drove them to excess. If life experiences had caused or aggravated a set of human behaviors, surely, for these youth, a healthier setting must be the cure.

When he wrote of the Orthogenic School students, "they all shared one thing in common: an unrelenting fear for their lives," Bettelheim generalized the thought to autistic youth. He continued, "the severity of their disturbances is directly related to how early in life these conditions arose, for how long they obtained, and how severe was their impact on the child."[5]

Because troubled youth, including young autists, may act as though they fear for their lives, Bettelheim deduced that something or someone caused them to feel that way, that their parents had behaved toward them in such a way as to cause them to be dysfunctional and unhappy. I think, rather, that autistic kids do not so much fear for their lives as they fear *being autistic*. They are often aware of their diagnosis and its implications for their future. Once self-aware—many autists I've known were cognizant—they fear for themselves and their ability to cope in a complex world.

As for their parents, it's not that they wish their children did not exist. It's rather that, for some, they wish their children were *not autistic*. This gets translated in the young autist's mind thus: *my parents wish I were different, and so do I.*

Yet what parent wouldn't become discouraged, distraught, impatient, withdrawing, or rejecting when faced, day in and day out, with an infant or young child who is unceasingly isolated and disdainful of human company? The young autist may then react to an understandable array of parental emotion as though it is yet one more burden to bear. But we must remember that taking the effect for the cause serves no one. The child's autism does precede the parent's reaction.

This book is about young autists who, at significant moments in their lives, are not merely diffident, solitary, and menacing, particularly when the world becomes too much for their vulnerable souls; it's also about how they can be keenly susceptible, unexpectedly attuned to the intent and feeling of others, desirous sometimes of expressing their feelings and searching for human company. You will become acquainted with some of these children—nine autists of the forty-five with whom I've worked over the years—in the pages that follow, depicting their dilemmas and interpreting their triumphs.

Diagnosing these young people does not do justice to their individual personalities. Nor do diagnostic labels usually include our personal responses to them. Every autist I knew forged a distinctive relationship with me, and as I became acquainted with each one, I almost forgot their ominous diagnoses and prognoses, often concentrating, as I would with any child, on each youngster's special, sometimes lovable qualities. They became whole people to me, living their lives as best they could within a meaningful, rewarding, prospective human connectedness. The narratives in this book illustrate a psychotherapeutic approach aimed not only at luring young autists out of their often impenetrable isolation but also at convincing them that they are worthy of the people world.

Many experts deem psychotherapy inappropriate for autistic kids. This is doubtless due to earlier, failed psychoanalytic or other psychotherapeutic attempts to reach these children. Or it may stem from the fact that there is no single therapeutic procedure that always works for them, nor a single unifying theory that explains their mystifying behavior. Yet this is hardly surprising: there is no single efficacious method to reach ordinary kids nor a universal theory that explains their troubles living in an unpredictable world.

Except for those written by their parents or by the autists themselves, many recent books on young autists tend to omit the complexity of feeling we may have about them and they about us. If we are to improve our efforts to help them, we must introduce ourselves to them with the most genuine commitment we can muster. The varied and highly personal perspectives that pervade their being reveal not just what ails them but also ways of approaching them. Communing with young autists, as I intend to show, helps ameliorate their most bizarre and antisocial behaviors and restores to them and to us the possibility of a warm friendship that, in turn, engenders the hope that the future is not as bleak as it once appeared.

Diagnosis and Experience

Diagnosis has become increasingly divorced from experience. This appalling state of affairs is particularly bothersome when it comes to assessing and planning for young autists. The trials and hard-won victories I have experienced living and working with these young people hardly prepared me for today's revised appraisal of autism—that young autists lack a theory of mind, that they experience only the simplest emotions. I believe this skewed evaluation of a significant human minority arises partly from a misuse of diagnosis. I say "skewed" because many experts who write about autism have never lived with or tried to help young autists, nor do they expect any real or long-lasting benefits from thoughtful efforts to do so. Autists have neither the wherewithal nor the interest to correct a misapprehension of their strengths and weaknesses. Rather than engage with us in any way—like a discussion of what's wrong with *our* view of *them*— they'd rather be left alone with their private reveries. What could be an interesting experience of the autistic youngster is not likely to emerge unless we reexamine and rethink our purposes in evaluating other people.

Diagnosis, whereby a physician identifies a patient's disease by its symptoms, originally consisted of the doctor's experience of the patient, mediated by his bedside manner. Even today a pediatrician presiding over a child's well-check acknowledges that the youngest of patients is likely to have his own agenda. To ignore it would conclude the interview, because the youngster would refuse to cooperate. Considering his needs and wants yields interesting information and permits the physical exam to continue.

All too often psychologists not only eschew the equivalent of the bedside manner, but they are also increasingly occupied by "objective" measures of human behavior. We are warned repeatedly of human subjectivity, yet the impact of the diagnostician's behavior and attitude upon the child is omitted from the report. To be truly objective, according to physicist Niels Bohr, one must focus on the measuring instrument as well as the subject of the investigation.[6] One such tool is the psychologist's own reaction, implicit in his observations and studies. Procedures and reports lacking these reactions create an unrecorded, therefore unknown, effect.

The pediatrician who asks during the well-check, "How's school?" or "What do you like to do with your friends?" comes closer to registering his own response to a child because he engages in normal discourse with her: he chooses, often on the basis of what he already knows, to ask her selected questions—and her answers sensitize the doctor to her individuality.

Likewise, the personal reactions of professionals who diagnose young autists ought to become part of their recommendations to them and to their parents. For example, if a diagnostician finds an autistic child appealing or occasionally responsive during the interview, the report to the parents ought to include the implications of these personal reactions for the child's treatment plan. The more the evaluating and diagnosing experience is mindfully used, the more likely the expert will be able to see beyond his nose. This is especially important in work with young autists who reputedly don't notice or react to other people. The diagnostic picture will only be more complete if it includes the autistic child's reactions to the person who is diagnosing.

In our technocratic society, we often feel that the last person we should consult about what's wrong is the person being assessed. Who can trust *him* to tell us what's the matter? But we must learn to trust autistic people and their often startling capacity to inform us about themselves if we are to help them. In the diagnosing moment the expert's experience of the person diagnosed ought to become explicit, the product of "us." Both participate in determining the category that unites behavioral minutiae.

The experts rarely make explicit the part of their own experience that leads them to classify others. "Psychoanalytic writing is full of nicknames for people—borderline, psychotic, heterosexual, narcissistic, obsessional" and "autistic," I'd like to add, "that in some contexts can sound immensely authoritative (diagnosis has always been the way psychoanalysts tell *themselves* who *they* are)" (italics mine), writes psychoanalyst Adam Phillips, who is skeptical of psychoanalytic orthodoxy.[7] The potential of diagnosis for influence over others is almost boundless for shy autistic people who often act helpless or violent just to evade being with others.

Implicit in diagnosis, Phillips notes, is a comparison of the diagnosed person to ourselves. We, unlike autists, are social, polite, articulate, responsive, normal, human. We are not withdrawn, diffident, isolated, menacing, mute, animalistic, or bizarre. If we force upon the diagnosis of autism the implicit or explicit notion that because autists are in important ways unlike us, they are in *all* ways unlike us, then we will try to shape their behavior toward some mythical, venerated norm that we supposedly share. If we learn to live and *be* with them as best we can, and they experience us as attentive and comforting, a human connectedness develops, and young autists behave more adaptively, more "humanly."

Ordinarily, the reductionist act of diagnosing distances *us* from other persons because it reduces *them* to a symptom checklist. I urge that we reconnect the diagnosing process to the experiencing process. If we attend to our personal reactions to autists and heed theirs to us, we can more accurately distinguish between autistic behaviors and actions that reflect a way of feeling, thinking, and being quite like our own. This would create a human context in which to assess what it is that impedes the autist from living a fuller life. And it would promote mutual understanding and greater compatibility between "us" and "them."

Remember: the diagnosis is not the person.

A Voice of Hope

My stance may seem radical given the commonly held view that not much can be done about autistic deficits once a firm diagnosis is made. Yet over half a century ago, the German physician Hans Asperger wrote one of the most humanistic treatises ever on autism. He notes the struggles autistic children have relating to others, and writes that the autistic condition "results in severe and characteristic difficulties in social integration." In fact, "in many cases the social problems are so profound that they overshadow everything else." Yet Asperger also opines, empathically and optimistically, "In some cases, however, the problems are compensated for by a high level of *original* thought and experience. This can often lead to exceptional achievement in *later* life" (italics mine).[8]

How prescient! Witness the exceptional achievements later in life of scientist Temple Grandin and writer Donna Williams, both childhood autists, who made spectacular contributions, respectively, to animal husbandry and human understanding.

Do we really know much more about autism than we did half a century ago? We have identified factors associated with autism, most not unique to the condition, including the Fragile-X chromosome, low IQ test scores, allergies, intolerance of milk products, infant inoculations, induced labor, sub-acute tetanus infections, and high serotonin levels.[9] But have we learned to think of autists as capable of human achievement the way Asperger did so long ago?

Asperger takes his argument a step further when he urges us to consider that, despite their difficulties, autists could "fulfil their *social* role within the community, especially if they find understanding, love, and guidance." He continues, "*Possibilities* of social integration which one would never have dreamt of may arise in the course of development . . . [which] gives us the right and duty to speak out for these children with the whole force of our personality" (italics mine). He concludes, "We believe that only the absolutely dedicated and loving educator can achieve success with difficult individuals."[10]

At the risk of being interpreted as romanticizing the autistic condition—a view that could falsely equate a balanced perspective with unbridled pipe-dreaming and that might inhibit people who wish to do so from imagining inventive remedies for the condition—I propose in the pages to follow, and following Asperger, that:

- we recognize and applaud the young autist's potential ability in particular social situations
- we speak out with the force of our personalities to augment the friendship of a retiring, eccentric, oppositional, or skeptical young autist with his inspired educator, parent, or friend dedicated to possibilities for a mutually satisfying life.

How different Asperger's prescriptions for autism are from those of today's experts, who write that the young autist lacks the expected range of human emotion as well as the normal cognitive ability to think reciprocally. Psychiatrist Leo Kanner's designation "disturbances of affective contact," promulgated in the 1940s as he studied socially isolated young patients, is still heeded today by those who assert that only the simplest emotions are available to autists (since when is *any* emotion simple?). Kanner also thought that the parents of the young autists he diagnosed were emotionally cold—hence the term "refrigerator mothers."[11] He later recanted and stated, as quoted by Clara Claiborne Park, the mother of an autistic girl. "Herewith I acquit you people as parents."[12]

Cognitive psychologist Uta Frith asserts that autists lack a theory of mind—their own and that of others. Because they may behave as though minds can't think or generate ideas, Frith assumes that autistic individuals lack a theory of the mind. The implications of this as yet unproven view are enormous. The assumption that others have a mentality reverberating to ours is the basis for much, if not all, conversation; how could we understand the other and be understood if we did not share the intention to communicate? Once we assume that autists cannot theorize about their minds or ours, we would likely cease trying to communicate with them. And how, then, could those who would work dedicatedly with autists come close to realizing Asperger's vision for them?

Much of the evidence Frith and others cite for a lack of theory of mind comes from these children's dismal performance on false belief or similar tests (to be described in Chapter 6). Impressed by consistent research outcomes for lack of theory of mind in autists, researcher Catherine Lord, formerly of the TEACCH center at the University of North Carolina,[13] warns, "Yet, in the end, their clinical and theoretical power will be determined by the extent to which they can explain the everyday social and cognitive deficits experienced by autistic individuals."[14]

Another group of researchers studying autism has adopted a more hopeful view. While recognizing that "autism falls into a category we would call 'affective or emotional communication disorders,' " the

Scottish researcher Colwyn Trevarthen and his colleagues differentiate between possessing emotions and expressing them. The disorder, in their view, is not in experiencing emotion but in communicating it.

This view is hopeful because it focuses on the diagnostics themselves, leaving room for an open-mindedness toward those diagnosed. Diagnostic and therapeutic efforts aimed at clarifying what makes an autist tick "tend to replicate what we see in autism itself, namely a propensity to conceive mental functioning cut into pieces. Problems are identified in 'cognitive functioning,' 'attention deficits,' 'language,' and 'communication,' not to mention all the physiological deficits found, such as gluten sensitivity, serotonin, or Fragile-X chromosomes."[15] I say let's put Humpty-Dumpty back together again despite the shortsightedness of the king's men.

The Autistic Spectrum

The term "autistic spectrum disorder," developed to account for the variation in the autistic population, is fertile and heuristic because it encourages the search for promising traits associated with autism that have been previously overlooked. Even though the causes of autism are likely to be biological, years of research on the condition have yet to identify a physical marker *unique* to the condition. According to Bryna Siegel, it is thus a "behavioral diagnosis." She cautions, though, "This is not to say that autism does not have a physical cause."[16] Causes are more likely than a single etiology, writes neuroscience researcher Terence Deacon: "The neurological basis of autism is still unresolved . . . there are probably many potential neurological causes for autism."[17]

Yet, except to exonerate child-rearing practices, it's not really saying much to note that autistic characteristics may be rooted in biology, since many human traits are; biological predispositions await the right surround to develop maximally. Perhaps some as yet unidentified trigger causes a susceptibility to the condition to erupt.[18] Pending clarification from neurology or biochemistry about the physiological aspects of the condition, parents and teachers of young autists need inspiring social, behavioral, and therapeutic methods especially designed to help them. Even with more refined scientific knowledge, I believe we will continue to seek procedures that keep these kids on track developmentally, help them adjust to school learning, and encourage them to reach out genuinely and optimistically to their peers.

Uta Frith also posits a biological basis for autism and Asperger's syndrome, noting that the difference between the two lies in the severity of the biological signs. Kids with Asperger's syndrome usually lack the language delay typical of the classically autistic. Frith concludes that "the two conditions may indeed be different expressions of the same basic defect."[19]

Investigators thus confirm the diagnostic utility of the term "autistic spectrum disorder." If it turns out, as many suspect, that neurobiological aberrations underlie all of autism—a frontal lobe dysfunction, for example, which originates even before the infant's frontal lobes are fully developed—then those who work and live with the isolated or violent autist could modify what has worked with the more adapted and willing group. Such a perspective would act as an antidote to a diagnostic impasse noted by Colwyn Trevarthen and his colleagues: "Because the category of 'childhood autism' in *DSM-III-R* [*The Diagnostic and Statistical Manual of Mental Disorders–III–Revised*] . . . if compared to their earlier forms, includes many more children under the category of 'autism,' both professionals and lay people have been led to regard the whole group of children so labeled as very severely and perhaps permanently handicapped, because of the connotations the term 'autism' carries."[20]

But autism's connotations need not be this damning. The idea that basic (neurological) causes underlie the entire spectrum could augur well for the least adapted group. A common neurological etiology for autism would imply fundamental methods for treating all autists. What's more, since all children on the spectrum show unusual behaviors in language usage, in social relationships, and more questionably in my opinion, in play development, intervention geared to assisting them ought to target these areas regardless of the severity of the condition— even though the least adapted autists would plainly test the ingenuity and stamina of those who would implement remedial efforts.

Once you've become acquainted with a few young autists, it's all too easy to recognize others with autism, even from afar. I've had this experience many times. I'd been at the beach, gazing abstractedly at the ocean, when suddenly my attention wandered to a family in which one youngster, isolated from the rest, seemed to be searching the horizon for something to appear. The others were rushing to and from the surf happily and noisily. I kept watching the family "loner." After about twenty minutes, a ship slowly emerged. Then the boy's face lit up as he gazed seraphically at the vessel while ignoring his family. It was as if he adored the distant ship but shunned the people right before his very eyes.

Another time, I witnessed a young autistic boy playing volleyball with his family and friends. He had an unobtrusive string attached to his belt that he would jiggle nervously between the serves, possibly to keep himself focused on this exciting but unnerving group activity. And there was the autistic nursery school student who grabbed me by the sleeve so that I'd usher her into the art room where she could paint her fingernails bright red. To me, these youngsters' behavior was unmistakably autistic, and I wondered whether the subjective certainty that a certain cluster of behaviors seems to signal autism has caused experts and others to perceive the autistic population as homogeneous and therefore untreatable.

These chance and brief encounters don't allow people to *be* with each other in such a way as to get beyond the first impression, the initial diagnosis. Such typical autistic behaviors as daydreamy spaced-out gazes or glassy-eyed stares, repetitive arm- and hand-flapping, frantic and continuous pacing and rocking, isolating behaviors like turning one's back on others, mutism, a strange use of language, an obsessional interest in one particular topic—all these are so conspicuous that many people, even experts, never get beyond these behaviors to know the nature of the autist's full personality. Taking "autistic spectrum" seriously might elicit curiosity about the autistic individual, if only to urge upon us to ask, "Just where on the spectrum does the young autist fall?" A mere step further and we are asking what kind of person she might become. The spectrum idea could replace diagnostic stasis with an attitude of hope, one that would spring from an appraisal of the autistic child's strengths as well as weaknesses.

Just how many children are being diagnosed as autistic? The preeminent expert on autism, Bernard Rimland, himself the father of a son he calls an "artistic savant autist," estimates that 4 to 5 individuals per 10,000 are autistic. The Autism Society of America estimates 15 per 10,000. Neurologist Oliver Sacks, author of the best-seller *An Anthropologist on Mars*, tells us the incidence is more like 1 in 1,000. A recent *Newsweek* article asserts that "autism is now thought to affect 1 person in 500," an estimate that doubtless stretches the diagnosis "autistic spectrum" to include Asperger's syndrome.[21] Yet a recent California study concluded that the increase in the incidence of autism is not due to a change in the diagnostic criteria, which remained stable for two cohorts in the 1980s and 1990s.[22]

Thus far, I've found no estimate of the proportion of autistic children with Asperger's syndrome or the relative proportions of "high-functioning" and "low-functioning" autistic children. Ozonoff and colleagues state that autism spectrum disorders affect up to 0.6 percent of the general population, and from two-thirds to three-quarters may be high functioning.[23] The incidence of autism may be four to five times greater in boys than in girls.[24] My group of forty-five young autists does not reflect this statistic: the ratio of boys to girls is less than four to one, but my group may be too small to reflect the true incidence.

Those young autists who are adroit, perceptive, and sometimes communicative obviously occupy the "high-functioning" portion of the spectrum. Many of these young people are gifted in one or more ways. They show "islands of ability," as did one of my autistic charges, Marcia, while singing and another, Stacy, while joking, impersonating, and punning. Some young autists maintain themselves in regular classrooms, both private and public; often their parents are encouraged to seek tutorial or psychological assistance for their children and counseling for themselves. The talented autistic young people often develop and refine their gifts throughout their lives, a fact that sometimes calls even more attention to their condition—perhaps an irony for some autists, since their often surprising abilities stand in such stark contrast to their social or other limitations.

A case in point is the talented autistic artist, Stephen Wiltshire, described by Oliver Sacks. Sacks comments that we have yet to find a theory that takes into account the impressive range of competencies Wiltshire displays. Sacks goes so far as to say, "[A]ll our models, all our terms break down before him."[25]

Yet when Wiltshire lost the companionship of his art teacher after graduating to a different school, and suddenly lost his initiative to do much drawing, the neurologist wonders just how much Wiltshire missed his teacher, because the boy talked about him formally and factually, "without any apparent emotion." If an ordinary child dropped a favorite activity in the absence of an important teacher, we'd take this behavior to mean the child missed, maybe even mourned, the adult with whom the activity was associated. Since Stephen Wiltshire evidently did not feel his loss (we don't really know *what* he felt), Sacks, like many experts on autism, gives less weight to the way in which the young autist *did* react to his loss. This sort of response illustrates the hazards of a "symptom list." The notion that autists typically don't feel the way others do could blind us to the full picture, which, if acknowledged, would create a context in which they could grow beyond their debilitating, straitjacketing condition. It is not idle to wonder how Stephen Wiltshire would have reacted had someone said to him, "Of course you don't feel like drawing anymore; you miss your art teacher."

When he witnessed Wiltshire's musical talent, every bit as commanding as his artistic bent, Sacks writes enthusiastically how Wiltshire, absorbed in a music lesson in which he seemed to come together as his own person, dropped his "autistic persona." "AUTISM DISAPPEARS," writes Sacks in his notebook, commenting on Wiltshire's "new mode of being." Reading Sacks's account, I remembered one of my autistic protégées, Marcia, who was also musically talented, and her perfect-pitch rendition of "Red River Valley." "From this valley they say you are going," she sang out in gorgeous, sonorous tones as I was about to interrupt our work together to take a trip. Did she wish the artistry of her song would persuade me to stay with her?

Delving into the nature of the autistic experience leads us to ask pertinent questions about it; for example, why do autists use language the way they do? Many of their utterances seem essentially poetic. I believe one reason Marcia chose to sing, aside from loving the sounds of song, was the cadence in the song's language. Another autistic child in my care, eleven-year-old Greg, was once playing with a poetry kit, composing sentences from words arranged on a magnetic board. He wrote, "I came and went inside that funny owl." Fond of and knowledgeable about animals from an early age, he now waxed whimsically about the earlier dead-serious alliance of himself with the animals that so fascinated him. Perhaps his use of language was not intended to communicate; rather it may have reflected how he perceived himself in the company of animals. His sentence was meaningful to me as I wondered: why talk or write enigmatically; what perspective does this reveal? He not only came to the owl but went inside it. What a playful, condensed, disingenuous way of expressing his affinity for animals!

I believe an autist's elliptical use of language means not just to arouse his own inner aesthetic reaction but also to provoke a sort of tease. "Just how interested in me are you?" the eleven-year old might have asked implicitly. "Enough to figure out my secret message?"

Greg, who imagined himself inside a funny owl, expressed the elated feeling he got from observing animals and pretending he was like them. His demeanor on showing me what he'd written was of a proud author. Moreover, in contrast to the recent past when he intoned animal facts to me endlessly and unemotionally, he now fully expected that I'd appreciate him and his sentence. For him it had been art first, communication second. Applauding only inwardly, so as not to come on too strong with this shy boy, I told Greg how much I liked what he'd written.

"Low-functioning" autistic youth—those who resort to self-injurious behavior like frantic or methodical head-banging or who dissolve into temper outbursts, screaming for hours about the slightest sensory discomfort or disruption of their routines—are generally suspected to be below average in intelligence or even mentally retarded.[26] They often do not speak. Some of these children have never said a word. Others begin to talk during their first or second year, but for some unexplained reason they suddenly or gradually cease talking at the same time they withdraw even further into their own worlds and innermost reveries.

Many of the "high-functioning" autists Asperger described nonetheless had a past studded with prolonged periods of hand-flapping, hair-twirling, and violent outbursts. I once knew an autistic adult who, as a child, had engaged in all these behaviors and more, but who seemed quite bright. Her parents took her for IQ testing when she was about nine. She told me that she'd tested mentally retarded, because she didn't like the examiner's frown. "She thought I was stupid, I guess," this autistic woman concluded.

Another autist, six-year-old Dirk, who never said "yes" or referred to himself as "I," yet who sang beautifully and drew intricate buildings, could not be tested because, according to his mother, he deliberately became mute when the psychometrist interviewed him. So he earned the label mentally retarded, which he plainly was not. When Dirk's mother asked him later why he refused to answer test questions, he asked her why he had to supply the answer since the examiner already knew it (see Chapter 3 for a description of Dirk's testing experience).

How many other so-called mentally retarded autistic children have forcefully turned away from testing only to be stigmatized as mentally deficient for the rest of their lives? None, according to psychiatrist Leon Eisenberg, who is quoted in a book that scorns attempts to help young autists. Dismissing the Panglossian notion that there is an intelligent child imprisoned within an autistic shell "with a philosophical shrug," Eisenberg said of autists, "Well, they're retarded."[27]

This uncritical generalization raises some important questions. Why even attempt to test young autists if it's known that every last one of them is retarded? Testing for IQ requires verbal responses, so why test near-mute autists, since no amount of testing will give us a reasonable cognitive estimate? Psychometrists are required by the intelligence test manual to establish rapport with the child and to make sure his attention is focused on the test procedures and questions before the exam begins. How many psychometrists are able to establish rapport and gain the attention of young autists, who are notoriously hard to reach and who have great difficulty focusing?

Standardized testing may be inappropriate even if we suspect that many autists are not mentally retarded. Since we know they dislike being distracted from their thoughts, why run them through a procedure the results of which cannot possibly be reliable? Even if autists comply with some of the test procedures and questions but refuse at other times, why assume they lack understanding when, at the very least, they have discerned precisely which questions they might not be able to answer? Perhaps they have a better sense of their own mental functioning than we wish to grant them.

Surely other ways of assessing autistic potential are available, including observing autists' behavior or conversing with them. These assessments may not be quantifiable, but this only begs the question: Should we risk an invalid test metric, or should we hazard a chary guess of their intelligence?

Behavioral Observation Is Important

As already noted, autism has been called a "developmental disorder," which means that the condition may not be present at birth but rather develops in the first or second year. Yet a 1999 analysis of infants' movements suggests an early behavioral marker for autism. Psychologist Philip Teitelbaum and his research team analyzed home videos of seventeen autistic infants, videos taken years before they were diagnosed with autism. Unlike normal infants, the autistic babies showed signs of movement disturbance between four and six months: there were asymmetries of the arms and legs while the infants were lying down or crawling; there were abnormal methods for rolling from back to stomach; and there were deviations from the expected gait while learning to walk.[28] This implies that the oft-noted eighteen-month critical period for autism to manifest reflects our historical inability to identify the condition much before a child is expected to speak. Were these results to be replicated, autism would seem to be present in very young infants—much earlier than originally supposed.

Another early marker for autism, reported by researcher Catherine

Lord, which discriminates reliably between two-year-old autistic children and their normal two-year-old peers, is the young autist's use of another person's hand as a tool. Similarly, many young autists do not point as normal children do; some show "instrumental" pointing, but none in Lord's group showed "social" pointing.[29] This means that although young autists may request desired objects by pointing, they rarely use this gesture to signal to or about other humans.

Although these observations are undoubtedly valid for some, maybe most, autists, we still need to observe carefully how each and every one uses our hands or arms as tools or in which particular ways they seem to point instrumentally, not socially. For example, the nursery school student who pulled at me in order to get into the art room did not simply use my arm as a tool to meet her needs. She knew from past experience that an adult must accompany her from where she was into the art room—and she also knew that the regular nursery school teachers wouldn't do so unless it was her turn to paint. She figured she'd try me out as an accomplice to realize her wishes. This required a *social* discrimination between me, a naive newcomer, and her teachers, who were more familiar with her habits. Likewise, if an infant points at a cookie or a toy rather than at his father as his mother holds him in her arms, we must make sure that the autistic infant is carefully limiting his visual range to cookies and toys, and that he is not including his father in his purview as he thrusts his baby finger forward. But early markers for autism are important to note; even earlier typical behaviors for autism than those at six months to two years would be helpful in planning for young autists. The earlier autism can be identified, the sooner parents, teachers, tutors, and other specialists can begin treatment.

No matter when the condition surfaces, if it is biological it might not be possible to treat the underlying neurological problem directly. So says neuroscientist Elliot Valenstein, who writes, "[M]ost investigators who have studied autism believe that this condition is caused by some brain defect, although there is no agreement on the nature of the impairment or the precise brain structures involved." He cautions, "even if a brain impairment were found to be the cause of autism . . . the best treatment available might remain psychosocial and behavioral."[30] Even if the biological causes were found to be heritable, a psychosocial or behavioral regimen might still be best since, according to scientist Stephen Jay Gould, "heritable" does not equate to "inevitable." "To a biologist," he writes, "heritability refers to the passage of traits or tendencies along family lines as a result of genetic transmission. It says little about the range of environmental modification to which these traits are subject."[31] We know far too little about young autists' ability to respond to their environment to assume that they would not modify some of their behaviors, especially if treatment were begun early.

These notions echo the thoughts of a number of parents who have written of the early identification of autism in their children (some younger than a year old) and who have described treatment efforts, lovingly and consistently maintained, that resulted in perceptible, sometimes lasting, gains. These parental efforts are particularly impressive since autistic children are, almost from the beginning, less interactive socially than ordinary children. The parents of young autists have fewer social behaviors to respond to. Parents may, in turn, respond less often and perhaps less enthusiastically. This would unwittingly exacerbate the social isolation of the already withdrawn, solitary young autist and might affect his parents' feelings toward him. They may pessimistically conclude, "Nothing I do works with this kid." Mothers in particular may feel upset, even guilty, if their efforts to draw out responses from their autistic babies and children fail. Even if they redouble their efforts to reach their child, parents might conclude that nothing works if the supersensitive young autist reacts negatively to increased pressure to interact. Acknowledging the biological component to autism may assure such parents that their infants' lack

of response does not stem from misguided parenting. Just as important, though, the biological correlates of autism should not preclude
determining the boundaries within which a young autist might learn
and communicate, nor should they obviate the need to flex these
boundaries with specific treatments.

Social Sensitivities

At the root of much of his reclusive anguish is the autist's uncommon, unpredictable reaction to *social* stimuli. Young autists are known
for their heightened sensitivity to many stimuli, yet they act incredibly
*in*sensitive to others—notably to unwanted social overtures. Over-
developed auditory and olfactory senses are common. Autists often
startle or wince at loud, sudden piercing noises or high- and low-
frequency pitches. Particularly abrupt noises signaling equally abrupt
events produce irritation or, sometimes, a strange excitement. Autists
sometimes rear back from bright colors and bold forms. They frequently recoil from another's touch even in the early infant weeks, so
that a mother's attempt to hold or cuddle her autistic baby, who stiff-
ens in her arms, ends up frustrating the mother and overwhelming her
panicky infant. Perhaps their hypersensitivity explains their wish for
sameness wherein not even the slightest detail goes unnoticed if it au-
gurs change.

Autistic sensitivity routinely permeates the lives of young autists; it
is a trait that is confusingly intertwined, in some, with their unusual
reactions to pain. Imagine your surprise upon recognizing a deep
wound covered with a large unsightly scar and not having the slightest
recollection of when and how the injury occurred. I've witnessed this
situation time and again. At one moment, the young autist is wincing
at stimuli, and the next he is unwittingly disregarding a bloody scar
as he nervously jabs his pencil into it. He must contend with this
existential discontinuity daily.

Often the stimuli autistic children find so unbearable emanate from other people. "[A]s a child, the 'people world' was often too stimulating to my senses," writes Temple Grandin in *Emergence Labeled Autistic*.[32] The sounds we call speech—noise to autists—spring from others. And grown-ups sometimes refuse to heed a young autist's unmistakable cue that he hates physical contact. In an effort to breach the emotional abyss that exists between them and the child, adults persistently try to hug and kiss him. But isn't any child disturbed by unwanted "affective contact"? Though their nonautistic peers might be so bold as to tell the offending adult to buzz off, autists appear to protect themselves by turning off their feelings.

Perhaps autistic babies withdraw even within families devoted to nurturing because of the eager relatedness these families offer. The risk for the young autist just may be too great. Warding off the most enticing human relationship could reduce the sensory stress. Is the cost of human relating, we may well wonder, worth the sensory agony these children suffer? Once they've realized that it is safer and more comfortable to avoid human contact, autistic children do just that, at their own peril.

People unfamiliar with autistic withdrawal cannot easily perceive that even the head bangers and the screamers are stimulus-sensitive. This seems egregiously contradictory to the uninformed. How could it be that stimulus-sensitive young autists overstimulate themselves by rocking, pacing, and flapping, yet cringe and wince when with us, so much so that they recede into sensory nothingness, a mental blankness? Bettelheim thought that it was by means of his own efforts that a young autist achieved a nonattentive state; by "his monotonous, continuous self-stimulation which arises . . . from his motor behavior . . . any stimulus from the outside is then lost, either by being blotted out, or in the concentration on inner sensations alone."[33] This implies that young autists deliberately stimulate themselves in order to block out the sensations coming from the social world. At its inception in infancy, their self-stimulation may not be deliberate, but once they recognize that they are able to block social stimuli this way, psychology joins neurology in providing them with a powerful tool to shun human company.

The simple example of an ordinary child who yells to drown out what he considers to be offensive demands or requests illuminates why autistic children bang their heads, bite their hands, or scream to the rafters. For the autist, such behavior helps obliterate the effects of the most unpredictable stimuli of all—that arising from other people. For autist and ordinary child alike, the insult is under their control, since their noise or pain is self-inflicted. Children doubtless think that if they themselves have initiated noise or pain, they can also put a stop to it.

Young autists have told me that they use pleasant sensory events to blot out the ill effects of noxious ones. Seven-year-old Stacy would sing "My Favorite Things," deliberately transposing the verbs "sting" and "bite"—just as she'd habitually transposed "you" and "I." She could manage the stimulation of the song blaring noisily on the record player by making it funny. She'd sing, "When the dog *stings*, when the bee *bites*, when I'm feeling sad . . . ," and would fall to the floor in gales of laughter as she did so, announcing, "That's funny!" Still giggling, she'd finish the song's phrase, "I simply remember my favorite things and then *I don't feel so bad!*" She was particularly fond of the line, "Girls in white dresses with blue satin sashes," which, I remembered, was exactly how she'd come to the Orthogenic School—in a white frilly dress with a satin sash. When I reminded Stacy of this, she at first looked blankly, then raised her voice once more in song, repeating, ". . . then I don't feel so *bad!*"

Donna Williams, too, remembers when she was three losing herself in "bright spots of fluffy color" (visual floaters) while people around her "gabbled."[34] She further describes being mesmerized more recently by a pink streetlight, so much so that her autistic friend had to plead with her to return to their shared world.[35]

Later developments in the hypersensitive child's life could be partly the result of his experience being autistic. Indifferent or inhumane care, our attitudes toward autists, a wrong treatment plan, the autist's own sense of failure—all might contribute to his pessimism about his future. Whether arising from autists or from us, their trepidation tends to ossify their condition, not just because innovative procedures haven't been tried, but also because those working and living with young autists may adopt the very attitudes that resonate to their own dejection: they sometimes accurately estimate, even as we do, the magnitude of the difference between themselves and others. Yet, perhaps no less significant, our resignation is, for them, like ignoring a rare plant, believing it would make no use of light or water.

When we appreciate that autists, like us, may develop progressively, we establish a human continuity between us and them that sensitizes us to these pertinent questions:

- What experiences challenge autistic indifference and engage young autists in their own recovery?
- Which of our attitudes enlist their participation in the social world?
- How will our spoken and gestural language influence them to respond?

To speak, for example, of twiddling one's thumbs when talking with a young autistic girl who is agitatedly waving her forefingers in front of her face, or "self-stimming," might establish a commonality between her and us. Though we don't "self-stim," we might admit that we twiddle our fingers when nervous. Common parlance inspires the idea in the autist that her experience is shareable.

No organism can survive without its proper environment. To adapt to their uniquely social world, human infants require a measure of responsible care from their families. Yet a call for human responsibility for autists may go against the grain of our society, which is at once sybaritic and conformist. Struggling consistently hard for one's child, whether autistic or not, is all too often a family goal worked at sporadically. And no child evokes the square-peg-round-hole adage more than a young autist. No amount of strenuous effort to fit and push that wayward peg into its circle will change its basic shape, but that doesn't mean that a niche could not be found for the square peg.

Categorizing people, whether or not they sort easily, seems to make their actions more predictable. If we know a child is autistic, we likely foresee that he will suffer problems in relating to others. And our society likes to know in advance what the outcome will be of a laborious effort on behalf of a particular class of individuals. Will they contribute to society, or will they be a drain on it? Outcome-oriented investigations and efforts thus present a problem for autistic youth. When the going gets rough, categorizing and predicting replace genuine thought, and this unnecessarily limits the treatment options for these young people.

Both the diagnosis and the treatment of autism need to be infused with human responsibility—*not* parental responsibility for its origin, but responsibility for its remediation. It is heartening to realize that autists themselves sometimes develop their own restorative strategies. Donna Williams, despite her sensory overloading and her "processing problems," was able to be introspective about her life and chronicle its progress movingly and meaningfully. "If the noise was too loud, too variable, or too high-pitched," she writes, "I could stuff my ears with cotton, wool or earplugs. If the lights were too bright, I could assume the uncomfortable role of an eccentric and put on dark glasses." About conversing with others, she remarks, "If people asked me what I wanted, thought, felt, or liked, I could appear generous and reasonable by putting the question back on them."[36] Besides describing her vulnerability to human communication, Williams's assertion reveals an exquisite understanding of how she might appear to others and how she could mischievously exploit appearances for her own gain.

Similarly, Paul McDonnell, the autistic son of Jane Taylor McDonnell, describes in the afterword to McDonnell's *News from the Border* his troubles making friends and his attempt to overcome his problems. The hurt that Paul felt didn't dissuade him from observing his behavior and feelings and comparing his experience to that of others. From these comparisons he learned he was not alone: "For a while I thought that I was the ONLY person . . . who got dumped by his girlfriend. I was glad to see that I was not alone." His compassion for others extended even—perhaps especially—to those who suffer the same condition: "I want to help other people who have autism. I know how they must feel sometimes, and I want to guide them in the right direction."[37]

Temple Grandin, too, helped herself transcend autism sufficiently to earn a doctorate and to teach and write on how to make the conditions under which cattle are slaughtered more humane. After noting her communication difficulties as a child, she reflects, as Paul McDonnell did, on making friends. She writes that in her forties she "grasped at last" an understanding of a friendship. Oliver Sacks's touching portrayal of his meeting with Grandin reveals her inclination for friendship. During his visit with Grandin they toured the countryside by car. Sacks describes how he was yearning for a swim and impulsively raced toward a body of water he thought was a lake. As he neared it, Grandin yelled, "Stop!" warning Sacks that before them was not a lake but water from a hydroelectric dam rushing toward him. "There would have been a fair chance of my being swept along, out of control, right over the dam," Sacks tells us.[38] Not only did Grandin save Sacks's life, she even permitted, perhaps reciprocated, notes Sacks, a hug upon parting from the neurologist.[39]

It simply will not do to assert that autists who make stunning recoveries were not autistic initially. This is like saying that an ailing plant that responds favorably to care was never ailing. The young autist, like any struggling individual who has finally achieved a measure of success, might well wonder about the expert who changes his mind about what was wrong with him to begin with. "What good is it," he might ask himself, "to work so hard when 'they' trivialize my struggles by arguing about my diagnosis? What about finding out what's *right* with me?"

The forty-five young autists I knew belong on a behavioral spectrum, the important dimensions being the ways in which they relate to people, including how *they* feel about others and how *others* feel about them. All had difficulties communicating and socializing. Only a few were regularly unable to play freely; most played intermittently with varying degrees of interest, imagination, and spontaneity. Of the forty-five, twenty-six behaved much like the individuals Hans Asperger described. They appeared intelligent, if eccentric; often showed giftedness in one or more respects; and communicated with others up to a point. Most of them did not show the language delay typical of classical autism. The other nineteen were generally less well adapted, although most, even when mute, appeared intelligent.

I refer to the nine children whose stories appear in this book as "autistic," even though the designation "Asperger's syndrome" (AS) is applicable to some of them. Given the cumbersome nature of the terms "autistic spectrum disorder" and "Asperger's syndrome," I'd like the narratives to suggest where a child falls on the spectrum. Likewise, whether a child is high- or low-functioning should be obvious from the depictions. Most importantly, the stories that follow represent an intimate unfolding of what autism feels like from within. I intend to show that young autists develop over their life spans. While they may not develop in ways precisely like their regular peers, develop they do.

Yet the ways in which the behavior of these nine children improved tend to attenuate neat categorization. Just when you think you've pinned down *the* crucial characteristics of the autistic condition—and this was true for almost all of the forty-five autists I knew—someone, the child himself or a perceptive parent or teacher, would describe a feeling, a behavior, an idea, that challenged the neat package.

I learned this lesson many years ago when a twelve-year-old boy, whom I'd believed to be hopelessly autistic, who talked in riddles in a high-pitched, deafening voice, when he talked at all, who refused to look straight at me, and who flipped his fingers wildly in front of his face and mine, typed out this message on my manual typewriter one day just before leaving my office:

SCBBCXZZZCBNJGFHELPMECZDFFF

CHAPTER TWO

Gregory's Journey

[No one] can ever express the exact measure of his needs or his
thoughts or his sorrows; and human speech is like a cracked kettle
on which we tap crude rhythms for bears to dance to, while we long
to make music that will melt the stars.

—GUSTAVE FLAUBERT

It had been some twenty years since I'd lived and worked with autistic
children at the Orthogenic School. Since then I'd been thinking about
autism and the problems of diagnosis. Five-year-old Gregory, referred
to me because of wild behavior in school, was a real puzzle. His facial
features were attractively chiseled even at a young age. Though bright
and alert, his countenance did not ordinarily relax or tighten into
typical childhood expressions—he neither smiled nor frowned. He
used language to communicate with others only when the conversations turned on one of his special interests. When his mother took him
for an evaluation just before his first meeting with me, he refused to
answer the doctor's questions and ran out of the office.

Although Greg had been suspended from kindergarten, he behaved
reasonably well at home and had adapted somewhat to family rules
and routines. Except when someone crossed him. Then he'd abruptly
and violently lash out at others, unnerving his parents and his brother
and sister, neither of whom was autistic. Greg's mother felt that his behavior could be neither predicted nor controlled.

Gregory did seem autistic to me as I listened to his mother's account
of his early history. While her son busied himself with blocks, she

described his isolation from people, his temper outbursts that often spiraled out of control, his impassive glances. She also lovingly described his artistic ability, beaming with pride as she told me about some of his drawings. "Greg can be quite affectionate sometimes," she summed up.

"Is this a wish?" I asked myself. Looking up from the blocks and glowering at me ferociously, Gregory hardly appeared loving.

Rather than concentrating on symptoms, I found myself reacting to behaviors of Greg's that were *not* typical of the autistic condition, if only to provide some relief from his rejecting attitude and from the miserably pessimistic prognosis that even today accompanies the diagnosis of autism. Most encouraging during my encounters with Greg was his responsiveness in conversation with me. To my surprise, I discovered a great deal about his perspective and his reasons for behaving in certain ways, which helped me understand, retrospectively, my experience with less articulate autists.

First Encounters

Not only did Greg wear an expressionless face much of the time, he avoided eye contact and refused to answer questions. "How are you today?" brought forth only a barely visible scowl and an almost inaudible mutter. He would only speak under his breath, chin down, his face covered by the collar of his jacket or his scarf. His mother, who had accompanied him to the first appointment, spoke of his unusual sensitivities to noise, touch, and bright and complex visual patterns. Years later, he explained that he also reacted instantly to odors. "Sometimes the smell even makes my nose *hurt!*"

To get a conversation going during our first meeting, Greg's mother reminded me of his collection of baseball cards and his inordinate fascination with animals, which she hoped would soften young Greg's rejection of me. As we began to converse, Greg spoke as though he had just learned to talk. There was a babyish tone to his voice, and he had several noticeable articulation problems. Even though he visibly relaxed while quoting sports statistics and enumerating many facts about animals, he still refused to take off his jacket or his scarf. He gave the impression that his clothing somehow contained him and his speech within a safe boundary, so that his overly clothed body would remain intact no matter how unusual or unexpected the situation in my office.

Meanwhile, Greg's mother was interspersing commentary on the circumstances of his suspension from kindergarten. When Greg threw a tantrum, he would thrash his arms and sometimes his whole body about so that he bumped into or appeared to hit out at others. He had hit his teacher, who then asked Greg to leave the class for the rest of the week. Gregory's impulsivity was indeed frightening, and he showed a split-second tendency in my office to explode when he felt thwarted.

Yet dour Greg perked up when he saw I had a toy that paralleled his interests. He shot me a brief, appreciative glance, making me feel his condition wasn't as hopeless as I had been led to believe and that his anger could be ameliorated if one met him on his own terms. I had shown him a box with twenty tiny drawers, each containing a small toy animal. On top of the box were pictures of all twenty animals arranged in a grid-like pattern that matched their layout in the drawers. If a child wished to predict which drawer held which animal, he could do so, provided he understood the picture corresponded with the animal's location.

I showed Greg this toy because of his interest in wild animals. I hoped he would communicate with me if he perceived that I shared his interests. But this was only part of my agenda.

I remembered that the Orthogenic School students were intelligent, even if mute or noncommunicative; they responded to human overtures if these were sensitively extended, and they understood what other people were about as long as they were viewed as trustworthy. In the intervening years before I met Greg, I'd read many works on autism that contradicted my early experience with young autists. I wanted to check my impression that Greg was intelligent, just as the Orthogenic School students had been, so I began to explore with him whether he understood the animal box set-up.

At the same time, I wanted him to reveal more about his interest in animals. I didn't want my questions to inhibit him from communicating his passion freely. I chose my words carefully so that he might learn to trust what I said. I hoped that the "crude rhythms" of speech would entice him out of his private world, that my voice might relax him with a kind of music that would melt his resistance to relating.

Greg soon emptied the drawers of their animals. "I wonder if you can figure out which animal goes where," I asked, suggesting that the pictures on top of the box might indicate the location of animals in their drawers.

Gregory studied the top of the box for a minute. Then he answered gruffly, "You can put them anywhere you want."

"Sure you can," I said, hoping to console him.

Greg started to force the animals every which way into their drawers, and then the drawers into the box. He muttered the names of continents as he did so. Then it occurred to me that he visualized grouping the animals by their continents.

I thought he did not fully understand that the grid atop the box matched the drawers of animals. But he surely understood that the grid signified a way of ordering the animals. His preferred organization reflected his interest in their natural environment. I praised him and commented that the way he arranged the animals could help us guess the ones that live close together. I got a brief glance and a little smile.

Greg began to play with the toy in earnest. He called it a "zoo" and talked with me about chimps for much of the meeting. When I agreed that the animal box was quite like a zoo, he again looked directly at me and smiled just a bit. Soon I had the eerie feeling that he began to smile not so much at me but at himself, basking in a setting that met his special needs rather than reacting to me, a specific person. This beatific, self-absorbed smile of Greg's reminded me of the way very young infants will smile, seemingly to or at themselves, probably responding to their own inner sensations. Could such self-absorbed facial expressions, I wondered, be a residual behavior originating in autists' infancies? In babies the smile evokes affection in the parent, an admiration of the adorable tiny infant who seems pleased with the world and herself in it. In autists of five years or older, it elicits a different reaction. Gregory's beaming face as he showed pleasure with himself was momentarily adorable, but because it wasn't social, it was bizarre and even irritating.

Greg soon began to name the animals, chanting their names loudly and slowly, announcing the continents on which they live. He made one mistake, saying that the armadillo lives in Africa. Hurriedly correcting himself, he cried frantically, "*Not* Africa. North America!" He could hardly tolerate mistakes, especially when he heard himself utter them.

He assiduously grouped the tiny creatures on my Oriental rug, pretending that the various shapes and patterns of the rug represented continents. As he chose one clearly outlined shape after another to be animal territories, he soon used up the entire rug, which meant he had to move ever closer to where I was sitting at one end. Finally, I had to get off my chair to give him room to arrange the Antarctica animals, which were at my feet. As he saw that I was bent on accommodating his play, he explained that the white fringe of the rug was ice. Gregory did not always show the infamous autistic tendency to avoid physical closeness, at least not when it suited him to approach me for his purposes. When he was finished grouping the animals, the young taxonomist sat back on his heels, pleased with his display, smirking and facing me.

When it was time for him to leave, Greg wanted to return all the animals to their drawers. He let out a high-pitched squeal when, not understanding his intent, I went to usher his mother and him to the door. He stood stock still, cramming the drawers with the animals, his body tense and resolute, as his mother and I stood by helplessly while he hurriedly nestled each one where he thought it should be.

When Greg came for his second visit, he didn't want his mother to leave. How well, I wondered, would he relate to me without his mother present? When I suggested that she might wait close by, he protested in a raucous, whiny voice, "No, no, no." I tried to comfort him by reminding him of his last visit, when he played happily with the zoo animals. Greg did settle down as his mother left, and began to mutter something about a "zookeeper." His syllables and words were muddled and hard to follow; his tongue got in the way of articulating. Yet he wanted to communicate with me. He wanted me to attend to the significance of a "zookeeper."

He might have imagined himself as the zookeeper, in charge of the animals he had classified according to their continents. Or, he might have likened himself to the animals and my office to a zoo, in which he felt caged or perhaps contained in a box by me, the "zookeeper." But I was wary of sharing these ideas with him. I wanted to get a better sense of what *he* thought.

I showed him a dollhouse doll, the one children usually designate as the "father" doll.

"Could he be the zookeeper?"

Greg chuckled slightly and murmured, "No, no, no." So much for that idea.

I was curious about his ability to answer questions in an environment that might appear different from the doctor's office in which he and his mother had been interviewed. Of the zoo animals, I asked, "Are there more African animals or animals?" Since I was quite sure by now of his above-average intelligence, I was interested in his ability to reason.

Greg replied that there were more African animals. This reply is not unusual for a five-year-old. Children this age are unlikely to distinguish set (animals) from subset (African animals) in order to imagine the latter group falling within the former. They think that because there are more African animals than American animals, there are more African animals than animals. I realized later that I should have asked Greg whether there *are* more African animals than American animals! My attempts to elicit conversation about the animals went nowhere, and like many autists who are questioned, Greg simply left the scene, as he'd done in the doctor's office, and ambled in the direction of my office door.

Surprisingly, he didn't try to leave the office. Instead he headed straight to another box of animals. Opening the box, he said, "You've got some farm animals in here." He seemed to say that I had both African animals and farm animals, so maybe there were more animals in all.

"More farm animals or animals?"

"More animals."

"That's interesting," I remarked. "How do you know?"

"Because you have only three farm animals," Greg answered tersely.

The manner in which he understood the classification question became clear only by implication. He implied that the number of animals was greater because there were only three farm animals. Because he had exerted himself strenuously in sustaining the conversation about animals, Greg began to behave impulsively. He toppled them all so they hit the floor with a soft thud. When I didn't react, thinking that he might want me to understand how unhappy he was about some aspect of our interactions or that he wanted to show me the animals could be grouped together in a heap, he retrieved them from the floor and lined them upon the table. He had the hippopotamus bite the zebra, glancing at my face for my reaction, with ever so slight a smirk. He grabbed an animal book, shouting excitedly, "Zoo, zoo!"

"You want me to understand what you're interested in?" I asked, referring to the toy animals and the animal book.

"Right!" he exclaimed, subsiding a bit.

Gregory was silent for a while. But when I asked, "How are things going in school?" he reacted as though it were an intrusive affront and ran behind a chair to hide. Out of sight, he explained, "I was hiding [in school] because I was afraid of the ball in soccer."

"Wow!" I thought. "Not only can he think reasonably, he can also talk about his feelings!"

Despite the abbreviated nature of his communications, Greg was able to express himself remarkably well, but it clearly fatigued him to interact with me for longer than a few minutes.

A child who can communicate but who fatigues easily is different from a child who can't communicate. What's more, Greg's behavior showed me that not all autists are unfeeling creatures, walled off from human emotion. Though I was somewhat taken aback by his admission of fright and his linkage of fear to hiding, I was overjoyed by his disclosure. I thanked him for telling me why he hid, and added that, by hiding, he was trying to show me how he felt both in school and in my office. Greg assented with a low growl, which I took to be a warning to keep my distance.

Silence followed. After a very long pause, he abruptly asked whether I have children. When I answered that I do, he leapt from where he was sitting and ran for the door. He was about to flee the office like a frightened animal when I explained, lowering my voice, that my children never came into the office when I was working, that only he and his mother and I would meet here. He spun around to face me and repeated, "never in office, never in office," trying desperately to comfort himself. His tendency to repeat phrases he'd heard—his echolalia—

occurred when he'd had a fright and sought to reassure himself by using some of the soothing and precise words of the other person.

Soon his mother arrived to pick him up. On his way out, Greg began to cover his fist with his jacket, mouthing and biting it. Observing him, his mother told me that he often tried to bite others and once bit her pillow. "At least he didn't bite *me*," she added cheerfully. In my office, Greg had opened his mouth wide, baring his teeth, and had made biting motions while staring at the tiny lion and cheetah in what appeared to be a near-total identification of himself with animal behavior. I wondered at the time whether Greg was "orally fixated" and whether he had become interested in animals because of their uninhibited, conspicuous "oral" behavior.

The psychological concept of fixation has it that young children under stress will regress to earlier developmental stages, to structures and modes of behaving that have become "fixed" in the psyche and that aid the child in defending himself against further trauma. The literature on autism in the 1950s and 1960s theorized that young autists couldn't progress beyond the "oral" phase because, as likely as not, autistic infants had not experienced oral gratifications from their "refrigerator mothers."

Greg's preoccupation with things oral, like imitating the biting behavior of animals, was to continue unabated until I met with him for a second series of visits five years later. I think now this behavior represents not his frustration with a rejecting, cold mother—his mother was warm and expressive, even temperamental—but rather the developmental stage he had reached and the ideas that were occupying his mind when he withdrew from the social world before the age of two. Because a withdrawal even from a conscientious and caring parent is so complete and seemingly final for young autists, it's as though the later stages don't register with them—they are not invested with emotional meaning. Or, if later stages do have an impact, they simply don't carry the emotional force that the first prewithdrawal stage held. If so, isn't it encouraging that a young autist wants to preserve a time in his life when he enjoyed some minimal but significant human contact?

Greg's work with me centered on his fascination with animals and his appreciation that I was willing, even eager, to follow his train of thought and the ways in which his animal preoccupation evolved. Imagine my euphoria when Greg one day began to make specific comparisons between animal and human behavior. He explicitly gave me permission to share his interest in animals at the very moment he expanded his animal kingdom to include people—the two of us!

Greg and I spent the rest of his kindergarten year in weekly meetings, during which he dramatized his many fears through enactments with toy animals or dolls. He listened to the information I gave to calm him. He had learned, for example, that some animals live relatively short lives. He concluded that because pets die within a decade or two, so would he. When I explained that human longevity and animal longevity differ, his worries subsided, and he slowly began to trust that I could help with his anxieties.

I explained to Greg's parents that his intelligence would enable him to understand their attempts to unravel his confusions. We had a series of parent meetings during which they described their son's every new worry. Soon we included Greg's teacher in the discussions, which focused on how best to deal with his feelings. His teacher and I believed that helping young Greg with his feelings about school would ameliorate the obstacles to learning that, paradoxically, his acute intelligence had produced. "He so desperately wants information about animals but is afraid of it at the same time," his teacher remarked. Greg was so frantic to escape the setting that made him anxious that he couldn't concentrate on what his teacher said or on the work she set before him.

Our combined efforts helped reduce Greg's fears, and he began to ask his teacher for help when apprehensive. This encouraged his teacher, who searched enthusiastically for new ways to present information, to make it less scary and more palatable to his young mind. Greg had adjusted well enough to his teacher to permit learning, and there were no more school suspensions. So Greg and I ended our work together, for now, though I did think about him often, wondering whether he would be able to maintain the gains he'd made.

Five Years Later

Ten-year-old Gregory returned to therapy because of school difficulties similar to those he had experienced when he was five. His impulsive and violent behavior had increased in fifth grade. His parents told me he'd had several good years since I'd last seen him largely attributable, they thought, to a few responsive teachers, but they were sorely frightened that this time he'd be suspended from school permanently. Greg defied his teacher, forbidding her to help with school subjects, and targeted his classmates with his so-called revenges. His bizarre behavior was often the stimulus for his classmates' taunts, which, in turn, brought forth severe, lengthy, vitriolic accusations and name-calling from Greg.

He had been tested and retested, diagnosed and rediagnosed. He'd had at least one promising testing experience in which the examiner took her time getting to know him before asking him questions. Greg earned a high IQ score (129 on the Wechsler Intelligence Scale for Children, or WISC, where a score of 100 is average) and, like so many other autists, showed uneven competencies, or subtest scatter. Some of his abilities outdid others. He excelled in tests tapping logical reasoning and factual knowledge. Two tests requiring visual-spatial organization confirmed the artistic facility Greg had shown ever since he'd been able to hold a pencil. Greg even got an above-average score on the test requiring an understanding of social conventions!

His examiner noticed that throughout the evaluation Greg tended to interpret material according to his own needs and wishes. Though she cautioned that this could be an impediment to school learning, during the testing she respected Greg's agenda, which was his ability to classify objects. He had shown this very ability when I first met him at age five. The examiner allowed him to express this openly so that she could assess what he had, in effect, taught himself. As a result, her report had a depth to it that other diagnostic write-ups of young autists often lack: it spoke of a whole person with real qualities.

When Greg wasn't daydreaming in class, he would protest strongly and loudly whenever his teacher tried to engage him in learning. Information coming from the outside threatened him, and he rejected it outright, either by storming out of the classroom or by turning his back to his teacher. He talked to her only when the subject was dinosaurs, his all-consuming preoccupation. He completed school assignments if they were about animals or if he had been allowed to choose the topic of study.

Math was a disaster. He hated thinking by other people's rules. He understood that writing essays or book reports permitted his ideas to flourish, but he couldn't bend numbers or formulas to fit his interests. It wasn't that he lacked math aptitude; he lacked the emotional fortitude to pursue it or anything else that appeared to arise from another's mind.

At first glance, I realized that many of the behaviors I'd seen in him at age five remained: avoidance of eye contact, a preoccupation with things oral, a habit of turning his back whenever he wanted to engage in solitary activity or protect himself from the onslaught of unbearable stimulation, both sensory and social. He was overly sensitive to olfactory and auditory sensations.

He reminded me of these one day when he said, "There's a kid who's always screaming on the playground, and it hurts my ears." Then he clapped his hands to his ears, completely covering them.

"Yes," I replied, "some people are like that; they have very sensitive hearing."

"I hate screeching noises, like on the blackboard," he continued, as he made a scratching motion to dramatize a fingernail on the blackboard, "and even thinking about it makes my ears hurt! I'm also sensitive to smell, some smells hurt my nose! I'm especially sensitive to the smell of dirt; I hate it when the vacuum [cleaner] is going!"

When he spoke of an absent person (the screaming kid) or of himself (his unusual sensitivities), Greg used language normally. When he was conversing with me face-to-face, he omitted key words to avoid acknowledging that he was talking *to* someone. He'd omit the pronouns "I" and "you" in conversation, because using them implied there were two of us talking. He'd mutter under his breath, "Want to play Hangman," without looking at me. It was as if he could handle only one channel of communication at a time. It was okay for him to speak to me without facing me; likewise, it was acceptable to look at me and smile, but not while talking.

By age ten, Greg had developed some additional behaviors typical of autism. He would pace back and forth across the floor, or when sitting on his knees, he'd rock rhythmically on his haunches, clapping his hands briefly but frantically, particularly during conversations when his emotions were aroused—for example, during a recitation on dinosaurs or chimps, or in response to a statement or question that got him going. The clapping occurred when I would comment, inaccurately from his perspective, about a topic on which he considered himself expert, or when I appeared to change the subject, which seemed to distract him from his chosen topic.

Greg's Animal Passion Deepens

Gregory began to sprint into my office like a fleet-footed animal. If he had to wait a few minutes for his appointment, he would roam the yard outside, like an animal on the prowl, searching for something.

Soon it became clear that he was mimicking specific animals. Sometimes it would be a chimp or a gorilla, as he'd scratch himself under his arms. Other times he would leap as high as he could, imagining, perhaps, that he was a deer in flight. Or he would tear at his snack with his teeth, ripping the flesh of a cut orange off its skin and chewing noisily.

One new way of behaving actually boded well for his future. Previously he would turn his back on me if he found my presence distasteful. Now he sometimes merely squinted at me or opened and shut his eyes rapidly, much the way Marcia would shut me out partially, not totally, as she gazed at me out of the corner of one eye. Paradoxically, this behavior appears when autists ready themselves for relating. Since they wish to engage with the other person but are still fearful of the other's reaction, they give only a partial glance toward the other, lest they discern disapproval, dismay, rejection, or other noxious reactions in the person's face or demeanor.[1]

In order for Gregory to continue to live at home and remain at school, he had to be reintegrated into the social world. I soon concluded that his outbursts were so uncontrollable, relentless, and frequent that our conversations had somehow to convince him that there were other, more auspicious ways of coming to terms with people. At first I was quite pessimistic about Greg because he had developed more, not fewer, autistic behaviors and because I met with him only once weekly, though I did consult frequently with his parents and teachers. Weekly meetings, even with consultation, did not seem a hefty enough dose to explore and understand Greg's perspective, much less to contain his outbursts and, most importantly, to convince him that the world was not an evil place that he needed to fend off at every turn. The unquestioned strength of his opinion that all other children were "bad," and the fragility of his control over his impulses, his hair-trigger nerves seeming to activate at the slightest provocation (a "look" from another child, a misstatement by his teacher about dinosaurs), all suggested to me that assisting Greg would be an arduous and long-drawn process, one that might not work at all.

In talking with him, I discovered some intriguing thought peculiarities. Complaining about his difficulty understanding fractions and launching into a tirade about his math teacher, he abruptly switched to self-criticism as he announced loudly that he probably had the lowest math average in the class. "And I think I have the lowest math IQ!" He went on to list his solutions to several math problems, estimating what his average math grade would be. When I remarked that he surely understood the averaging concept, he smiled briefly, only to harangue himself yet again about misunderstanding fractions. "The trouble with fractions is they never say one-third or one-thousandth of *what*!" he concluded miserably. I said his observation was a very good one, and I was sure if he asked for help, his teacher could assist him. He looked skeptical, so I explained that in some fraction problems the student is to determine the fraction of a certain number, as in "What's one-third of nine?" In other problems, I told him, the student is to determine how many thirds make up a whole. Probably because I was too wordy, he brushed off my attempt to clarify with a wave of his hand and irritably demanded that we play Hangman.

Playing the game of Hangman, Gregory chose words for me to guess that paralleled his interests: dinosaur, ibex, jerboa, and anaconda. Perhaps he chose words that I would find difficult to guess but, at least initially, he seemed to concentrate solely on himself and his imaginings of animal behavior. He seemed casually disinterested in me and in whether I would find it difficult to guess or spell these words. "Some of these words are hard," I once said. He replied, "They aren't *words*; they are *names!*" I started to explain that names were indeed words, but all words weren't names when he interrupted me to proclaim, "I like science a lot!" I thought at first that he turned the conversation away from any and all ideas forthcoming from me so as to refocus what we talked about solely on himself. Perhaps, in professing his attraction to science, he was thinking of taxonomic schemes, specifically those encompassing his Hangman "names."

I gave up trying to converse reciprocally with him, since he seemed to find it so offensive, and chose for my next word his own name. After guessing the letter *g*, Greg quickly surmised what the word was and flushed with excitement as I praised him. It seemed I had in this one conversation accomplished one of my goals: I was able to engage with him when I catered to the details of his perspective. He seemed to listen, still smiling, as I said, "You know, Greg is both a *name* and a great *word!*" Perhaps he would even contemplate the idea that names are a subset of the word category even if he had never thought of it before. I was thinking of the literature on autism describing how autistic children can hardly tolerate ideas that are not their own.

Yet there is an alternative interpretation of his behavior, one that occurred to me weeks after, prompted by my realization that Greg had always been interested in animal classification. Could the communication breakdown between Greg and me have occurred because I was thinking of only linguistic classification and he was thinking of only animal classification? In our conversation I referred to the fact that names (nouns), like verbs and prepositions, are all words, parts of speech. Greg referred to categories of animals as he chose one animal name after another to illustrate subset and set: dinosaur for the category reptile, ibex for goat, jerboa for rodent, and anaconda for snake. Then he tried to alert me to what he was thinking by exclaiming how much he liked science!

At the time, perhaps, I had a subconscious understanding of Greg's message as I chose his own name, the verbal marker of his identity, to spell in the game of Hangman. Then rapport was restored as he smiled and flushed with excitement. He may even have concluded that I understood his communication; why else would I have chosen his name to spell, implying a similar relationship of subset to set, Greg for the category human?

Interpreting Greg's statement as evidence of a developmental delay not only shut down our conversation in an important way, it also revealed that I was unduly preoccupied with a possible deficit in Greg's thinking. I believed that, unlike most ten-year-olds, he was still struggling with set/subset distinctions when he actually implied a set/subset distinction different from mine. At the very least, it would have been interesting to hear how Greg would have responded had I tried to engage him in an etymological discussion of the word *name*, which he had so ardently championed. "Teachers need to help autistic children develop their talents," writes Temple Grandin. "I think there is too much emphasis on deficits and not enough emphasis on developing abilities."[2]

I think now that when he said that words are names, Greg tried to convince me of the worth of his *ideas.* If so, it was I who was unable to integrate his meaning and not he who was unable to assimilate mine. At the time, I was so convinced that Greg must be led to countenance the opinions, knowledge, and viewpoints of others that *his* was the message that got lost.

Greg's Lectures

Before Gregory could become comfortable talking fully and directly about his problems with people, he had to establish a friendship with me. Initially, it turned out to be a one-sided arrangement. He had dropped his interest in baseball cards, saying they were babyish. But he delved ever more deeply into animal lore and displayed his new expertise proudly. He would lecture me as I listened attentively. He was the teacher, I the pupil.

As I listened, I realized that his command of biology was astonishing. Not only that, the cognitive processes by which he had organized the vast amount of material he'd learned were similar to those of any preadolescent. He had mastered classification structures and concepts, and he had learned how to order events. He once held me transfixed for the entire fifty-minute hour by his discourse on the evolution of the dinosaurs.

Occasionally he would answer my questions. When I asked if any of the books he'd been reading explained the extinction of the dinosaurs, Greg became excited by extinction theories and wanted to trace for me the history of these ancient reptiles. He had grouped them not just by their physical characteristics but also by the eras in which they lived and their regional habitats. He did not merely list facts. He fashioned his dinosaur lecture into a compelling narrative, introducing each new age of the gigantic animals as a new chapter and announcing their biological names and where they lived.

I began thinking that we experts are so busy identifying what children like Greg lack that even if we admit they are capable of classifying animals, we denigrate this achievement by believing something like, "This is an island of ability. These children use it to avoid human contact."

I began, mentally, to list Greg's capabilities. His pronunciation of dinosaur names was perfect; his knowledge of biology and geology, impressive; his understanding of taxonomy, exquisite. He indulgently and politely inquired whether I knew the difference between phyla, genera, and species. Occasionally he'd include other species and their biological relationship to dinosaurs, once interrupting his narrative to comment that scientists still do not agree on whether birds are related to reptiles.

He gazed closely at me for my reaction after he made a particularly important, emphatic point. His voice was passionate, reflecting his love for and fascination with the monstrous animals. From the beginning he built a sense of continuity and tension into his story, matching events to chronological time and dinosaur eras. Did he imagine communing with dinosaurs the way Flaubert envisioned tapping crude rhythms for bears?

I began to imagine someone other than me, Greg's parents or a favorite teacher, listening to his lecture. Might they notice only his repetitive pacing? In his excitement he roamed my office, head down in serious thought, his methodical gait delimiting areas that cordoned off my chair with an invisible boundary. I mused whether this behavior might discharge the energy he felt emanating from his mind and body. I wondered if it was also an attempt to locate me psychologically, to hold my attention, to differentiate speaker from listener, him from me. Perhaps his pacing allowed him to tolerate my questions, a few of which he anticipated before I had a chance to ask them.

"Now, about that extinction," he reminded me, humorously. "We have six more stages of dinosaurs to go through before we get to that part!"

Perceiving that I was truly engaged by his monologue, Gregory foresaw that I was most interested in the behavior of the dinosaurs. He informed me that these giant animals didn't just prey on smaller animals. "They also cohabitated. They managed to coexist compatibly even though they were aggressive!" he clamored zealously.

He occasionally checked my level of dinosaur knowledge. "Have you ever heard of tyrannosaurus?" he asked earnestly.

When I assented, he replied, indulgently, "Yes, that's a very well known dinosaur."

He showed how much he understood me, my interests, my level of knowledge. Social nuance came easily as he anticipated what I personally knew and differentiated common knowledge from the esoteric. He concluded that I would not know many technical details of dinosaur history, as I was neither a biologist nor a paleontologist.

Almost imperceptibly, he shifted the conversation to animal intelligence. He began by talking about the size of the dinosaur brain. I had no idea where his lecture would lead and was quite amazed and delighted to hear him say, "Being stupid is when people do things they know they're not supposed to do. The dinosaurs weren't stupid; they were dumb." He referred to the difference between being aware of acting stupidly and acting "dumb" without being aware of it.

Greg began to draw other animal–human comparisons. He was fond of discussing the ways in which chimps and humans are alike and different. He peppered this discussion with provocative dramatizations of antisocial primate behavior, assessing my reactions as he went along. He picked up a toy animal and began to imitate its spitting.

Soon he switched to the social behavior of animals and told me that chimps are really smart, unlike dinosaurs, whose brains didn't allow them to act intelligently. About chimps he added tersely, "Not as smart as humans, though." He then said thoughtfully, "But I trust animals more than I trust humans, even if they aren't as smart, because humans are tricky, and they can be tricky because they have more intelligence." He pondered this statement silently and then remarked pithily, "But if the IQ test were about how animals survive in the wild, they'd do better than humans!"

He returned to the topic of spitting animals. I wondered aloud whether animals spit when they are upset. Gregory took the discussion directly to a problem he had in school. He described how he had misinterpreted another boy's attempts to help him, how he'd gotten upset at his classmate, and had spit at him. He implied that he hadn't picked up on the social cues needed to react appropriately. "I thought he was treating me like a baby," he said. Stopping and starting his sentences, he finally blurted out, "How can I tell if a kid is trying to help me?"

Deeply impressed by his direct request for help, I told him, "You might try looking closely at the boy's face, just as you would observe a chimp at the zoo. Surely, you would understand the boy just as you understand chimps by their facial expressions and by their gestures.

You can tell when a chimp is friendly; so you can tell when a kid is, too."

"Yes, I have a problem," Greg admitted. "A girl in my class called me a monkey." Sensing that I would counter with the fact that primates are smart, Greg continued, "So if she calls me a monkey again, I can just say monkeys are smart. Or maybe I should just tell the teacher," he added doubtfully.

"Those are both good options," I replied, impressed by Greg's amazing understanding of his social problems and his earnest attempts to remedy them.

Toward the World of Humans

Greg eventually focused more on his interactions with people than on extinct dinosaurs, those huge beasts of the past. The link between prehistoric animals and humans was his new interest in apes, the animals most closely related to Homo sapiens who, like us, populate the earth today. He displayed a typical autistic naiveté as he admitted not always comprehending the implications for others of his behavior—his animal impersonations, his terse communications.

But I thought his social awkwardness was not so much a disability as it was a sort of social atrophy. Shy and isolated children like Greg enjoy little commerce with others. They don't usually build a social repertory that feels familiar or dependable or predictable. Nor do they develop the comfort and assurance that comes with repeated, daily human interactions that turn out well.

Yet, Gregory was aware of his social malaise, an awareness that was critical to his emerging ability to use his therapy visits. In the following months he and I concentrated on improving his school adjustment, a rocky therapeutic road that tested our patience and our stamina. Because Greg had attuned himself to his family, I thought him capable of relating to his teacher and of socializing with his peers more adeptly and congenially.

My encounters with Greg energized me to stay the course with him and others like him. I was motivated to reconsider my experiences with the Orthogenic School students. I yearned to distill the ideas I'd formed in living and working with Marcia and Stacy, to integrate them with what I was learning from Greg, and to impart my exhilaration and optimism about young autists to others.

CHAPTER THREE

A Meeting of Minds

It is only through her encounters with doctors that she
becomes either a hopeless case or an evolving person.

—ELIO FRATTAROLI

Writing of a young girl deemed "impossible" by one of her doctors, psychoanalyst Elio Frattaroli shows us in his interesting book, *Healing the Soul in the Age of the Brain: Why Medication Isn't Enough*, how the same individual can have opposite impacts on her two doctors. One doctor becomes dismayed by the patient's refusal to swallow her medication; the other understands her refusal, as there's no reason for her to cooperate with medical procedures that appear to be inimical to her well-being. Frattaroli stresses how differently these two attitudes, emanating from two presumably well-trained physicians, affect their patient when he writes, "The difference in what they are able to see in her and how they react to what they see profoundly influences the way she in turn is able to see and react to them."[1] With this in mind I'd like to paraphrase the opening quote: *It is only through a young autist's encounter with other people that she becomes either a hopeless case or an evolving person.*

The following questions ran through my mind as I became acquainted with autistic young people and tried to help them: "*Is* he hopeless?" "*Is* he developing?" Sometimes at war with myself, the setbacks of young autists or their victories either agonizing or elating me, I'd determine to plow ahead no matter what, certain that succumbing to despair would confirm my worst fear—that they could not be helped. Nothing like a pessimistic attitude, I quickly learned, to bring out their most troublesome and troubling behaviors. But would a different mindset, a guarded and informed hopefulness, create just the interpersonal setting to bring forth their attempts to relate, to adapt, to evolve?

This is a book about what can be done with autistic kids, what a "team" can accomplish with them. The team consists of everyone committed to helping them with their autism: their parents, their teachers, specialists, neighbors, friends—and the autistic children themselves. The coordinated efforts of those interested in providing a helping hand characterize such a team.

In this chapter, I introduce the remaining eight autists who are the subjects of this book. I focus on the issues and concerns, both educational and psychological, that have occupied me in my work with these children. I describe how I invite the child to join me in a friendship and how we are able to discuss or share his experience in which we approach a meeting of minds. I hope these portrayals will vivify both the dilemmas and the delights in helping autistic kids speak to us, explore their minds and their feelings, make friends, and accommodate to the learning and socializing required in school.

Marcia

One of the first autistic youngsters I lived and worked with was Marcia, a subject of Bruno Bettelheim's 1967 book on autism, *The Empty Fortress*, and a student at the Orthogenic School. Marcia was almost eleven when she was admitted to the School, and I only twenty-three. At the time I had another autistic preadolescent in my group of eight girls. I'd become fascinated by the condition and challenged by the interpersonal puzzles it presented. I was not entirely keen about undertaking the care of yet another young autist, but something about Marcia was particularly appealing. She was obviously intelligent, though she hardly ever *did* anything. She'd spend hours sitting rigidly at a table around which her dormmates would gather, having jammed herself up to its edge as closely as she could. Nevertheless, she'd gaze at me carefully but surreptitiously. It was her subtle attempts to hide her interest in me—and in the others with whom she convened silently (after all, she could have retreated to her bed)—that convinced me she was smart. Several times a day I'd catch her eyeing me appraisingly, glances that I later surmised were meant to assess her ongoing survival odds. After all, she'd been shipped off to a totally unfamiliar and, to her, alien environment. She could not have had the slightest clue as to its value for her.

Marcia was a beautiful child, as many young autists are, her face graciously formed and harboring limpid, sometimes searching eyes, though much of the time she stared at the ceiling, her eyes rolling upward. She'd shake her two forefingers sideways, rapidly and excitedly, then drop her eyes to gaze in a sort of trance at the colorful, shiny metal top of a container that often held cookies or other snacks. She ever so occasionally looked directly at me or burst into song, possibly trying to communicate something to someone, her voice strong and sonorous, exactly on pitch. I fancied she somehow knew I'd been a music student in college barely a year before.

Years later, when I read psychiatrist Robert Coles's impression of autistic youth, I thought of Marcia. I remembered that she seemed to be waiting for someone to rescue her, and that someone often seemed to be me. About autistic children, Coles writes, "It is not that such children are without enough intelligence; some are very bright. At first glance they may appear merely shy and a bit odd. . . ." He continues, "For some reason they frequently seem particularly thoughtful—when they are not wild and menacing. It is as if they are under a spell . . . waiting only for the 'right' person to come along."[2] This was Marcia.

She was shy, more than a bit odd, sometimes even menacing, as when she would fiercely rip off her clothes and tear them to shreds; she was often deep in thought, under a self-imposed spell. And I imagined that she indeed waited for just the right person to come along.

I have already noted that experts today designate three problem areas for autistic children: language, sociability, and the capacity for play. Marcia and the other autists I lived and worked with were clumsy or wanting in the first two domains, but most could and did play intermittently, even before I began to work with them. Their variable expertise at play before therapeutic assistance calls into question the experts' assertion that young autists don't or can't play. As we shall see, this belief is linked to the experts' view that autists lack the ability to conceptualize *mind*—either their own or that of another. Whether they are scholars who concentrate on the theory of mind and show little interest in helping young autists, or whether they are experts who do try to help, the majority assert not just that these children cannot play, pretend, or imagine, but also that they lack the requisite cognition to impute motives and intentions to imaginary figures or inanimate objects. Though Marcia did not initially speak to me or socialize, she *did* sit close by while others socialized. She was careful to watch the actions and possibly to surmise the intent of others, if for no other reason than to estimate how she would fare in her new environment.

Recently some researchers have challenged the thesis that autists lack a theory of mind and that they have no capacity for play. In their book *Autism As an Executive Disorder*, James Russell and his colleague Christopher Jarrold assert that pretend play may be problematic for these children, but not impossible.[3] In fact, encouraging the idea of pretense, they suggest, may help such children surmount some of their difficulties, a notion that is borne out by my experience with young autists. They can be enticed to observe others at play and will occasionally, seemingly despite themselves, join in the fun for a short while.

A word now on what I mean by "therapeutic assistance." I'm referring to the therapist's, tutor's, or even the parent's healing attempts to grasp the child's *own* way of perceiving things—even though parents, being closely, intimately, and continuously engaged with their child, are not therapists in a technical sense. Yet surely parents' efforts can be salutary. The therapeutic requirement to search out the young autist's own perspective may seem simplistic and patently obvious, but given a second thought, it plainly is not. Many professionals believe that young children lack the ability to formulate views and that even if they do so in some rudimentary way, they lack the ability to communicate their take on life sensibly and reliably.[4] It is not difficult to guess the opinion of such an expert when confronted with a young autist. If ordinary children remain largely unaware of their own perspective, surely the young autist who is believed incapable of registering his emotions and who may lack the capacity to recognize his own mind's workings would not be aware of his viewpoint—or even that he *has* one. Hence the futility of seeking it out, explaining the paucity of data on the autistic perspective.

Once I've understood the youngster's own perception of the world and his place either in it or removed from it, I explain to him how I understand him. The young autist's response, whether he speaks or only acts, confirms or denies what I've said. It's simply untrue that autistic children do not react at all to what you say and do. They may not react in a comprehensible or conspicuous manner. Yet I've found that searching for meaning in the slightest, subtlest turn of the head, flicker of the eyelids, or in the more obvious and disagreeable increase in rocking, pacing, daydreaming, or hand-flapping, helps the interaction along—just as it would if a parent overinterprets, perhaps, the

early prelinguistic vocalizations of her baby. If my hunches turn out
to be off the mark, I try again. If I've at least partially understood the
young autist's dilemma—which in many, if not all, cases consists of
his awareness that he is "different," even autistic—I then attempt to
enhance and expand our mutual understanding, which, if genuinely
felt, implies that something can be done about his troubles. Otherwise,
why would I go to all the effort of detecting and verifying them?

A mutually acceptable therapeutic plan for the young autist is not
easily arrived at. For him, it may not consist of his adapting to society
at all. It may be that he wishes I would listen attentively to scores of
discourses on dinosaurs; or tolerate his silent repetitive activity at the
washbasin, running water over his hands interminably; or provide him
with countless drawing materials without expecting him to say one
word to me about his art; or remain empathic when she executes, once
more, a routine 180-degree pivot so that I'm invariably staring at her
back; or retain my affection for her despite the utter chaos and terror
she creates around us; or respond immediately and graciously when,
to my face, I am addressed as "she." For therapeutic efforts to be
effective, the young autist must perceive some gain accruing to him
from adapting enough to converse or to interact. But isn't this true of
everyone?

The process of getting to know one another is much slower with
young autists; conversations occur at first with galling infrequency.
Most important, though, it is the *exchange* of *ideas* between *us*—
rather than *my* advocating behavioral change in *him*—that leads the
young autist to expand his horizons, to alter his repetitive behavior,
to converse meaningfully, eagerly, and reciprocally, to socialize enthusiastically and genuinely, and to play freely.

Marcia and I began to build some sort of clandestine relationship
around our mutual interest and pleasure in music. She'd often express
how she felt by an uncanny choice of the very song that put her feel-

ings into words perfectly. As a novice therapist, exhilarated by this insight, I thought, "How clever to find a way to communicate without seeming to." She could give voice to her emotions without claiming, necessarily, that the feelings she sang about were her own. She would, for example, sing about her mother when she heard others around her talking about their mothers. One day she burst forth with "Why Can't the English Teach Their Children How to Speak?," a song from the musical comedy *My Fair Lady*. I found this particularly significant, because Marcia and her caretakers had worked diligently to find out why Marcia hadn't learned to speak. She seemed to tell us that it was her mother who found it difficult to teach her. When we remembered that her mother was English, the choice of this song made perfect sense. And it made sense in the larger context of what I have come to think of as the "Orthogenic School mystique," which, as many distressed parents who read Bettelheim's book on autism doubtless remember, viewed the mother–child relationship in the lives of young autists as wanting. Marcia tried to join the children with whom she lived in their comments and complaints about their mothers.

Yet the point is not simply that the mystique led Marcia and me astray in viewing mothers as unresponsive (as many parents who read *The Empty Fortress* were also led astray). It is rather that songster Marcia was attuned to her environment, an attunement she seemed to flaunt subtly by her musically evocative rendition of the very lyrics that told her story. She may also have suggested to us that we, too, would have a hard time teaching her to speak.

The appeal music itself had for Marcia led her to communicate with me. Gifted as she was, how could she have evaded enjoying her splendidly sung melodies and how could she have completely avoided realizing that others enjoyed them as well? In their 1996 book, *Children with Autism*, child psychologist Colwyn Trevarthen and his research group remark that music therapists to autistic children believe their participation in musical endeavors and their "being influenced by [the] *aesthetic properties of music itself*" (italics mine) help young autists gain a sense of relatedness to others with whom they are singing (or otherwise making music) and acquire an increased sense of themselves.[5] With Marcia, I felt it was art first, communication second. She usually liked to sing alone and would stop abruptly if I tried to join her, but she would smile and produce more melodious lyrics if I sang back to her after she finished singing, as in a musical conversation. And for all I knew, she'd played singing games with her mother!

Trevarthen further reports that music therapists have found that musical improvising between therapist and young autist appears to replicate the emotional bonding and intimate communication that occur normally between mother and baby. If Marcia's mother had sung to her when Marcia was little, she may have hoped she'd be able to communicate with me by singing. She may have wanted to create an emotional closeness by attracting me with her beautiful voice. And in an important way Marcia *did* speak to me through music.

I realize these thoughts represent my fond hopes, but I think it not unreasonable to infer that the songs Marcia chose to sing were directly related to what was going on between us. She showed me just how much she understood the nature of our psychotherapy meetings by warbling the dwarfs' song from *Snow White*. "Hi-ho, hi-ho, it's off to work we go!" Desperate to relate to Marcia, I was only too eager to impute a grand significance to every song she chirped. But isn't this quite like a mother who delights in every small advance her little one makes? What the child gains is the mother's enthusiasm, overinterpretations and all!

Marcia's putting words to music seemed to help her over her awkwardness with syntax. Though she had quite a few nouns and some verbs in her spoken vocabulary, syntax bedeviled her for years. Songs provided the words she found so difficult to utter and to order. If she'd spoken to me directly, she'd have had to supply the verbal connectives herself.

Do Marcia's mutism and her verbal awkwardness mean she'd had no one at home to speak to who cared about her? Not at all. Marcia was clearly important to her parents; otherwise, they wouldn't have gone to the effort and expense of seeking help for her. If we are able to help young autists in today's world of ever-sprouting diagnosing and categorizing, we must prove to them that *they* are important to *us*. We professionals must document with our impressions of autistic children the ways in which they affect us personally; we must document how our actions, interests, inclinations, motives, and yes, our *feelings*, affect them. This would give the diagnosed autist the sense that she is a real person.

Stacy

Stacy, too, was a student at the Orthogenic School. She had just turned five when I first met her. She was a small, pert, rather well-coordinated little girl whose intelligence impressed me the minute I witnessed her little body in motion. Her behavior showed singular purpose—for example, she attacked only the eyes of other children. Years later she said to me, "Know the reason why I scratched out eyes? Because I wanted big blue eyes, not little teensy brown ones." By then her typical reversal of pronouns, calling herself "you" rather than "I," had moderated somewhat, and she would agree to call herself "I." She wished to look in the mirror and see big blue eyes, as she said, not tiny brown ones; this is yet another instance of a young autist being wary of some stimuli but drawn to others in a way that reveals strong preferences.

Stacy's symptom list included pretending she was a record player. Tirelessly she would sing the same favorite tune, "Mary Had a Little Lamb" (the benign rhyme a strange choice, given her penchant for attacking others). She would repeatedly and resolutely march circularly, mentally tracing, I thought, the shape of the record as she sang. Later she told me she imagined a singing motor inside her. The words to her song were enunciated perfectly; her melodious high-pitched voice hit all the song's notes effortlessly.

For all her precise articulation, Stacy nonetheless exhibited the well-known autistic "pronominal reversal." Like many other autists, she replaced "I" with "you," but never the reverse. Just as autists avoid the affirming "yes," their use of "you" to specify themselves reflects an aversion to an "I" that socializes, that communes with other people. I think Stacy avoided calling herself "I" because she often lived a solipsistic existence in which she didn't view herself engaged in any human encounter. In such a world, the child does not interact, so why use those parts of speech that denote one's own social acts? Why give the lie to a self who doesn't, perhaps refuses to, exist?

Yet Stacy would sometimes mock the other person as she called herself "you." This occurred when she was asked to do something (like accompany her dormitory group to supper) or not do something (like refrain from heaving her toys across the room). Then she called herself "you" to stress that her compliance—if indeed she *did* comply—was not her own idea. It was not "I" but the adult "you" who had made it happen. There was a distinctly accusatory tone to her voice when she said such things as, "*You* ate supper," or "*You* didn't throw *your* toys around anymore."

Stacy was not as withdrawn as Marcia but rather had established a reign of terror at home and tried her level best to create the same kind of menacing regime at the Orthogenic School. Just before she was admitted to the School, her care had been given over to one or two maids to soften the impact of Stacy's temper outbursts on her family. She would stare at people with glassy, expressionless eyes, a look that gave me the willies. Like Marcia, she showed a distinct distaste for human company, preferring toys. She had an urgent need for everyday situations to remain exactly the same. This, in addition to her relentless rejection of my efforts to take care of her, nearly drove me to distraction.

Amazingly, her inclination to converse thrived as I tried to figure out how she perceived daily events. Language came much easier to Stacy than to Marcia, and this linguistic fluency allowed me to grasp more readily her take on life. From the beginning Stacy, unlike Marcia, was well-spoken enough to correct me when I had mistaken notions about her.

Sometimes she'd behave as any very young child would—for example, by playing happily in the bathtub, squealing delightedly and splashing water on herself, on the floor, or on anyone who happened to pass by. Yet she would abruptly cease playing the minute I came too close to her, eyeing me blankly or downright angrily, chanting some indelicate and unkind made-up word with the intent, I felt, to persuade me to keep my distance. She once called me "Halloweeny" to signal that she thought I was bewitching her. What I wanted most to do was to wrap small Stacy in her bath towel and cuddle her on the way to her bed where I had laid out her pajamas. Recognizing my intentions, she would have none of it. She seemed to sense, faultlessly, when I felt affectionately toward her; furthermore, it seemed to make her furious. For years, every time someone around her found her fascinating or lovable, she would react by tossing a chair across the room or by throwing the nearest object to the floor where it landed in smithereens. She could tolerate the idea of human feeling only in dramatic enactments in which she would impersonate the full range of human emotion without, necessarily, claiming these feelings as her own.

What kind of experience had Stacy suffered that made her behave this way, I wondered, still under the sway of the then-popular notion that autists had been reared by unloving, distant parents. Now I ask myself what kind of internal bind Stacy had created for herself, one that was doubtless reasonable to her, yet caused her to become agitated or downright phobic by the threat of human interaction?

Stacy's partial recovery turned initially on our conversations about natural phenomena, especially those she so desperately wanted to fend off or to control. Because she was afraid of rainstorms—especially the bright sudden lightning flashes and the loud thunder rumbles, which she dubbed "rumble-bumble"—she became interested in the natural world and hoped that the information I gave her about it would help her protect herself. Our meeting of minds first occurred as I shared pertinent facts, which meant to her that I would protect her. Since she was so bright, I found myself exhilarated by watching her mind grow as she grappled with concepts about controlling and predicting the weather. It was rough going, because she could spin magical ideas about control and prediction faster than I could decipher them or look up in the encyclopedia the technical knowledge she required. The processes by which she came to apprehend and understand weather facts gave me the opportunity to refine some ideas I had about how children's minds mature. Stacy's interest in the natural world was serendipitous for both of us.

Much later, she expanded her investigations into the natural world to include the social world—an absorption equally attractive to me. Her inventive, witty use of language—punning was not beyond her—cemented our relationship in ways that hadn't occurred in my work with Marcia, attached to her though I was.

Stacy enacted many dramas during her early years at the School and personified aspects of reality that frightened her. She tried to gain control over her surroundings and her scared feelings in one inventive stroke. When she was afraid of drowning in the University of Chicago's swimming pool (the children went swimming twice a week), she invented a pretend person named "Pool." She bossed Pool, articulating precisely what he was to do, and once filled a balloon with water, saying it was Pool. With a mischievous smirk, gazing straight at me, she burst the balloon with a pencil and declared, "Pool, you are a bust!" I thought she meant that Pool was a bust at teaching her how to swim, implying that the person who was actually a bust as a teacher was me.

Marcia finally spoke after many years of silence, but she never found conversation easy. What's more, I was never entirely sure that I understood accurately the meaning behind Marcia's truncated speech. For all our joint efforts at communicating nonverbally, the difficulties in conversing with Marcia and the relative ease with which I discerned Stacy's meaning proved to me just how important language is when communing with young autists.

James

Two-and-a-half-year-old James came to see me in weekly consultation some thirty years after I had lived with Marcia and Stacy. Jamie had been severely frightened since about age one, and by the age of three he had developed so many fears that it was almost impossible for his parents to take him anywhere or to comfort him. The fears and worries of many young autists are much more intense and long-lasting, so different from the usually transient, understandable anxieties of ordinary children.

James's parents brought him to see me, hoping I could help them entice him out of his isolation. They had read accounts of young autistic children (Jane Taylor McDonnell's News from the Border, Catherine Maurice's Let Me Hear Your Voice, and Russell Martin's Out of Silence).[6] They had also heard of special home tutors and sensory playrooms for autistic children. They were particularly interested in learning how to help their son with the feelings he experienced while playing.

Jamie did play, hesitantly and infrequently, using tiny dolls to dramatize events he'd witnessed at home or at school. Yet he became inordinately frightened by his own enactments, not surprising since their purpose was often to express the angry and sad feelings that bothered him so. He was able to instigate playing scenes but was unable to bring them to a reassuring conclusion. He seemed unable to use playing for coping.[7]

As I became acquainted with Jamie, I began to advise his parents how to gauge when their son's play became too frightening. I suggested that they take charge of his play resolutions when he seemed overwhelmed by anxiety. Since they were familiar with many of Jamie's play themes, they could intervene directly to bring about a happy ending. Soon Jamie began to mimic his parents' imagined denouements, which reduced his anxiety and led him, eventually, to play more freely.

Jamie was a beautiful child with dreamy, dark round eyes that would widen enormously when he was looking at someone. Gazing back at him, I discovered he wasn't just vacantly staring at my face but was enthralled by the environment surrounding it. Sure enough, when later I stared at myself that way in the mirror, purposefully trying to take in more than my reflection, I saw that I had reproduced the famous "autistic look." I appeared to be strenuously not committing myself to anything, staring out into the vast emptiness of space, totally oblivious. Then I recalled that when I first met Stacy, she, too, had a blah look that told nothing about what was going on in her mind—that is, until she went into action.

Sometimes, when James looked at me this way, he appeared mesmerized by the rainbow colors of the poster hanging on the wall behind me or the highly visible striped pattern of darkened wood in the old cabinet to the side of me. Could it be, I wondered, that he wasn't simply avoiding my gaze but was absorbed by pleasing visual stimuli and was as committed to them as he was to human qualities, perhaps even more so? I thought of Marcia's hypnotized reaction to the bright red and yellow flowers on the shiny top of the snack container. When we conclude, often reprovingly, that autists' indirect gaze signifies a rejection of human company, do we not ignore that their wide-eyed gaping might indicate an appreciation of other sights by which they are particularly captivated?

James was a sweet-tempered child, alert and competent even in infancy, but withdrawn and scared much of the time. He spoke in his first year and could nest graduated blocks as soon as he could sit up, at around seven months. Like Stacy, he seemed to find himself frequently in a high state of intense stimulation. When I first knew him, he was interested in everything that shines. He could spot a shiny substance a mile away and was drawn to it as by a magnet. And yet he would hide from other sources of stimulation, especially those emanating from other children. He would devise elaborate mental systems, turned into contracts with his parents, by which he sought to protect his possessions whenever another child came to visit. He identified strongly with fictional characters in movies, stories, comic strips, and TV shows. He told me that he often dreamed about these personalities. Once he even said, "In my dreams, I *was* Garfield!" And many months later: "I used to transform myself into other people in my dreams."

James, unlike Stacy, never referred to himself as "you." When I first met him, though, he did talk about himself as "he." "He wants a cookie now," he would intone methodically. His parents responded by asking, "You mean James wants a cookie now?" to which he'd answer echolalically, "James wants a cookie now." But his echolalia occurred only when someone pressed him to change the way he spoke, to identify himself as "I."

Stacy's use of "you" and Jamie's use of "he" to refer to themselves reflected a different existential dilemma facing these two young children. While they both wished to express the psychological distance they felt from themselves, Stacy mimicked the other person, imagining she was the very person who was talking to her. Jamie seemed to talk *at* himself as though he were only another "he." Similarly he would refer to his mother and father as "the parents." "When are *the* parents going to pick me up?" he'd ask as he nervously waited for their arrival. Neither child behaved as though it was *they* who initiated action as long as they used the pronouns "you" and "he" to refer to themselves.

James's version of himself as somebody other than "I" abated when he began to admit to his intelligence and to own his actions.

At roughly the same time that James began to refer to himself as "I" and to his parents affectionately as "Mommy" and "Dad," his countenance changed from vaguely gazing to concentrated looking. He even made eye contact with me on occasion. Yet at other times, he approached my eyes as though they were a subject for scientific investigation. He told me once that he was trying to see what colors were in my eyes and how they looked behind my glasses. This did give me the spooky feeling that I was a mere object to him. But then he would back off, smiling. Once he said, charmingly, "What beautiful colors there are in your eyes!" He had isolated all the hues, finding each sensorially compelling. Like the childhood autist Donna Williams, James showed distinct preferences for some sensory stimuli at the same time that he retreated from others, like the noise produced by pesky children.

Maintaining the illusion of stasis was of utmost importance to Jamie. Anything unexpected, whether physical or mental, was rigidly eschewed. This meant that my office had to be arranged in precisely the same way each time I met with him. And I had to speak in a certain way, no other way. He would ask questions to which he knew the answers just for the security of predicting how I would respond. If I arranged my office differently or said something surprising, he would replace objects in their familiar places or correct my speech and my ideas pedantically. Board games, which soon caught his fancy, at first had to be set up and played exactly the same way, week after week, so that he knew beforehand who would win and how.

Remarkably, James displayed at the young age of six a sense of guilt at being different—essentially at being autistic. Quite possibly he knew how concerned and worried his conscientious parents were about him and so wished to spare them further discomfort by imagining himself to be like other children. His guilty feelings arose from his realization that he would always be somewhat different, and therefore somewhat of a problem for his beloved parents. In the pages that follow, I'll describe how sensitive young autists can be to their parents' and teachers' wishes and hopes, especially when these children begin to feel better and thus have less need to isolate themselves from their families and from the reactions of others.

As James matured into a robust seven-year-old, he remained apprehensive but not phobic, and his competence grew apace—in schoolwork, board games, even in manipulating people to get his way. He often acted competitively with peers over school grades and with me during board games. He developed a broad spectrum of knowledge that he'd recite precisely and pompously, much like a little professor. His mental processes, revealed in conversation with me, became better organized. He continued to be mildly diffident to others. Since playing board games gives the players the opportunity to refine their social negotiations with one another—for example, by arguing about the rules and procedures—the board-game format offered Jamie and me many fortuitous occasions to come to terms with one another.

Paulie

Compared to working with their talking peers, comprehending what a totally mute autistic child is all about is taxing, arduous, mystifying, and often frustrating for everyone involved, and often equally unpromising. Even if such a child chooses to reveal himself to others, he must rely on expressive modes other than language to make his needs, thoughts, and feelings known. The mute autists with whom I worked invariably reminded me of Marcia, because she was so often and so inexorably silent. When I began, after I'd left Chicago, to work with completely mute young autists, I was passably prepared to deal with the enormously disconcerting yet curious experience of being face-to-face with intelligent silence. The saving grace in such a situation is that some mute autistic children will express themselves through the arts, like drawing, mime, or music, as Marcia did.

One very small autistic boy, Paulie, who was about five and who had never said a word to anyone, had the most discerning countenance I'd ever seen in a mute autist. Yet the minute I spoke to him, even though I said a mere "Hello," he would turn his back on me, slowly and methodically.

The simple words "hello" and "How are you?" apparently overcame Paulie with such a rude feeling that he would cringe and turn away. He may have hoped I would then cease talking to him. If so, he got what he wanted, because I *did* lapse into silence, wondering why a mere "hello" would prompt him to rotate his body. My words seemed only to increase his solitude, possibly because he felt monstrously insecure about his ability to talk and therefore to communicate.

Sometimes I would proffer a little toy to this fragile-looking, thin little boy with enormous, vacant eyes, but only a toy he had touched briefly the week before. And sometimes he would accept it, his tiny flabby fingers working lethargically to grasp it while he stared, glassy-eyed, at the ceiling or out the window next to where I sat, conspicuously looking off to the side but not directly at me. He would engulf the toy with his tiny hand cupped casually, lest I think he was truly interested in it. Maybe he feared what I would expect of him if he took the toy. I might expect him to talk.

When Paulie was about two, his parents had noticed that he was very different from his siblings, who, they said, behaved normally. Paulie was withdrawn and mute, engaged in repetitive arm and finger movements, and refused to look at anyone directly. They thought, like so many parents with autistic children, they must be doing something terribly wrong with Paulie, else he would behave more like his brothers and sisters. They brought Paulie to see me hoping that as I got to know him, I might be able to instruct them on how to care for and help their son.

I soon felt that Paulie and I were playing a silent game in which we both pretended the other was not there. Since I sought to keep my distance to avoid offending him, I felt I was colluding with Paulie in not acknowledging his presence. All the while, though, I had the weird feeling that he knew as well as I did what our little game was about: his continuous silence had the aim of making me disappear, in order to lighten the effects of my presence on him. I felt in a psychological bind rather like the one I'd experienced so many times with Marcia. Being intrusive with a child like Paulie wouldn't work—I knew that. Since I began to meet with him soon after I left the Orthogenic School, I had not yet formed in my mind what one *does* do with a totally mute, withdrawn young autist. I had to find a way to encourage relatedness without being overbearing, especially since the merest suggestion of an overture from me seemed to provoke Paulie's redoubled efforts to return even more steadfastly to his inner world. I hadn't yet figured out that it was my speech, not my intentions or my attentive silence, that caused his withdrawal.

Initially I had no idea that Paulie had a particular talent. How could I, since he said nothing and did so little? I was astonished one day when he abruptly began to draw. Now his fingers and hands worked energetically and masterfully. He must have noticed all along that I laid out paper, pencils, and markers, together with what I inferred were his favorite toys. These items had been plainly visible, though he gave not the slightest hint that he saw them. Perhaps my silence, resonating to his, or my offering a small toy from time to time, encouraged him to *communicate without words*.

Paulie and I came to a meeting of minds of sorts when he let his line drawings fall off his hand onto the table, where I was sitting just close enough for me to see them without getting up to approach him. They depicted the physical aspects of the building in which we met;

astonishingly, the details were so accurate that I was instantly able to decipher them. The cartoonlike pictures—he'd framed them rectangularly with bold, dark lines—represented the weekly sequence of coming to see me: the first frame showed the office building and its front door; the second, a hall that led to the stairs that he climbed to my office; and the last picture showed the toys he had played with and the plate of snacks I always laid out for him, even though he never ate a single bite. I was inspired by his little story but afraid to show too much emotion lest I overwhelm him. Then he might never draw again.

More than any of the other autists I knew, Paulie's behavior seemed to typify the autistic dilemma. He so desperately needed my help, but my very act of providing it seemed to create such agonizing inner turmoil that he had to withdraw. The only way out for us was to pretend that I wasn't doing very much. Incommunicado Paulie did not want to recognize that speaking or the expectation that he speak was at the root of his troubles. I believe this is why he refused to eat in my presence. Using his mouth for eating would reveal that his oral apparatus was functioning. If this were so, he'd be expected to talk or, worse, be sanctioned if he wouldn't or couldn't talk.

Thinking about Paulie, I realized that psychoanalytic theory in an important sense had it backward when it came to the mute autist's silence. At the Orthogenic School, we theorized that if one could just liberate the use of the young autist's tongue, teeth, and lips, the child would be free to speak, having regained or gained anew the use of the mouth in slurping, mouthing, chewing, and the like.[8] We encouraged young autists in psychotherapy to engage in these activities freely in the hope that mute autists would start to talk.

Now I think it is the mute autist's realization that he *does* use his mouth for functions other than language that leads him to defend against speaking by pretending he has not the slightest interest in *any* mouth functions, exemplified by Paulie's studied disinterest in the very snacks his mother told me he enjoyed. Paulie knew, I thought, that I wanted him to speak with me. Because he *didn't*, he felt ever so strongly that he *couldn't*. Couldn't *communicate*, that is. What better way to "prove" it true than by pretending his mouth had no functions whatsoever? Mute Paulie's autistic dilemma, then, might have been ameliorated if we'd worked out together how he could communicate without talking.

Burt

Things were much different with another mute autistic boy who was not graced with any particular talent. Burt made expressive noises that gave some hint of his feelings, but he never put a name to any of them; nor, for that matter, did he name any thing or any person. He was four and a half when I started working with him, and for more than four years, he never appeared to recognize me the way ordinary children do. I'm sure he knew who I was, but he never had that expectant look of recognition, that glad-to-see-you demeanor. He was never surprised to see me when we happened to meet under circumstances other than his scheduled appointment. It was as if events just occurred mundanely in a steady stream before him without any personal significance and without any implication that he should react to happenings or initiate them.

For years I tried to concoct connections between what this nice-looking, somewhat awkward boy was doing and the noises he made. He would flail his body around, seemingly aimlessly, often uninhibitedly grabbing his genitals, picking his nose, and generally behaving as if decorum did not exist. And even if it did, he couldn't have cared less. His eyes would sometimes light up in recognition as I spoke, but more often he would gaze dreamily to one or the other side of me or widen his eyes into gigantic circles at nothing in particular. There was no pattern to his activity that I could ever detect. For a long time, Burt never singled out any of the toys or equipment in my office, never focused on any specific play activity in even a diluted, indeterminate manner. How hard it is not to project onto a flagrantly uncommunicative mute autist one's own thoughts and feelings! Burt, unlike Paulie, had no apparent resources nor the interest to make his meaning clear. For all I knew, I was so off the mark when I spoke to him that I actually discouraged him from talking. Why speak if what you might be persuaded to say is so vastly different from what the other person expects?

For a time I believed that Burt deliberately made himself as inconspicuous as possible. But why? I soon realized he wished to hide his longing to dash off at the earliest opportunity from other humans, to be alone, away from human stimulation. In fact, all Burt did that one could reasonably interpret was to run away from his family every chance he got.

Young autists often separate themselves from other people by distancing themselves physically. Many of them roam about or wander away from their homes or out the gates to their yards, sometimes to get away from people but other times to pursue their solitary interests, like counting fence slats. Paul McDonnell, whose story is recounted by his mother, Jane Taylor McDonnell, in her book *News from the Border*, explored how far the telephone lines went.[9] Fortunately, young Paul allowed his mother to accompany him.

Since Burt rarely ran from either school or his appointments with me, I made some headway when I asked him why he would run from home, of all places, when he seemed okay with his teachers and, perhaps, even with me. At this, he began to slap his thighs vigorously, which I took to be a signal that he'd been slapped when he disobeyed his parents' sincere and frantic remonstrations that he not endanger himself by running to the freeway. At last, I thought, there was a link between action and talk. I knew from Burt's parents that they had slapped him for running out recklessly, but it also occurred to me that Burt might have it backward: perhaps he thought he ran because they slapped him when, in fact, they slapped him because he ran. If so, he displayed, at age seven, a delayed mental habit common in younger children who believe that if A causes B, then B causes A. Young Stacy, fearful of storms, displayed similarly immature reasoning. She believed that going outside would make the rain stop because we come inside when it rains.

It belatedly occurred to me that Burt didn't run from school or from my office because these sites were farther from the freeway than his home was. I could hardly be sure that he was reacting differentially to people in his life, that he preferred his teacher's and my company over that of his parents. He simply did not know how to get to the freeway from school or my office.

Runaway Burt's tenuous connection to me and the meaning of our work together was so elusive that I fear there was none. He did start to signal to his parents that he intended to flee by acting increasingly agitated, providing them with enough warning to protect him more effectively. Their anxieties about Burt lessened somewhat, and he finally began to play regularly and deliberately with water, letting it run warm and cold over his hands for hours on end. Burt perhaps wished to explore this facet of nature, but he never invited nor permitted me to join his water play. I was only an observer, never a participant.

Dirk

For most of Dirk's young life he had been remote and silent, but suddenly, in his sixth year, he became "hyperverbal" and vigorously protested the testing procedures his mother had scheduled to determine the cause of his erratic behavior. Dirk seemed painfully aware that he was being scrutinized for deficiencies and became restless, even defiant, during his psychological evaluation. Years after I knew Dirk, I read in Russell Martin's *Out of Silence* of eight-year-old Ian, Martin's autistic nephew. Ian reminded me of Dirk because, as it turned out, Ian had understood he was different since early childhood. He had begun to communicate by typewriter, describing his feelings in a way he had not been able to before. One day he was about to refuse to go to school when his mother reminded him that his best friend would miss him if he were not there. Young Ian typed a denial that he *was* a best friend. His mother asked why, to which Ian typed that it was because he was autistic. Martin concludes of the mother–son exchange, "Ian *knows he is autistic* and believes it makes him different."[10]

I had thought Dirk's protests over the evaluation represented his attunement to his mother's anxiety about the test outcomes. It happened that Dirk, too, was afraid of the results, of the diagnosis "mental retard," as he called it. Dirk, like Ian, sensed that something awful was wrong and concluded, not unreasonably, that he must be cognitively deficient. He had all too often overheard his parents and others who knew him well question his mental potential.

Because he refused to answer test questions, the results could hardly be interpreted reliably. He garnered a host of diagnostic impressions and conclusions that suggested to me that his doctors were nonplussed by his behavior and really didn't want to deal with him. Words would rush out of Dirk's mouth so his thoughts were indeed hard to follow, but with a little time and patience they began to be strung together in a narrative that made sense. His mother sought my advice for Dirk, who was reeling from the impact of testing. She hoped I could "use the right words" to explain the outcomes to her son.

Dirk's mother had become distraught by the lack of clarity and the innuendo in the doctors' reports, much like Beth Kephart, who wrote of the trials surrounding the psychological evaluation of her son, Jeremy, diagnosed with "pervasive developmental disorder." Because of its vagueness, this notoriously blurred nomenclature thwarts parents in securing professional counsel on what to *do* about the child. "And though it should have been helpful to have a name for the thing that was so deeply troubling Jeremy," Kephart writes, "a diagnosis is far from a cure. The fix for children like Jeremy is, I have discovered, a baffling admixture of trial and error."[11]

And so it was trial and error for Dirk, his mother, and I as we tried to piece together what had been so upsetting and what to do about it. Refusing to say a word in answer to the psychometrist's questions, Dirk would not even point to pictures to show that he understood what was required. Dirk's later query of his mother gave some clues: "Why does *he* [do I] have to point to the duck, *she* [the tester] knows where it is!"[12] Dirk used the third-person pronoun to refer to himself, but he revealed much more by his pithy question. He showed in a flash that he had all along known that "duck" was the correct answer but had declined to supply it. Dirk's mother and I speculated that far from showing mental deficiency, Dirk's answer revealed he had a pretty good idea of his tester's intent and her estimate of his intelligence. She wanted him to point to something whose whereabouts were known to her but presumably not to Dirk. Dirk verified not only that he knew what he allegedly did not, but also that he had guessed his tester's surmises. A year or so later he started to complain to his parents and to me, "People think I'm soooo stupid," and "They call me 'stupid' in school."

As Dirk's behavior shows, it is sometimes irrelevant in a situation with a savvy child whether the subject complies with the test instructions. The idea that the testee must come up with the conventional answer whatever the circumstances unnecessarily limits the diagnostic procedure, especially with autistic children about whom one is as likely to learn from noncompliance as from compliance. Things get a lot worse when the examiner concludes that an unusual response, even if it's well reasoned, indicates not the mutual understanding of a fact (where the duck is) but an inability to adapt to the test situation and thus an incapacity to adjust to society.

While his doctors were arguing about his diagnosis, Dirk's teacher produced a splendid description of him. It not only suggested he was autistic, but it also intimated that Dirk did not wholeheartedly reject social overtures but rather had mixed feelings about them. "Dirk shows sporadic rotating behavior," she wrote, "running and twirling and sometimes seems withdrawn into his inner self. Much of the time, he crawls on the floor or runs around the room on his tiptoes." By the time I met Dirk, he had stopped rotating and twirling but would often crawl on the floor, pretending to be a dog, barking realistically, though he still would not say much. "He covers his ears, turns his back on others and only talks with them when asked a question about what he's doing and then maybe he will answer a soft yes or no," Dirk's teacher continued. With me, too, Dirk would only respond monosyllabically with the word "no" or a muttered "uh-uh," or he'd repeat what I said mechanically and monotonously. It wasn't until I'd worked with him for about a year that he would say "yes" or answer a terse "not yet" if I asked, for example, whether he would like to play with me.

"It seems like all things divert his attention," his teacher wrote. "Too many crayons on his desk, noises, all sights and sounds bother him. When he stops daydreaming he seems to get too many messages at once and he can't shut any of them out and focus on the important ones. He must be reminded or refocused to continue with the task he was called upon to do," his teacher concluded. Dirk's social ambivalence was evident to his teacher when she noted that he would respond, albeit briefly, when another child spoke of what Dirk himself was doing. His ambivalence was evident to me when he didn't outright reject my invitation to play, only postponed it as he said, "Not yet."

Still, Dirk's doctors bandied about several diagnostic labels, popular during the time Dirk was tested, including "minimal neurological dysfunction" and "hyperactive," but without specifying which of his behaviors had led to these diagnoses. One doctor flatly asserted that Dirk was "certainly not autistic."

His teacher's description of him, though, is quite similar to Donna

Williams's portrait of her childhood self. "I was three and a half," she writes. "My parents were visiting some friends, and I was standing in the hall outside the living room. I was giving myself the whizzies— arms outstretched, spinning around and around."[13] Williams resorted to physical activity to diminish unwanted stimulation. She gave herself the "whizzies," just as Dirk twirled or ran around the classroom. Two descriptions—Dirk's teacher's and Donna Williams's—imply that the activity these two children engaged in served to protect them from *human* stimuli—from her parents' friends in Williams's case, from the other children in Dirk's—not just too many crayons, sudden and loud noises, and unexpected events.

Williams also recounts her experiences in a "special school," including her problems staying on task, because she was caught up in sensory experiences that transfixed her, as she was to write time and again in her memoirs. Similarly, early in my work with Dirk, he could not focus on anything while a song was running around in his head. Instead he often burst out in high-pitched, piercing tones that were at once excruciating and exquisite. He not only pushed away offensive stimuli but also surrounded himself with the stimulation to which he was most drawn—musical sounds. Dirk selectively rejected some stimuli and had an intense appreciation of others. Describing her fondest memories of school, Williams writes, "I loved the heavy oak doors of the school church, the polished floors, the colored glass up so high. I loved the way it all smelled and the trees that hung over into the playground." She continues, "I loved cream buns at recess. I loved my metal school badge, which was sewn on to my blazer."[14]

When not overwhelmed by intrusive stimuli she could not control, the young aesthete Donna Williams reveled in the sights, smells, and tastes associated with school, just as Dirk got himself through the day by improvising the most appealing of melodies. When his teacher, like many a teacher or tutor to young autists, responded to Dirk's frustration at too many bothersome objects on his desk and removed some of the crayons to refocus him, Dirk showed himself to be something of an artist, creating a colorful picture of a small boy singing, running, and jumping, revealing a discernible effort to alter the boy's posture to capture his various activities. Far from being altogether and routinely unresponsive to their surroundings, autists can be particularly sensitive to them, delighting in the sensuous pleasures they give.

Not surprisingly, my first connection with Dirk was in my humming along with him. He must have thought my singing was intrusive at first, because he would cover his ears with his hands, pointedly grimacing and frantically gesturing for me to stop. So I softened my voice and worked diligently to improve my pitch. Eventually Dirk tolerated our singing together when he began, like a conductor, to guide our chorus by thrashing his arms around dramatically. I dared not hope too much, but it did seem as though a bond was forming between us. I showed him the toy musical instruments in my office, whereupon he began to match the colored keys of the xylophone with their counterparts on the music pages and put words to the notes, eventually asking me "who made" the songs, mostly nursery rhymes.

Though I was interested in getting Dirk's attention so that we might do something together—I could hardly stand the ease with which young autists ignored me—I wasn't at all invested in making him attend to a preplanned agenda. I wished to support the integrity of his chosen concentration on singing and humming. From there, we branched out into the shared world of music. Taking advantage of the autistic child's interests as I tried to join his first timid and sometimes awkward ventures into a social world had yielded intriguing results before. As urgent as it is to introduce the autist to heretofore ignored aspects of reality or to get him back on developmental track, the therapist—or tutor or parent—must on occasion act as if she's got all the time in the world for waiting until the right moment. An interested nonchalance can beguile a young autist to make those small, tentative, and first social moves so necessary to the inception of a friendship.

Much later, Dirk and I came to a meeting of minds on the "good" and the "bad" in the world. He became obsessed with such superhero characters as Superman and Batman. The way he talked about them led me to understand that he sometimes truly believed he lived in a superhero universe. Our discussions often had an almost philosophical quality to them, much like the many talks I had with young Stacy decades earlier. Like Stacy, Dirk was fascinated by "good" and "bad" people. For him, cartoon characters and real people could, in an instant, stand in for one another. He evolved many complex but confusing schemes for classifying fictional characters (in movies, in comics, in his imagination) that, surprisingly, helped him relate better to real people. Yet his personal criteria for good and bad could advance superhero Dirk only so far as he tried to adapt to actual social situations.

Wendy

Before I met with eight-year-old Wendy, her mother told me that Wendy often did not gaze directly at people and had preferred, since early childhood, to entertain herself alone in her room for long periods of time. When other people would talk to her or interrupt her solitary activities, she'd frantically tear at her eyebrows or twirl her hair so forcefully that it would come out in small fistfuls. Wendy's parents brought her to see me because she was prone to lengthy and tempestuous outbursts at home and had begun to dissolve into angry tears at school. She was a skinny, gawky child with beautiful dark eyes framed by the longest eyelashes I'd ever seen. Her eyes appeared to have a film over them, seemed to cloud up whenever she looked at me. She seemed more interested in her private thoughts than in people, her thoughts appearing to dance intriguingly before her. At first, Wendy was disinterested in how I might react to her. She seemed to absorb the entire environment around my face as she enlarged her eyes abstractedly and talked to me in a dreamy voice. Hypersensitive to noise, Wendy would inquire suddenly and urgently for the source of all sounds in my office. Likewise she was exceedingly sensitive to touch, whether it be a tactile affront arising from scratchy or wrinkled material against her skin or from another person hugging her or otherwise getting too close physically.

By the time I got to know Wendy well, I'd been thinking a great deal about James. For both children, the setting immediately encompassing a person was as important to them as the individual within it. For them, people were part of the natural and physical world, whether these two autists were outside among the trees and flowers or whether they were inside reacting to the physical details of my office. Given that some autists appear to be more *in* and quite literally *of* the world than we are, the expert view that they are disconnected from reality seems simplified or downright wrong. Both James and Wendy wished to see me *in* or *of* the world instead of to look merely *at* me. Isn't it just possible that the sensitive sensoria such children exhibit enable them to be a part of the natural and physical world in a profound, intimate way? Wendy and James fancied certain stimuli much the way Donna Williams was attracted to cream buns and her metal school badge. James was drawn to shiny objects, Wendy to my shiny bracelets. Both children headed straight for anything in my office that twirled or rotated—but only when they were feeling mellow. Otherwise, they would reject much or all of their environment as forcefully as they would dismiss overbearing or intrusive people.

James would often bump into me or step on my toes as though I were a piece of furniture; Wendy would sometimes act as though my body or clothing weren't mine personally but could be automatically appropriated by her. She would grab or fondle some of my beads or a scarf around my neck for the pure pleasure of touching something smooth or soft. This didn't seem to me to be a lack of ego boundaries as some experts have suggested; in their view the young autist, lacking a sense of herself as a subject, blurs or imagines merging her being with that of another person.[15] While I thought Wendy perceived me not as a subject but more as an object, like a toy, she always considered *herself* as a subject.

The trouble with psychological theory that fails to ground itself in careful and diverse observation and that does not inquire directly of another's perspective is that it can conflate two seemingly related but actually distinct phenomena. It is possible for a person to treat someone she doesn't want to acknowledge as an object, yet have a robust sense of self. When Wendy consented to make my acquaintance, she acted reciprocally, as though the two of us were conversing or drawing or playing a board game. Her sense of ego and body boundaries—that is, her recognition of the limits of her being—functioned well. Yet Wendy avoided referring to herself as "I." Whereas James would substitute "he" for "I" in the sentence, "He wants a cookie now," Wendy would intone, "Still hunnnng . . . gry," asking for snacks indirectly and conspicuously omitting her personal pronoun.

At first Wendy said almost nothing to me and answered questions monosyllabically, referring only to facts, never to feelings or ideas. She would chant in a high-pitched singsong as though she were on stage. Again like Jamie, she came across as an erudite little lecturing professor, informing me of fact after fact but only those that consumed her. At other times, she would roam about my office, picking things up, only to stare at them scornfully and briefly, hurriedly releasing them from her hands as though they hadn't the slightest significance for her—as though they didn't exist, really. Then she'd continue wandering. I got the feeling that she couldn't think of anything to do. Perhaps this was so because the objects in my office didn't match her preoccupations closely enough. I soon realized she might have another reason for pacing aimlessly—perhaps she wanted to test whether I'd accept and respect her desire for solitude. Or would I expect her to act like other children?

Wendy was remarkably talented. When, at long last, she consented to talk to me, she displayed a prodigious writing gift and, later, an artistic facility. She would even speak of her story characters' feelings as she typed her tale. Or she'd include cartoon captions in her drawings, indicating how the characters felt. At the same time, she shied away from anything admittedly linked to the companionship we were slowly building. Gradually and shyly, she would *imply* that we did things together, because only belatedly had she acknowledged to herself and to me that we *were* together.

Wendy's stories and poems were imaginative and fanciful. The story plots were quite solid for such a young child, and she experimented with many genres, including fairy tales and some fable-like creations. She was reluctant to show me what she'd written and would bashfully explain that her writings were "private." To earn her trust, I had to accept her need to hide her stories and assure her that I would not intrude on her mental activity unless she gave me permission to do so. Still another reason, I thought, for experts to believe that autists have no theory of mind: they often act as if they don't, so fearful are some of revealing their thoughts to others. A brief reflection, though, would vouch for Wendy's theory of mind since the attempt to conceal something requires the kind of mental activity that accounts for the wiles of the other.

Once I chanced upon a slip of paper on which Wendy had printed just a few words. She instantly understood that I had read them and became distraught and angry, roaming and pacing the floor tensely and frantically for the rest of our meeting. Warily I inquired whether she was angry with me for looking at what she'd written, wary because my question might be interpreted by her as still another intrusion. To my surprise, scribe Wendy responded with a boisterous and noisy, "Yessss!" Her fury didn't abate, though, and she stormed around my office stamping her feet until it was time to go. Yet there was a subtle change in her demeanor, and I thought I detected a bit of staged drama on her part, as though my identifying how she felt led her to playact her anger even more. She could have been toying with how it felt to get angry in my presence, testing, as many a young child will, whether I would retaliate. Or perhaps she wished to hang onto the angry feeling for as long as she could for some other reason—maybe to impress upon me once more that I must always ask first before I read anything of hers, or maybe, simply, to study her own angry reaction. A young autist I was to observe several years later appeared to do the same. He'd register a feeling and turn it over and over in his mind; he once said to his classmates of a humorous skit he and they had produced, "It's funny, funny, funny!"

Wendy soon began to draw in earnest. Her drawings often consisted of people who were busily doing something, "not just standing around doing nothing," she explained, now relaxed and eager to show me her work. The fact that the people in her drawings were doing something seemed to reflect that she, too, was no longer "just standing around doing nothing." It was not at all difficult to discern the activities of the people she drew. She could capture a person's facial expressions explicitly and amusingly.

Sometimes she asked me to join her while she was drawing, and much to my chagrin, she soon realized that I have little artistic talent. She began to tease me, especially about my inability to draw people. How ironic, I thought, that Wendy, an often solitary young autist, was more adept at depicting people than I was—with feelings and in action to boot. Supposedly limited in her ability to notice and relate to others, this young autistic artist was manifestly accomplished in portraying human qualities.

Wendy would coach me how to draw people, and soon I realized she was an excellent teacher, so much so that my clumsy drawings began to improve, much to her delight. Not to be missed was her obvious enjoyment of my embarrassment and frustration at being unable to render on paper what I wished. It was as though Wendy had provided herself with a safe laboratory in which to observe my display

of emotion right before her eyes. And some of the emotions she detected in me were precisely the ones that had caused her own distress.

Our meeting of minds occurred when I recognized that Wendy was
showing me just how much she reacted to, understood, and was engaged by both social realities and the natural world. For her, drawing
was a conscious attempt to portray those aspects of an increasingly
appealing world that caught her interest. In this particular apprehension of reality she was more adept than I. Her exquisite eye for detail
revealed just how attuned to her surroundings she could be. Among
the many ways of perceiving reality, Wendy found the one to share
with me that suited her best.

Nathan

Some years after I finished my work with Wendy, ten-year-old Nathan was brought to see me because his parents were disturbed by his
angry outbursts, which seemed to occur when daily events did not
turn out perfectly. Something would go wrong in school, or he would
fall down at the bus stop, or a favorite book would be missing from
the library, or his younger brother would fail to follow Nate's learned
commentary—all these mishaps would send him reeling into a consummate frenzy, lasting for hours. His parents told me that he didn't
speak until the age of three, when he began to utter full sentences,
many of these echolalically. "I wish you'd stop repeating me," his
parents would say, only to hear Nathan predictably respond, "wish
you stop repeating me." Like many autists, he could hardly bear the
slightest change in his routine. He hated crowds and would avoid
family outings for this reason. When nervous, he'd display rapid, repetitive arm and hand movements, all the while eyeing me to see if I
noticed them and trying his best to blend these movements into something more ordinary, like picking up a toy and exploring it by rubbing
it on all sides. He suffered from repeated nightmares, which never
woke him and which he did not remember the next day—except that

he had experienced some unspeakable anguish during the night. About this, he said flatly that he didn't want to remember his dreams and was startled, then pleased, when I remarked that Freud once wrote a book on this very topic.

On more than one occasion, I saw Nathan deliberately turn away without turning his back on another person. This was unlike Paulie and Gregory who would unabashedly turn their backs to me whenever they felt like it, usually to diminish the stimulating effects with which my mere presence burdened them. Instead Nate would watch what was going on out of the corner of his eye so as not to let on that he was observing; he was relying on what specialists call "peripheral" vision. Nate's behavior reminded me of the times Marcia had declined to turn her full back toward me and had compromised by watching me askance without really seeming to. In this way, she expressed her deeply felt ambivalence about my person. It took years for Marcia to reach this compromise. Nathan had developed it when quite young, and it had served him well when he experienced mixed emotions about being with people and knowing what they were about. He also did not want others to know what *he* was about.

Nate wished to conceal from me that he was observing; he didn't want me to know that he knew I was watching him. Marcia, on the other hand, used peripheral vision to express her mixed feelings about recognizing my presence just after I'd returned from an absence. She may have been relieved or even glad to see me upon my return, but she was also angry and wished to deny my presence. By denying my presence, she may have felt she could deny my absence. Peripheral vision was a handy way for her to solve her conflicting feelings. But Nate did not want me to know that he was cagey enough to observe me without seeming to.

Nathan seemed aware that he often isolated himself from others, and so developed a formal demeanor to modify his diffidence. He had the motions of social graces down pat, but he ran through them swiftly and with little apparent feeling. Similarly, bookish Nathan exhibited his vast store of knowledge on certain topics in a formal, scholarly, high-pitched monotone. When I first met him, his recitations consisted of facts, hardly ever feelings about the facts or reasons for adumbrating them.

As we got acquainted, I might ask how he came to be interested in the origins of the universe or in medieval times. He'd occasionally smile directly at me and reply that people are not required to have a reason for what interests them. I thought of Greg, who once told me in disgust, "I'm just interested in animals—*that's it!* I always was and always will be!" Perhaps these two boys thought my inquiries into the origins of their preoccupations meant I wished they would relinquish them. Perhaps they believed I viewed an unabiding interest in the universe or in the animal kingdom as a "symptom," something to be overcome or eradicated.

Nathan was a handsome boy and, when not upset and distraught, a sweet-tempered and loving child, especially toward his parents and a few favorite teachers, who helped him through his tantrums and otherwise went to great lengths to meet his many needs. When he saw that I was genuinely interested in what he made of science and history and that I didn't object to such repetitious behavior as his selecting the same board game week after week, he began to chat with me about his view of the world and his place in it. I soon discovered that, of all the autists I have known, Nathan had a splendidly attuned psychological sense, both of himself and others. His mother told me that she and her son had frequent discussions about people's feelings, including Nathan's own. In effect, she taught him how to resonate to himself, how to be sensitive not just to others but also to his own feelings and moods. He had also learned to anticipate his mother's reactions to his troubles and to his successes. Though he had engrossing scientific conversations with his father, the empathy he displayed in my office had developed in conversations with his mother. He could read my intent and emotions in an instant, especially, but not solely, those that had to do with him. Sometimes he would mock me unsparingly by refusing to allow that something was on his mind, knowing how interested I might be in it, leaving me dangling, his eyes sparkling with mischief, finally relenting with a broad grin and, in mock submission, releasing some small bit of information that he knew would please me. He had to test many times how long I would be patient before he came forth with earnest answers to my questions. Both Nathan and Stacy, who had asked interminable questions about the weather, knew full well that their developing minds intrigued me and would satisfy my curiosity whimsically.

Nate knew exactly why he was brought to see me. His accurate analyses of himself and his family dumbfounded me. Once he held forth on the unanticipated consequences of "time-outs," an isolating strategy his teachers had used to help him contain his anger. He told me that time-outs did help him at the moment, but that his feelings would burst later. "Now I know," he mused, "that feelings don't vanish with time-outs; in fact, they just erupt even stronger after school is over."

Nathan's description seemed a textbook analysis of the ill effects of suppression—a perception that took me completely by surprise. When he saw how exhilarated I was by his psychological prowess, he began to display this ability in areas other than direct conversation. For example, he would analyze the strategic significance of particular board-game formats or speculate on his own reasons for making a certain move in checkers, finishing up gleefully by guessing at my probable game gambits.

The communion Nate and I established turned on his intuitive gift and his willingness to share with me the very commitment to understanding oneself and others that I had made almost four decades before.

• • •

If there is a single precept that is most effective in working and living with young autists, I believe it is this: conceding that autists are able to receive and use our help enables them to reveal or develop their true, natural psychical repertoire. Nathan exemplifies this most poignantly. The serious impediments to adequate functioning he initially presented almost completely masked the remarkably diversified and advanced spectrum of adjustments he was able to execute under favorable circumstances. It was Nathan's own determination that energized his return to sociability. The extent to which those of us working and living with young autists can reactivate their own efforts to adapt, not just to the world but also to themselves, is the measure of their success and ours.

CHAPTER FOUR

I Can See Me in Your Eyes

> . . . I no longer craved being swept away . . . in the all-consuming
> tide of total mental and sensory blankness. . . .
> —DONNA WILLIAMS

What invigorates autists under the age of ten who have the physical and mental wherewithal to converse meaningfully with others? They must be reenergized to take some action on their own. They must be convinced that talking will benefit them in some way. After all, it will be through their own prodigious efforts that they will strive to transcend autism. However egregiously wrong Bruno Bettelheim was about the parents of autistic youth—believing they had somehow caused or aggravated the autistic condition, that parents may themselves have brought about the autist's inattention to the social world, including the words of others—he was correct when he emphasized that unless the caretakers of young autists can persuade them that their efforts to adapt to and affect the social world will be rewarded, they'll be consigned to a life without substance, without rapport, without hope. "[Young autists] came to life only when we [at the Orthogenic School] were able to create the conditions, or otherwise be the catalysts, that induced them to take action on their own behalf," writes Bettelheim in *The Empty Fortress*.[1] Whether it be a mother who joins her son in tracing the origin of telephone lines, or one who permits, even encourages, her little boy to use his bright chartreuse woman's hat in any way he wishes, or whether it be parents who use any technique or device they can think of—tape recorders, typewriters, or computers—to advance communication in their children, the common thread in all these endeavors is the parents' hope and conviction that somehow, some way, communication with the wary, isolated, unwilling young autist is possible.

We know now from parents' remembrances of their autistic children and from autists themselves that their troubles often stem not from lack of arousal but from overarousal. Donna Williams describes her childhood need to be unbothered by the world and her need to "disappear" from it, which continued into her adulthood. The disappearing seemed automatic in her early years, but later it "shrank in length from hours to minutes to seconds. . . . I no longer craved being swept away like this in the all-consuming tide of total mental and sensory blankness, where 'the world' stood irrelevant and uncountable leagues away."[2] Since she no longer wished so desperately for social distance, Williams was perhaps more attentive to the impact others had on her, including their communications. Reading of Williams's craving for nothingness, an unspace that seemed safer than the confusing, buzzing boom of an overstimulating world, I was reminded of Stacy's riveting need to have daily situations exactly the same, including what people *said* to her. She'd play word games for hours, just to hear me voice precisely what she expected. For example, if we were talking about kitchen cleansers, she'd chant "Ajax," waiting menacingly until she heard me say, "Comet" or "Lestoil." If I had already said "Comet" in response to her "Ajax" just seconds before, to cover all cleanser bases she now required me to respond, "Lestoil"—and heaven help me if I didn't! If I delayed my response by a split second, she'd mobilize into a fury, tossing chairs across the room, or she'd withdraw once more into a kind of nothingness, rolling beach balls around the room by the hour. I thought she chose beach balls because their soft pliability invited her to rest her head on them when she was tired.

At age five, Stacy had yet to lapse completely into that seemingly serene, otherworldly, dreamy state Williams describes, typical of Marcia, Burt, and Paulie. Their disinterested mien seemed impenetrable. No matter what I did or said, the trance would continue as they didn't listen, didn't look, didn't move, didn't care; or as they frantically shook their hands and arms; or as they appeared captivated by an inordinate study of internal bodily sensations.

Yet to this day, I perceive intelligent deliberation in that daydreamy look, in that torpid turn of the body that renders my person efficiently, just barely, yet ever so irritatingly out of their sight, the dead silence following my words, all of which say to me, "To hell with the world; I will not be bothered by it." How to converse with such a child? Indeed, why try?

> Things *don't* heal; *people* do!
> We *don't* fix people; we fix *things!*
> —STACY

So said Stacy at age seven, after two years of living, playing, and talking at the Orthogenic School. She had become wondrously expressive, sometimes impishly so, witty and loquacious, a child philosopher of sorts. She was working on a problem a younger child has likely solved—one nevertheless important since autists are said to treat people as if they were things. The problem was the difference between healing and fixing, between animate and inanimate, whereby Stacy used the actions *healing* and *fixing* to distinguish between people and objects. It was the kind of childhood conundrum, once perplexing but now resolved, that hardly needs further explanation for many a young mind. But Stacy had only recently come across the notion that not only could questions be answered, but they also could be asked. Earlier she had habitually assumed that the offending world was a given, including its maddening unpredictabilities. To her mind the world could not be changed in any happy way, certainly not by her, except when she wreaked revenge upon it for its perceived menaces to her. Then she appeared to turn the world upside down in her rage.

At seven years, she had learned by the force of her own promising activities that she could affect the course of daily events in a safe, sometimes hopeful way. Those staffers who lived and worked with her had striven to persuade her of this essential truth. Having been more intensively convinced by others than an ordinary child need be, Stacy sought desperately yet proudly to remark on it, incredulous sometimes at her own insight that, say, toys can be fixed, but people must be healed. She was willing to share this exciting news with anyone who would listen.

Not nearly as immobile or withdrawn as Marcia, Stacy ferociously attacked others, intending, as she told me years later, to scratch out their eyes. As I described earlier, the reason for her assaults was that she wanted big blue eyes and not tiny brown eyes. She later tried to control her impulse to grab for others' eyes by redirecting this need. She carefully tore out the eyes of animals and people from her picture books. Decades later, I read in a *Newsweek* article of an autistic six-year-old who "is so afraid of open eyes that she doesn't look at people. She even blacks out the eyes of the figures in her coloring books."[3] Although her own eyes were glassy and expressionless, revealing nothing of her own true being, strangely enough Stacy occupied herself with the "windows to the soul." Her attacks, though, were so specifically aimed that I couldn't help thinking there must be a compelling reason for them. Guessing there was helped me maintain a modicum of sanity as I tried to fathom and withstand Stacy's attacks. At least she didn't try to blot out my presence by incessantly flapping her arms or twiddling her fingers as Marcia did.

Stacy tried hard to tell me what was on her mind, what scared her, what enthralled her. About her absorption with everyone's eyes and now their eyeglasses, she told me one upbeat day, "Remember when

I used to scratch out eyes? I wanted to grab them. I wanted big blue eyes, not little teensy brown eyes. Now I'm interested in glasses. Now I grab glasses, not eyes."

When Stacy told me why she grabbed for the eyes of other people, she was reflecting on her behavior in much the way a person, replete with a theory of mind—at least of her own preoccupied mind—analyzes herself in psychotherapy. But Stacy did not stop there. She went on to flabbergast me with one of the most exquisite observations of sensory reality I have ever heard from a young child. Gazing deeply into my eyes, her face but an inch from mine, she spoke in a low, confidential, almost hypnotic whisper: "I can see me in your eyes, you know." Then she widened her eyes as much as she could so that I could see my own image reflected in them! Could Stacy have thought that one's image in another's eyes meant that one's self inhabited another person? If so, she may have grabbed for eyes to reclaim her shadow.

Now I understood why she continually said to staff and children alike, "Open your eyes real wide." She was checking and rechecking her discovery that her own shadow was visible in the pupils of others' eyes. Implicitly, she may have wondered whether identifying her image in someone's eyes, just like her habit of calling herself "you," endangered her sense of who *she* was. In reaching for the eyes of others and for their eyeglasses, she may, quite literally, have been grasping for self—to get herself out of someone else. So I told her, "No wonder you poked eyes; you wanted your own self out of there." With an uncommon gentleness she sighed, "Yes!"[4]

Soon Stacy would ask others if she could try on their glasses. Pity the unfortunate person, though, who didn't comply or who, from Stacy's perspective, didn't have a good or interesting reason for refusing. Time and again I heard glasses-bearing staffers (I didn't wear glasses at the time) explaining to Stacy why they couldn't honor her request, the most reasonable to her being that they couldn't see her if they didn't wear their "lenses," as she called them. Despite her aversion to people, she seemed taken with the idea that others were interested in her and in what she was doing. It was also to Stacy's advantage that trusted adults knew of her whereabouts; then they could protect her from life's dangers. Yet she maintained an air of silent suspicion as she listened to the discouraging reply, all the while glaring impertinently at the other person's every move and facial expression.

Living with Stacy made me aware not just of her intimidating behaviors but also of her natural gifts, linguistic fluency among them. She perfected a fine sense of humor expressed by inventive neologisms and clever puns and by her side-splitting cartoonlike drawings in which she depicted comic faces with exaggeratedly happy smiles or sad frowns. These qualities, together with her growing acute appreciation of how the world worked, led me to ponder whether received human wisdom could be expanded by getting to know how Stacy, and others like her, transcended autism. Stacy's way with words blossomed as I tried to fathom the perspective underlying it.

Her neologisms and puns, funny and shrewd, sometimes prophetic, sought at first to alert me to her needs or anxieties. Since she liked the toys provided for her at the Orthogenic School, items that allowed her to manipulate as well as cuddle (nursery push-and-pull toys, stuffed animals), she used to call her dormitory her dormi*toy*. Anything that touched upon her worries about the eye's functioning usually set her going. References that hinted at, or words that merely sounded like the verb "to see" caught her in a frenzy of excitement that only slowly abated as she told me what she was experiencing.

No surprise, then, that she perked up when she heard the song "Beyond the Sea" on the school's jukebox. Thereupon she widened her eyes enormously and demanded of others that they do the same so she could, like a doctor, examine whether their eyes seemed to be working. We were all puzzled by her reaction to a song about the ocean, until someone realized that Stacy thought the song's title was "Beyond the *See*."

Perhaps she interpreted the song to mean that some objects, people, and events were beyond seeing, so she checked people's eyes.[5]

Much later, she created a pun, transposing the words "sea" and "see." Sarcasm dripping from her voice, she announced to those with whom she was angry, "You're bee . . . yond the see . . . ee!" She banished others from her view when frustrated by their actual or expected rejection.

As her inquiries became more sophisticated, I was eager to hear what she would ask me next, what new, ingenious, and unexpected idea she would surprise me with. So now she wasn't just trying to describe her needs and worries, but she was also trying to amuse me. In a single ten-minute conversation she could run the gamut from suddenly realizing that Joseph and Guiseppi are different language forms of the same name to exploring systematically the all-important distinction between people and things.

"Things don't live. People do. People don't ruin in the laundry like socks. Things ruin." Now, *sotto voce*, "Things *don't* heal; *people* do! We *don't* fix people; we fix *things!*" Breathlessly, "Things heal? *No*, they *don't.*"

I thought it remarkable that Stacy began to include people in her world, vigorously seeking to differentiate them from objects, including imagining reliable markers allowing this differentiation. To accomplish this, she had to abstract concepts from what had been haphazardly strung-together visual experiences. She had to understand that seeing or sensing something is different from conceptualizing it. As she began to mark this difference, she turned to problems in understanding nature and in understanding her relationship to me.

One question that could not be answered solely by observing was Stacy's query about the setting sun. "Where does the sun go?" I explained that it is the earth that moves, hoping she'd think out the solution by herself.

"But does the sun go down?" Stacy asked, enunciating her words precisely ("But duzzz it go dowwnnn?").

"It looks like it does."

"It always shines, do you mean?"

When I didn't answer her directly, Stacy may have thought I was being evasive for some obtuse reason. So urgent was her need for plain sense that she resolutely searched our conversations for honest confusions or my ulteriorly motivated subterfuges. Then she enunciated her words precisely and exaggeratedly so as not to confuse me about her stated intent, persistently rephrasing my statements with "do you mean?" tacked on at the end. Attributing a misunderstanding to my mentality is evidence that she assumed I had one. Looked at closely, her statements did not represent echolalic repetitions either. By following my lead in asking me (as I'd asked her) "do you mean?" at the end of many statements, she was flagging her need for *us* to get *our* communications straight. In this benchmark endeavor, she wasn't mimicking or opposing me; rather, she was fighting her way out of autism.

What's more, Stacy may well have been accustomed to camouflaged messages. Perhaps people had been loathe to talk sense to her for fear of further alienating or harming her. She may have heard, for example, the words, "I love you" but understood quite another implicit message ("Mommy says 'I love you,'" Stacy would say). She may have understood something like, "I love you, and I must not let on that I am angry at you for misbehaving." Autistic children are invariably perceived as handicapped in many ways. In an effort to protect them, they might be more likely than their peers to be told things insincerely. Wouldn't they, even more urgently than other children, want to get through the verbiage and down to brass tacks?

Stacy soon threw herself into the task of proving my sincerity. She began to anticipate so accurately what I would think, do, or say that it felt for all the world as if she were reading my mind. She had decided that if she explained the reasons for her misdeeds she'd stand a better chance of making them palatable to me. So she would describe her mischievous shenanigans in detail. "The red paint is on the ceiling for a *rea . . . son*," she once singsonged with a smirk, mocking the Orthogenic School's We Do Things for Good Reasons maxim. How sincere would I be in allowing that she had a good reason for what to her was the bad act of hurling paint to the ceiling?

If she didn't want to talk about getting angry at me, she would cite every other adult she could think of at whom she'd ever gotten angry. Finally, she would dramatically relent, satisfying my eager inquiries with tongue literally in cheek. "Yes! I am *angry* at"—followed by a deep breath—"one, two, three, four, five, six, seven, eight, nine, *Karen!*"

Another time it was, "Ladies and gentlemen, boys and girls, I am very *maaad* today!" I found it hard to keep a straight face, and in fact, things usually worked out best if I dropped my psychological stance and simply enjoyed her humor and laughed along with her.

Stacy was by now eight years old, just the age when pondering one's own thoughts and trying to discern those of others is developing apace. Long ostracized for her attacks on others, she had, like her peers, begun to benefit from bouncing ideas off other people. The factual minutiae she accumulated began to be organized more deliberately. It's not far-fetched to say that she was building a loosely knit paradigm capable of ordering the many small truths she would continue to come across. Like other young autists I have known who acted as though people were unimportant to them or simply not there, Stacy began to set forth hypotheses to test aspects of the world, especially those she considered dangerous, and to argue her case with the very people she had previously disqualified from her purview.

Sometimes the autistic imagination can be a cosmic one. Stacy's questions about the world went beyond what is typically expected of children her age. Far from being empty-headed or concerned solely with the objects of a static world, her mind could encompass a surprisingly broad range of reality.

Stacy wanted to know, "Do rivers and lakes boil?" By now I was very sure there *was* a good reason behind her questions, so I asked, "Do you mean from the warm sun?"

"Yes," she assented nervously.

"No." I said. "The sun may feel warm, but it's not boiling the water. Remember the temperature of the lake water?"

"Yes. Not boiling." She seemed to have trustingly accepted my answer even though it was patently incomplete. If the sun "boils" in the sky, she may have wondered, why does it not boil the earth's surface?

James, quite a bit younger than Stacy, asked whether the fiery plane crash was the result of the airplane's traveling too close to the sun. Maybe this kind of morbid questioning doesn't occur to ordinary children because they feel safer generally—although its analogue did occur to the mythmakers who gave us the story of Icarus!

Consider what might be termed Stacy's "rain phobia." For months, as soon as the clouds began to darken or it began to sprinkle, she would become frantic and, of all things, ask to go outside. Despite the anguish they caused, the thunderous noises and sudden light flashes did not deter her from heading for the door. It seemed to me that she was attributing a magical power to her own behavior in regard to rain. I thought she reasoned that if we go inside when it begins to rain, we can stop the rain by going out. "Maybe you think it will stop raining if we go outside," I said warily one day, "since we come inside when it rains." Excitedly, "Yes!" "Well, no wonder you wanted to go outside, then."

As she got a little older and as the pelting rain would subside into a soft pitter-patter, Stacy often said bravely, "But the ducks *love* the rain! They *love* the water!" Note that the hallmark of robust reasoning in children is their awareness that events can be viewed from a perspective other than their own. How could Stacy have concluded that her opinion of rainstorms differed from that of ducks had she been mired in the no-man's-land of a mindless brain?

As Stacy matured, her probes into the workings of the world did continue to center, and increasingly so, on facets of her life she found troubling or distasteful. She revealed she was as subject as any child to the hazards that come with more mature cognition. The more intelligently a child thinks, the more problems she creates for herself. This is because her precociously developed intellect brings her to dilemmas that her emotions are not quite ready to appreciate and to resolve. This is especially a problem for young autists, because when difficulties increase, parents, teachers, and tutors mistakenly conclude that their treatment plan is ineffective. When autistic children begin to socialize more, to think out problems more systematically, and to share their thoughts with others, their minds and emotions begin to function in a way they had not before. As a result, the children must adapt to their own new way of being, a halcyon circumstance; it means that those who take care of young autists must not get discouraged by the dilemmas caused by development.

Formerly a deep sleeper, by the age of nine Stacy experienced a sudden fear of drowsing off. She seemed preoccupied with the remnants of the day, loose ends that, despite her best efforts and mine, couldn't be tied up neatly. Or so I thought.

One evening at bedtime, Stacy sat on my lap for a long time asking questions. "What happens if you leave milk out overnight?" (Note she used the colloquial "you.") I began to explain about food and the need for refrigeration, describing what happens to ice cream, one of her favorite foods. "If you leave ice cream out, it will melt."

"What happens if you put ice cream back [in the refrigerator]?"

"It will refreeze."

"What happens if you put sour milk back?"

Stacy seemed to wonder whether refrigeration would return sour milk to its sweet state. If so, she wished to know which processes reverse themselves when something is returned to the refrigerator. So I told her that melted liquids can be refrozen but sour milk cannot be resweetened.

Muttering to herself, "What happens if you leave chairs out overnight . . . No! They *don't* spoil." Then to me, "Why don't oranges spoil overnight?" Since oranges and milk are both food, she queried, why doesn't the same rule of spoiling hold true for both?

Stacy appeared to be conducting a complex analysis designed to reveal what she urgently needed to know about nighttime's effects on animate and inanimate objects. So in every question she paired *overnight* and *spoiling*. In her mind the night itself, not just the absence of refrigeration, caused food spoilage. I thought she assumed it was the dark that caused the food to spoil. Though she understood the difference between herself and a chair, she may have thought she was "spoilable" like milk and not sturdy like oranges. And it could be the night itself, acting upon unrefrigerated animate items (foods) and beings (herself), that caused the deterioration. But in specifying *over*night she may have referred to the passage of time, which does lead to spoiling in unrefrigerated foods. When I said, "Although you are very much alive like the oranges and the milk, you will not spoil overnight," Stacy rolled over in her bed and fell asleep.

At the time, Stacy's felicitous response seemed like magic. It occurred, though, because she was by then aware that she could use her mind to make sense of the world, thus reducing her apprehensions about the integrity of her body. She also realized that her thoughts often interested and amused me, which strengthened the affectionate bond growing between us. There is probably no more comforting thought to young children than their recognition that much of what they think, feel, and believe is comprehensible to beloved adults in some important, albeit familiar or even ordinary way. This is just as true of young autists as it is of other children. After years of very little psychoanalyzing and a lot of attentive caring, including structuring question-and-answer conversations so that Stacy might recognize what she wanted to know about the world, she told me, "I just love you, Karen!" I got this welcome news when, instead of leaving her with another Orthogenic School staffer, I stayed with her for the better part of twenty-four hours (as parents do), which perhaps convinced her that I must have loved her, too.

Stacy's progress came in spurts, but when it occurred, its quick and ready course startled and inspired me. I thought young Stacy might have a chance for a full recovery. Her infectiously beaming face, cheeks red and shiny from the winter's cold, eyes sparkling as she looked up at me fondly while hanging by her arms on the snowy jungle gym a short year after being admitted to the Orthogenic School, made me think she was the picture of normalcy. Helping her up the stairs from the dining room where she had made a meal of bread, butter, and milk (mostly butter!), Stacy leaned back against me for bodily support, her six-year-old sneakered feet playfully kicking at the steps as we went along. I wanted so very badly to hug her. But Stacy didn't tolerate hugs even if they came from a trusted person. I had to remind myself repeatedly that what I took for "normalcy" in six-year-old Stacy was actually the behavior of a much younger child.

Yet when she was eight, she ran perfectly normally to me for a hug when she spotted me playing catch with my husband on the University of Chicago's campus. I was off that day when her dormitory group happened to be taking a walk. Stacy left her group and ran to claim me as her special person before the eyes of my husband. How like other children, I thought, as I ran to intercept her from crossing the street alone. She wanted to make it plain that, although she didn't know him, she was as important to me as my husband was. How very "oedipal" of her!

When she heard, some two years later, that I intended to leave the Orthogenic School to join my husband in Boston, she implored, "Take me with you, Karen!" Pulling at my heartstrings, "Karen, *take* me!" she cried.

As I explained that she must stay at the school and continue working on her problems with her counselors and her teachers, I thought how sad it was that Stacy had worked so hard for so many years to fashion a relationship with me and how discouraging it must be that her labors would come to this. I reassured myself that she'd surely form other attachments upon my leaving, and I also thought how much I would need the kind of milieu the Orthogenic School provided to "take Stacy with me"—even if that were feasible. As every informed parent of an autistic child knows, Stacy and others like her need multiple services to grow, not just one promising relationship, but the consistent care of many: devoted parents, trained teachers, tutors, friends, and yes, sometimes even psychotherapists.

Even a bright, responsive autist like Stacy is vulnerable if she loses the very part of the holding environment that allows her to converse with me the way she did. That holding environment for Stacy meant my attending sensitively to her intelligent thoughts, many of which unfolded with incredible, if sometimes confused, logic. I say "incredible" because at that time I was just learning about the logical development of all children. Stacy did take notice of my affection for her, but she could not have failed to notice, as well, how interested I was in her thinking, since her developing thoughts were the basis of many of our interactions.

In the chapters to come, I show how Stacy's inner world, populated by "pretend people," gradually gave way to a social world occupied by the people with whom she actually lived. During her early years at the Orthogenic School, her dramatic enactments with imaginary characters evoked in her the feeling that she, too, might be "pretend," that she might not be real. To show her that she was not pretend, that she was a *real* girl, I had to join her in her pretend world. I did this by talking to her imaginary people when she would let me or when she had them address me.

In time, she began to use her imaginary figures to comfort herself; they became friendly and loving, a source of pleasure and also of knowledge. They had shed their berating, provoking, punishing personalities. She had previously been afraid of people's affection, but now she could safely imagine a "pretend person" taking care of her, teaching her, even loving her.

You'll read in Chapter 7 how Stacy impersonated her esteemed male teacher as she pretended to talk to him through a benevolent character. In Chapter 8 I describe how Stacy learned more versatile ways of negotiating the social world. Her imagined conversations came to be based on real kids. This led to lasting friendships, associations that were a source of frustration *and* fun. Her peers sometimes talked to her imaginary friends, as I had done, but only if she permitted it. More often, her companions urged her to leave her make-believe world for the real world, to join in with them. It was only then that Stacy allowed herself to be mentored by an older girl who taught her how to read, how to learn willingly from another person.

Thirty years later I began to work with James, who was even better endowed than Stacy. He had the benefit of attentive and forgiving parents, who helped nip his encroaching autism in the bud. During the years I worked and lived with Stacy, she had only brief visits with her mother in the Orthogenic School's front parlor. She also had to watch staffers leave the School and knew that one day, inevitably, she would suffer similar losses of the people to whom she had worked so hard to attach. The brief visits with her mother did not reassure her that someone would take care of her if her counselors or teacher—or Stacy herself—left the School.

James would never have to undergo such a loss and he knew it.

Despite his anxious moments while waiting for his parents to pick him up from my office or from his school, he was and would always be a cherished member of his family. Jamie's parents had found him a private school that welcomed him eagerly and whose teachers adapted to his eccentric ways. Moreover, his parents and teachers were wonderfully receptive of my counsel based, in large part, on my years with Stacy.

> *I* know how birds migrate. I just wanted to see if *you* know it.
> —JAMES

Four-and-a-half-year-old James made this concise statement about two years after I began working with him. It revealed his certain grasp of the *mind* concept—he knew what *he* knew and wondered if *I* knew it, too.

Jamie, like Stacy, would often act as if he were at the mercy of sensory stimuli, often the very sensations he particularly liked, not just the ones he found distasteful. He would rivet his eyes on revolving lights, like those on police cars and other emergency vehicles. Since safety barriers set up by the police and construction crews often have stripes, everything striped in my office commanded his attention to the exclusion of everything else. When James would say he *was* Garfield of the comics, not merely *like* him, I recalled Donna Williams's accounts of her imagined personalities, "Carol" and "Willie," who had taken over her waking life, not just her dreams as Jamie's Garfield had done. Williams was the victim of punitive parenting.[6] Perhaps she transformed herself into two other personalities, hoping that by being someone else she would gain her parents' approval. Jamie's parents, in contrast, encouraged their son to be himself. When he would dream he was Garfield, they responded by enumerating his real characteristics. They were able to combat Jamie's autistic tendency to dissociate from the self, whereas Williams's parents only reinforced it. So it seems

Donna Williams's urgent writings of and for herself freed her to *be*. I wrote in Chapter 3 of Jamie's need to control my office and its furnishings as well as the way we interacted. Once, when he got an answer to a question about birds migrating, he exclaimed like an exacting didact, "*I* know it. I just wanted to see if *you* know it!" A little over four years old, Jamie was comparing one mind to another—his to mine.

Now he was just as interested in dealing with facts as he was in fantasizing. His play revolved around what he'd learned from science shows on TV and from his teachers, as well as from board game rules and procedures that he mastered in his meetings with me. These activities seemed safer to Jamie than did fantasizing about real or imaginary events, which invariably aroused feelings he feared he could not control. At home, too, he reveled in the board game format. His attachment to his father flourished as they competed, safely and pleasurably, within this structured context.

Although he loved playing board games, Jamie could maintain to himself that he hadn't actually chosen to play by insisting that I get the game from the shelf while he wandered casually about. One day, waiting for me to set up Parcheesi, he picked up some small toys while perambulating, carelessly letting them drop to the floor, as though they had not the slightest significance for him. Yet he watched me closely to assure that I did precisely what he expected. I was enthused by his interest in games because they require social negotiations and, inevitably, agreement on the rules and procedures.

Jamie soon began to assert that the colors of the game's playing pieces represented degrees of meanness. After specifying which color was the least mean, the second least mean, and so on, he exclaimed, "Red is the meanest color of all! Which color do you want to be?" My answer, irrelevant to him, that I didn't at all want to be mean, naturally fell on deaf ears. He didn't grace it with the slightest acknowledgment. So I reluctantly picked the "least mean" yellow color, unaware just how involved I had become in his game plan. My choice was greeted by a scornful guffaw and many loud hoots as he said, "I *knew* you would pick that color!"

Then James fell silent and thought for a long time. "You picked yellow because it was the least meanest. So it's in your imagination that yellow is the least meanest [color]."

"Yes, I picked yellow because you said it wasn't as mean as the other colors. But *I* didn't say colors can be mean."

"Oh yes you did! You picked the color yellow and that means it's *your* imagination that says yellow is the least mean."

Just as Stacy confused two very different concepts when she heard "sea" as identical to "see," and thus thought the song "Beyond the Sea" told of something being out of sight,[6] James blended the idea of color with feeling. This is yet another instance of preconceptual thinking in children, in which two or more ideas are, willy-nilly, connected to one another, where the associations are puzzling to us but quite real to the child. This is another example of childish behavior that is not unique to autism.

Jamie had inveigled me to buy into his world completely. He had arranged it so that the only way I could play the game was to become part of his personal scenario. Jamie knew I was eager to play a game with him, though he may not have known that my reason was its implications for social negotiations. It wasn't just his need to control things, as when he asked just those questions to which he knew the answer so as to predict my response. This time I had the feeling he wanted to create a new reality out of our interactions. Either I had to agree that the color yellow is mean or decline to play the game. So it's not that autists invariably have no theory of mind. Rather, for some autists, *their* theory of mind predominates over *yours*.

In Jamie's case, once he admitted people to his world, the same domineering trend that had governed his actions with objects came into play toward people. To the autist, the most unpredictable stimuli emanate from other, often noisy, humans. It was as though his ability to control people and to predict their actions acted as a buffer to the onslaught of his sensory sensitivities. While Jamie no longer jerked upon hearing a sudden sound, like the cycling of my office refrigerator, he did startle at the unexpected resulting from human interaction. He used his mind to attempt to control his peers' minds when they wished to play with his toys. First he tried to talk them out of wanting to, and then he prevailed upon his parents to persuade his companions that his toys were not interesting. Once he acknowledged other people's existence, Jamie could hardly help redoubling his efforts to command their actions, their wishes, even their thoughts.

Jamie did acknowledge me as a person, finally. He did so in an amusing fashion reminiscent of his earlier tendency to call himself "he." Now, when playing a board game with me, he would mutter to himself, "What is *she* going to do *now?*" "Who is this 'she' you're talking about?" I asked. Calling upon the mental process that cognitive developmentalists term "logical necessity," Jamie replied, "It's *got* to be *you,* because you're the only female in this room!" His answer was logically necessary because there were no other choices—zero degrees of freedom. In this instance, I thought he was playing with pronouns, comically referring to me as "she" rather than "you." Before, he was dead serious that he was just a "he" and not an "I."

James began to understand that his capacity to comprehend was virtually unlimited in that he could access social know-how at any time. In contrast to Stacy's attempt to "read" my mind and manipulate my responses, which usually centered on charming me so I would not get irritated at her wrongdoings, James was more interested in reading me to prove he was always right. By the time he was seven, he was strongly motivated to show that he could predict my actions better than I could predict his. He assumed, egocentrically, that I was thinking the same way he was. His mental maneuvering pervaded practically every conversation we had.

Once, he brought his collection of police Legos to my office and proudly displayed them, commenting that he thought he had more Legos than I had. I was about to agree that he probably did have more when he turned to me, asking with an impish grin, "Do you think you have more Legos, or do you think I have more?" I answered that I really didn't know for sure, because I hadn't counted either his or my Legos.

Unabashedly he quizzed, "But do you *think* I have more?"

"What do you think?" I countered, pleased that he was asking for my estimate but also getting the feeling that Jamie had involved me in a wild, upwardly spiraling guessing game.

"I asked you first."

"I asked you second"—my lame attempt to be funny. To this Jamie giggled and put his hands emphatically on his hips, giving me a sarcastic look.

"Guess which policeman goes with this police van."

"I really can't guess because to me all the policemen look exactly the same." By this time I felt I was being programmed like a computer rather than being asked for my personal opinion.

"Go ahead and pick."

Reluctantly I chose the policeman nearest to me, knowing, though, that he had set me up for some kind of whimsical test.

"You're wrong!" he shouted gleefully. "Pick the police officer that goes with *this* vehicle!"

"I bet no matter which one I choose you're going to tell me I'm wrong."

Blushing, Jamie hid his smile behind his hands but still insisted that I choose one of the Lego policemen. Just as I did so, he exclaimed triumphantly, "You're right!"

A mind game this surely was. But what did it mean? By judging my last choice correct, Jamie deftly falsified my generalization that he was trying to find me invariably mistaken. His was merely the innocent task of judging me wrong or right based on some as yet unstated criterion. Later I realized he also might have been testing my ability to withstand wrongness. Would I dissolve into frustration, anger, and tears the way he sometimes did when things didn't go exactly his way?

I had read the theory of mind literature on autism when James and I had the previous conversation, in which I was taken by his capacity to finesse another person when it served him. At the moment I was more interested in his thinking processes than I was in what he may have tried to express about his emotional state. Perhaps he would have listened had I tried to express that, though I didn't really like being wrong, everyone has to learn how to accept correction and guidance. In an important sense, this is a universal human dilemma.

I did wonder what he thought of my interpretive statements, those geared to the way he thought and felt. He tended to correct me about my musings, or even make fun of them.

James was once setting up the game of Monopoly and worked hard to get his piles of dollar bills just so. As he was organizing the piles by denomination, he mumbled about his choice of a game piece, whether to be the dog, the race car, or the briefcase: "I don't know who I am yet."

This time I tuned into his feelings about himself—his young identity—as I said, "It takes some time to figure out who we are."

Jamie gave me a quizzical look and replied, "I'm talking about the *game!*" Thus he showed how much he understood what I meant. He had to have comprehended in order to dispute it and assert what *he* was talking about.

Again, he was no different from the multitude of other children to whom I have talked. While appreciating my interest in what they say, they make it plain that what they say ought to be taken the way *they* mean it. Little Jamie had previously refused to look at me, had backed himself up against the physical boundary of my wooden bookcases with a glazed, shell-shocked stare that made me want to envelop him in my arms and tell him everything would be all right. He would only consent to nest some blocks methodically to calm himself and, perhaps, to demonstrate his three-year-old intelligence. Now he was quite prepared to debate with me the proper confines of a therapeutic encounter. Good for him!

Several weeks later, James told me he didn't dream he was other people anymore. I thought of our abbreviated conversation in which I suggested that our sense of identity evolves. He had been clowning around, taking on the comical gestures and postures of his favorite movie and TV personalities. At first, he simply lapsed into these impersonations with no explanation. But he anticipated that I would wonder who he was imitating, and so he preceded these episodes with one-word entrées, usually the name of the mimicked actor. Then he'd begin his pantomime. Yet in his dreams he felt he was himself.

Gradually these episodes occurred only after I returned from an absence. After one of my vacations, James greeted me by grimacing, scratching himself, jumping around, and hooting like a monkey. Another time he leapt out of my line of vision, only to emerge suddenly with an instant new personality, that of a TV talk-show host. Maybe he thought I had left because I didn't like who he was so he pretended to be someone else. When I asked him whether he thought he had to be different to get my undivided attention, he insisted with a wide grin that he was *only* playing. Perhaps he felt secure enough to test, in play, his true identity against the sham of fictional characters.

Before I had begun to work with James, I'd been unsure just what the benefits of fifty-minute psychotherapy meetings would be for young autists. Stacy had responded propitiously during our conversations at the Orthogenic School, but I was able to attend to her needs around the clock. I wondered whether once-weekly meetings would be enough, even for a well-endowed child like James—that is, until I realized that his parents were providing the kind of home environment conducive to his growth. Though not a therapeutic milieu, James's home setting gave him the structure and nurturance he needed to continue developing and to make use of our conversations. His parents helped him with his anxiety about the unexpected and his need for sameness by writing his daily schedule in bold, colorful, easily readable lettering so that he could predict the day's events more readily. When he isolated himself, his parents enticed him back into the family by gently sitting him on their laps, talking softly to him, offering him his favorite snack. They invited him to play with his favorite toys while sitting among them as they read the morning newspaper.

Despite his progress and his parents' skilled attentiveness, Jamie and I sometimes seemed to rush headlong into one dead end after another. By the time he was almost eight, his opening gambit had become oppressively routine. This was because he had integrated the inception of the therapeutic hour in a way that would maximize his control over it. When he wondered aloud what he might do, for example, I'd respond that it was his choice. In saying "It's up to you" or "It's your time" to the children with whom I meet, I hope to encourage them to use their visit in a way that suits *them*, not me or their parents. Jamie would invariably ignore my statements. Probably his idea of control did not yet extend to new behaviors but only to those that had been successful before and that therefore must be repeated unchanged.

Eventually Jamie and I would settle on a shared activity, but he insisted that I begin the interaction by setting up the board games or getting out his favorite Legos. That way he could maintain to himself that our shared activity was my choice, not his. He had not really initiated a social contact.

Yet Jamie did know that in everyday life people take turns. He talked with me about kids having to take turns in school. He could have asked himself, "Why doesn't *she* take turns? Why do *I* always have to choose?" Jamie didn't openly protest my invitation to choose; other children do say, sometimes heatedly, "It's your turn; *you* pick something today!" But not Jamie. Ironically he may have wished *I'd* drop *my* routines, that I'd participate more in selecting shared activities. Perhaps the young autist wished and hoped that the therapist would be more of a social partner!

I believe my lapse in understanding Jamie harked back to my experiences with other young autists. His silent behavior made me think of the many times I had so carefully approached Marcia or Burt or Paulie, sometimes arousing in them a glimmer of interest only to have my hopes dashed by their return to solitude. Even though James was much less diffident than they were and, by age eight, appeared quite "normal," I couldn't help worry that he would withdraw or be faced with some developmental impasse that he couldn't surmount. I thought I might have to start all over again should his progress stall. I believe it's the "Oh no, not again!" feeling that we who work and live with autists experience that makes it so difficult to persist, a feeling that is not lost on autists who, despite their indifferent demeanor, may conclude, too, that all is lost if their favorite people become discouraged or give up on them.

We must find ways to contain these feelings, or we risk acting on them. We must realize that progress in autistic relating is not linear, that it will have its ups and downs just as the progress of any child has. One pitfall may result from the inner autistic vulnerability that, perhaps, no amount of patient, dedicated care can ever eradicate. Or an impasse may result from our own limited patience. Though Jamie's recovery is significant in showing how far an autist may go to approach the social world, the inevitable uncertainties must be reckoned and coped with respectfully and resourcefully.

• • •

James still had to pull back from our conversations and interactions. He would find any excuse he could think of to leave the scene with me and would flip through the pages of a book or silently rotate a top by himself. I asked myself whether he was really that different from other children who withdraw from therapy occasionally. Did his behavior still have that relentless, irrevocable feeling when he seemed to shut down routinely when conversing got to be too much? Was he really as fragile as I feared he was?

When he'd withdraw to a solitary activity, I'd say to Jamie that perhaps he was not ready to do something with me right now. He would distance himself from me even more, his behavior becoming intensely repetitive, so much so that I found myself straining to detect the slightest variation in what he did—*any* variation. I concluded finally that my strained efforts only increased his belief that he was somehow being manipulated to act a certain way—a way that could be unremittingly alien to him.

I tried another tack. When he would get up from a shared activity— a game, drawing, or Legos—I would do the same. I wondered if Jamie needed reassurance that two people could be together pursuing their own separate interests without remorse or implied recrimination. I'd straighten up the office or look up a word in the dictionary.

James immediately noticed what I was doing and once exclaimed with a big smile, "Hey! What are you *doing?*"

"The office was a mess," I'd reply, or "I remembered I had to look up a word in the dictionary."

"But you're supposed to be playing with *me!*" Hands on hips and with an appraising glance, he soon gave me the dice so we could continue the Monopoly game.

Then he began to confide in me again. He told me he had begun, once more, to "play around" with his emergency vehicles, but he seemed embarrassed by this admission, as though he should have grown beyond his engrossing preoccupations. Since he had volunteered that he'd returned to police-car play, I felt comfortable asking him, "Are there any emergencies in your life?"

Jamie laughed, then fell silent.

"I know there have been some changes lately," I said, referring to a recent change in schools.

Emphatically he replied, "Yes, it's different. It's *too* different!"

"Do changes seem like emergencies?"

"When they are *too* different, they *are* emergencies!" So James deftly clarified for me the difference between something seeming to be true and something being true. Big changes were emergencies, period.

I thanked him for explaining his feelings and asked whether he would like to talk about it further. Sighing, he said he'd rather play chess, adding, "At least I know I'm good at that!"

I replied, "Yes, you are very good at chess, and you're good at talking about your feelings, too."

"I've started to play chess in school, and so far, I haven't lost a single game," Jamie replied immediately. Playing chess comforted Jamie more than did thinking and talking about how he felt.

James's absorption with emergencies represented his feeling that disasters will occur as the result of life's unpredictabilities. Before, he had imagined being protected from emergencies as he marshaled the support of the toy police cars to resolve them—"to fix them," he had said. Now he knew he could cope with at least some changes by talking about them and also by reminding himself of his competence, which he did as he played chess. He perhaps had a sense that his competence would assist him in tolerating novelty. In admitting that he had associated change with an emergency, he now considered only major changes to be emergencies; thus, he could master some other adjustments quite well. He could risk losing to other children in chess games. This is what psychologists mean when they say that, as the result of talking things over, the child is better able to cope. Having relegated some of life's novelties to the manageable, Jamie was able to meet at least these situations with renewed vigor and hope. A new lease on life evokes still more coping attempts in the young autist, just as it does in any child.

Playing chess with his contemporaries was a major step forward in James's social development. Because his "little professor" behavior struck the other kids as strange, sometimes as offensively pompous, James found it difficult to maintain friendships. At first he had no inkling that his know-it-all attitude turned kids off. With a casual, blasé wave of his hand, he'd dismiss their faulty chess moves as "stupid." His befriending attempts were impeded by what he did to others, not merely by his fear of what they would do to him.

As he became friendlier in therapy and realized that making friends with me held no particular danger, Jamie became friendlier toward children. In our talks, he was able to understand the stumbling blocks to friend-making that he himself had erected. He had insisted, for example, that he knew my mind better than I knew it myself, saying it must have been my idea that a color equals a feeling. I'd countered with what I actually thought: I said the idea was his, not mine. I meant to communicate that different minds have different ideas, which encouraged him, on occasion, to compare his mind to that of others. He'd often tease me, telling me he was the smartest person of all, eyeing me gleefully as he anticipated that I'd mount a mock protest.

I hoped that this type of conversation would assist Jamie in adapting to his peers. When he was a little older, he'd talk directly about some problems he was having with classmates. When words failed him, he acted out his difficulties as we played his favorite board games, invented Lego set-ups, or drew pictures together. In Chapter 8 I explain how I tried to capture what another child his age might do or say in response to Jamie's impish oppositions and monkeyshines. He understood implicitly what I said and my intent. He'd trump my ideas with his own, so as not to be outdone by someone who may have seemed to lecture him just as he had declaimed to others.

Given Stacy's and James's responses to conversation, it's worth asking whether autists like runaway Burt and mute Paulie form basic human mental connections, those between acting and feeling or those between thinking and doing. These connections are essential if an autist is to profit from psychotherapy. Although he didn't speak, Paulie did seem aware of a link between thinking and doing. And even though he didn't voice it, he seemed aware of the connection between his memories of our weekly meetings and his depictions of them as he studiously worked on drawing the office building in which we met. He seemed to anticipate my reaction to him, that I would be glad—overjoyed actually—to receive his drawings, which he, however listlessly, delivered to my open hands. Burt briefly appeared to conjoin his acting (running away) with my speech (when I wondered why he would run from home of all places). Perhaps through the therapist's language, these boys learned that their feelings and actions originated somewhere and that it would not only be possible to track their origins but it would also be unexpectedly helpful to do so.

Hel . . . llooouuuw . . . Karrren . . .
—BURT

These were the first words Burt ever said to me, after I had finished working with him. He'd come to visit me during his several-year residency in a special program for autists at a local state hospital. His words were said in a low monotone—Burt was by then thirteen and pubescent—and he elongated the vowels and the letter r to form a kind of low moan that was at once anguished and mechanical.

During the four years I worked with Burt, I had no doubt that, though he ignored words and conversation, he was nonetheless attuned to those facial expressions and bodily gestures—probable precursors of speech—that foretold his immediate future. He would gaze apprehensively in his mother's direction when she shook her finger at him, promising him a swift retribution if he ran to the freeway. He would stare vaguely and tentatively in my direction when I invited him into my office, perking up just the tiniest bit when I reminded him there would be a snack waiting for him or that we could play his favorite water games. Since he didn't actually say anything in response, to either his mother's remonstrations or my invitations, I couldn't be sure that he *did* link our speech with his actions.

Is Burt's apparent intuition, his obvious receptive understanding of language, enough to grant that his mind is able to conceptualize itself? Can a mute child's limited repertoire allow him to advance beyond intuition to reach the lauded conceptual status? We could answer with a qualified yes if we analogized mute autists to the deaf-mutes studied by psychologist Hans Furth, who found that his group of nonautistic, nonspeaking children, though lagging somewhat behind hearing, speaking children, *do* proceed from the intuitive to the conceptual, albeit belatedly.[7] Since mature concepts are formed and tested in social discourse, perhaps the deaf-mute, like the mute autist, is hampered by restricted access to the very interpersonal turf that nourishes rational thought.

Not that speculations such as these mattered much when it came to Burt. The minutes in which he may have begun to connect my words with his actions were just not numerous enough to prevent his behaving hazardously. He was eventually enrolled in the twenty-four-hour contained program for autistic youth. There he was trained by behavioral methods to speak social inanities. His words appeared inane to me because they sounded utterly devoid of meaning. When Burt was brought to see me after spending two years in the program, his mother was understandably hopeful and even elated by his first words. "Burt can *talk* now; he says *words!*"

Indeed he did. How she hoped he would, through some small attempts to speak to her, bridge the awful abyss that had existed between them. And how she wished his first few words would undo all those terrible years when she could not connect to her son, or feared that she could not, years when she complained desperately not about Burt's running away, but about the fact that he *could not say words.*

With his mother watching, Burt moved his lips mechanically to say hello in a stentorian tone. What stayed with me were the pathos on his mother's face and the unexplained hurt in Burt's eyes and voice as he mouthed those syllables. Although Burt and his mother had been communicating after a fashion for many years, it hadn't carried the weight for Burt's mother that his actual words did.

On the day mute Paulie first portrayed our meetings in line drawings, I had no clue how to respond. I still earnestly hoped that he would speak. I thought if only I could find the right words, he would relax his vigilant stance and release from his lips some secret, arcane, maybe even prescient news. In my initial attempts to help Paulie, I had limited my search to language, the very modality that seemed so distressing to him.

Moments of silence ensued as I surveyed his drawing of my office. Then I began to slowly trace with my forefinger the first cartoon frame to the last, saying nothing, not even venturing a single comment that I thought his picture was about our meetings. Nor did I remark interpretively that though objects were depicted in his story, there were no people. Not that I didn't want to. I wanted so much to start a real conversation that I had to remind myself of the first time I met Paulie, when he turned his back as I said hello. So I didn't dare talk, much less about people.

Paulie seemed interested in my silent frame-by-frame acknowledgment of his story; he gazed dreamily at me with a slight smile. I offered a few words. "The door and the hall." Then, "The stairs." Finally, "Now my office." In referring to my office and not to me, I hoped to avoid personalizing our meetings too excitedly. I got an appraising, curious look from him, so I wondered aloud, "Maybe this is a story of you coming to see me?"

At this, Paulie went to work in earnest, drawing assiduously without stopping until our time together was up. His new drawings seemed to be about events and places other than our shared times. My careful phrasing of questions to elicit a hoped-for yes or no or even a nod brought forth nothing. Paulie simply never acknowledged that he heard my questions. His unresponsiveness wasn't due to hearing loss, because he would instantly attend to noises that transfixed him, like fire engines screaming outside or the quiet shutting of doors in the building. His mother corroborated my impression of intact hearing; testing had revealed no auditory disability. Perhaps his drawings of other places and events were his attempts to share more of his life with me than just the little bit we had when we met together. I guessed that he had drawn his classroom, since there were desks and chairs. I guessed he'd made a picture of his home, since he had produced a roofed house with what looked like a garden. Maybe he was drawing all the places his attentive mother took him to, logical from his perspective, since his first drawing was the very place in which he met with me. He would react with a slight smile, but he never committed himself to a yes or a no. He would sometimes cock his head at my suggestions, staring at the ceiling, appearing to be mulling over what I had said. Finally, it seemed to me that he was willing to commit himself to *communication* but not to *language*.

Unfortunately, I was not to work with Paulie for much longer. One day his parents accompanied him to my office—they usually let him run up the stairs by himself—and told me they would be moving soon and so this would be our last visit. Immediately, Paulie set to work on his final drawing. It was another cartoonlike sequence in which he showed a small boy entering the office building, climbing the stairs, and entering an office—the very first time he had drawn a person, obviously himself. There were also the toys and the plate of snacks. But this time, just as he was about to leave, he handed his drawing to me, perhaps as a goodbye gift, letting it drop into my hands impassively as a token of the times we had spent together. His intent to communicate mutely was obvious. His silent message imparted his sense of what I wanted from him—his recognition of our meeting, of my existence—and his resignation over our separation given the listlessness with which he symbolically said good-bye.

On the basis of his overt behavior, I have hypothesized that Paulie understood my intent in some small but significant way. Rigorous proof of Paulie's theory of mind would be hard to imagine, but neither is there a test thus far that can prove the contrary. Just as we cannot at present know for sure that a young autist possesses theory of mind, we cannot know with certainty that he does not. So can we be sure that Paulie wasn't reverberating to my purposes with his own understanding of them? Just because he did not articulate what he understood does not mean he didn't comprehend. Maybe his parents or I could have persuaded him to communicate by writing or typing. To see if Paulie could or would write some of his thoughts, I had planned, just as his parents informed me of their impending move, to introduce some written words on my own cartoon drawings—my "answers" to his unspoken messages.

Although my work with Paulie spanned only a few months, my work with Stacy, James, and Burt was extensive. These experiences allowed me to understand just what could be accomplished in a lengthy relationship with young autists. Burt's progress often faltered, notwithstanding his belated use of words or short phrases. I'd become disheartened about his inability to accept the friendship I offered to him. He seemed to be a one step–forward, two steps–backward kid. When he encountered people or said hello to them, he became so anguished that he'd retreat even more determinedly into his solitary world, stubbornly refusing to acknowledge even the most careful, calm, softly spoken befriending invitations.

Playactor Stacy and "little professor" James reacted auspiciously to my efforts, but in puzzling, confounding ways. I was exhilarated by their unexpected responses. It was a challenge to fathom the puzzle of their behavior, the conundrums embedded in their language. What they said often seemed a fascinating, impenetrable code that I was determined to decipher.

My conversations with these two brilliant young autists sometimes took on a battle-of-wits character, which I clarified by asking them outright if I'd understood what they said. Both children delighted in correcting me, in setting me straight about themselves. I was amused by their antics, which appeared to communicate to them that I truly enjoyed being with them, that I enjoyed them as people.

CHAPTER FIVE

From Solitude to Sociability

Dolly eat up a bottle.
Give *me* a bottle!
—MARCIA

Songster Marcia was fourteen when she made the statements that open this chapter. By the time she had been at the Orthogenic School for three years, she at last permitted herself to play and to set up tea parties for her favorite doll. It might not be surprising to hear a young child request a bottle, but a wild statement erupting from a teenager about a doll eating up a bottle took me completely by surprise.

Because they have lived longer with their autism, older autists like Marcia are different from younger ones. The longer these children live apart from people, the less likely their ideas, fears, dreams, and wishes will be amended by others. Conversational give-and-take encourages kids to rethink their attitudes, opinions, thoughts, and feelings. Without this social stimulation, autistic people—indeed, all of us—are subject to the perils of solipsism—not just the loneliness of it, but also its hollow boredom. Yet even older autistic kids will respond if they find themselves with people who appreciate them, who offer them a soothing, interesting solace.

Marcia behaved quite peculiarly and impersonally when she fed her doll. She'd hold it at arm's length, the fingers of one hand carefully squeezing the doll's cheeks so the liquid would pour in a steady stream from the baby bottle into the doll's mouth without spilling. She seemed intent on getting every last drop of water out of the bottle and into her baby doll. While at first she didn't volunteer anything about this odd behavior, she'd briefly answer my questions about it. "What's the dolly *doing?*" I'd inquire incredulously, wondering whether Marcia imagined the doll to be such a repugnant creature that she wished to distance herself from it as much as possible; wondering, as well, whether she thought the feeding experience itself was disgusting. Then one day she mysteriously explained that the doll was consuming the bottle itself: "Dolly eat up a bottle." As though the two thoughts were naturally and necessarily linked, she seemed to justify her first sentence with the second: "Give *me* a bottle!" The most I could make of this was that Marcia imagined the doll's consumption of the whole bottle deprived her of *her* bottle. When I tried to put this thought into words, Marcia began to intone joylessly, "Wait, wait, wait . . ." No amount of consoling her that the dolly's bottle was hers to do with as she pleased, including drinking from it herself, changed her tune. For some reason, I thought, she just wanted to drone endlessly the word "wait."

Years later, mute autistic children like Paulie or Burt reminded me of Marcia, because she was so often implacably quiet, just as they were. When she did speak, it appeared to be torture for her, just as it seemed to be for Burt when he said hello to me. How to activate Marcia when she was withdrawn and hostile to the slightest suggestion that she act; how to put into practice Bettelheim's notion that we could bring Marcia to life only by being the "catalysts that induced [her] to take action on [her] own behalf"?[1]

Yet the fact that Marcia spoke at all was encouraging. Her age two-to three-year old language provided the building blocks, it turned out, to more advanced communication, where meaning became more fully nuanced. Eventually she could be persuaded to converse if she felt safe and in rapport with the person to whom she was talking and if the topic near-perfectly matched her interests. She would even talk to a favorite dormmate if her friend discussed with her the proper way to feed and cuddle a baby doll.

"No, no, no!" this younger, nonautistic girl once said to Marcia as she was suspending her doll midair and as far away from her body as she could. "You're supposed to hold your baby like this," the girl explained, taking the doll from Marcia and cuddling it. "Then you're supposed to sing to it and rock it in your arms," Marcia's friend said softly, moving closer to Marcia so that she could talk with her intimately and confidentially. This girl believed, as did I, that in order to persuade Marcia to alter the way she behaved toward her dolly one had to painstakingly teach her the basics of human care.

To me, Marcia's withdrawn silence implied at least a partial recognition of the social world. Why else turn her back on it? This deployment of will, I thought, is all too often ignored or denied by us because it's easier to think that the autist "can't" when she "won't." She must be deficient when she turns her back to us or does absolutely nothing in the real world, because to concede that she deliberately turns away or remains inactive insults us and arouses anger. When she was well into adolescence, Marcia and I had quite a few conversations about how she felt about herself and about me. When asked why she turned her back on me, she would reply, as if it explained everything, "Karen angry." She may have thought, accurately, that I was irritated at her for incessantly turning her back on me.

About herself, she volunteered, "Marcia is a strong girl."

"Strong to do what?"

"Strong to do nothing." Then, as though it followed as the night does the day, she queried, "Why you talk?"

Autists, like the rest of us, can deliberate in some situations, but in others they find themselves so woefully inadequate that it is almost impossible for them to take advantage of our offered assistance. The abbreviated "Karen angry" showed that Marcia understood the connection between her behavior and my reaction, though she found it difficult to say just why she behaved as she did. This makes it all the more imperative to seek out what young autists can and will do and say, what they are prepared and motivated to accomplish. Without any difficulty whatsoever, Marcia asserted she was strong to do nothing. She also apparently found it easy to ask me why I talked to her, why I asked her questions.

With Marcia, I could invent all sorts of communication tactics to ease her difficulties with speaking. After all, I spent more than seven years of full days and many nights with her, while I only met with Paulie and Burt once weekly. Early on, saying an entire sentence seemed beyond her; she spoke mostly monosyllabically or in short phrases. I thought of starting the sentence for her, hoping she would "fill in the blanks." If I wished to know what she wanted to do that day, I'd say, "Marcia wants to . . . ," waiting for her to specify her wishes. Often I had to add other words so that she had to add only one more: "Marcia wants to go to the . . ." would prompt her to finish the thought with "store" or "playground."

Whether to wait until Marcia was ready to communicate and interact or whether to press her to do so was always the operative question. A similar concern occupies Clara Claiborne Park, who writes of her young daughter's autistic withdrawal and Park's attempts to draw almost three-year old Elly out of it. In a curriculum especially designed for her daughter, Park invents little games to encourage Elly to play, but Park does not insist too much. By tossing rocks into a pool, she invites some small action from Elly that young children do naturally. She hopes that Elly will pick up a rock to throw in the water. "No, she won't. Not today. I do not press; I know the answer is final. My immobility is a mirror of hers. I have learned to wait."[2]

In much the same way, I tried to interest eleven-year-old Marcia in some aspects of nature. She sat cross-legged on a lawn near the Orthogenic School, an invisible boundary seemingly surrounding her as her legs nested akimbo under her upper body. Sitting with Marcia on the green was like waiting for an Armageddon that seemed never to arrive. Slowly each silent battle we waged over whether she would acknowledge the grass—or better yet, me—built up inexorably to a tortuous and unendurable peak. Shattered though my nerves were, I tried to remain as immobile as she, lest I disturb some delicate balance in her universe. Her implicit no was crashingly final.

Yet, I did wait until Marcia showed some tiny interest in her environment before I made my move. Soon I noticed she was fingering blades of grass, one by one. Abruptly she started to rock back and forth, toward and away from the grass, but on the forward thrust she carefully observed each blade. Then she smiled when I said, "One, two . . . ," so I continued counting until I heard her soft voice join mine in enunciating, "Five, six, seven, eight, nine, ten," the last number in her series voiced in hushed, squeaky excitement.

Suddenly it dawned on me that Marcia had been waiting for *me* when I thought I'd been waiting for *her*. She was waiting for me to sit silently and calmly, tolerating her endless inaction with an equanimity matching hers. If so, her matter-of-fact complacence about doing nothing while we sat together was not only intentional but also evidence of a careful reading of me: that I so much wanted her to respond for my own reasons, including a curiosity about what it took to get autistic youngsters like Marcia to respond appreciatively and vocally. Shortly after this thought hit me four decades ago, I heard myself saying to at-a-standstill Marcia, "What is it you're *not* doing now?," soon followed by, "What is it you're not *saying* now?"

By then she had begun to create tea parties for her favorite doll. Hearing my questions, she hopped to it and began to set up the cups and saucers for her doll, filling the cups with water and carefully pouring the liquid down the doll's gullet. Perhaps the do-nothing, say-nothing stance was the best Marcia could muster during the blackest moments of her life, including the interminable waits she had to endure to be attended to when she was an infant. Marcia's mother had recounted how busy she was when Marcia was little, and how she did everything in a hurry for her. This may have convinced Marcia that doing nothing—not complying with her busy mother's requests—would require her mother to attend to her more regularly.[3] The waiting I had to endure was a replay of Marcia's own waits, her perception that she was waiting endlessly to be taken care of, which she expressed by saying of the playacted feeding with her doll, "Wait, wait, wait . . . ," on and on.

What were parents to do before they knew that autism is probably a neurological condition? Marcia's mother may have thought the most sensible plan for her dreamy, recalcitrant daughter was to convince her that adapting to the exigencies of the real world was Marcia's best bet.

Teenager Marcia, often inactive and withdrawn, needed a gentle but firm prod to go beyond an immobility that appeared to counter her mother's hurry to get things done. Marcia wanted to slow her mother down, so she did nothing in order to get more of her care. Marcia's inactivity with me had the same intent—to slow me down. Since I did slow down, often to a standstill, Marcia might have imagined inflicting on passive me what her hurried mother had seemed to inflict upon her.

My questions about not doing and not talking implied that Marcia had something in mind when doing and saying nothing. The questions seemed to release her action in regard to her dolly in much the way a pithy statement to a person in psychoanalysis seems to lift an inhibition. I hoped that in asking her what she was not doing or not saying, she'd become more in tune with what she *was* doing—namely, thinking. I hoped to connect her refusal to act with thinking. Then she might risk acting. Since thinking about serving her doll pretend tea had no untoward consequences, perhaps acting overtly would be safe as well. And she just might use words to tell me what she was doing. She was arranging things so her dolly could "eat up a bottle."

As I attended to what Marcia actually said, she became sufficiently comfortable with her thoughts to share them with me, especially her wish, heretofore submerged, to be with people. Her mysterious linguistic code was often accompanied by telling actions that spoke more loudly than her words. She sought physical contact from those she trusted most—for example, being carried around by me or hugs when she was caught by one of her counselors during the "chase" game. I fervently watched as her personality seemed to blossom. I'd scan her words for clues as to how she felt about herself and how she felt about me. Although her condensed language revealed much about her sense of herself in the company of others, her silent attachment to me more clearly revealed her budding persona and signaled the progress she was making in emerging from behind her protective "curtain."

I continue Marcia's story (in Chapter 7) by describing her attempts to connect to me, her startling way of hugging, and her struggles to get straight the personal pronouns "you," "me," and "I." To my chagrin, I realized during Marcia's word struggles that I'd gotten unduly accustomed to her practice of referring to both me and her as "you." So when she began, quietly, shyly, and subtly, to refer only to me as "you," I had to rethink who this ethereal but circumspect charge of mine really was.

The meaning of Marcia's speech was still hard to decipher. It seemed to arise full-blown from another, quite subconscious realm, alien to me but strangely familiar to her. Young Greg spoke in that strange way for a while, but his use of language had adapted to everyday conversation and had broadened sufficiently to make his meaning more accessible. Marcia's meaning seemed forever open to multiple and often reckless interpretation—one reason I long ago surmised that the best starting point for understanding an autist's spoken communication is to interpret it literally.

> The other kids are mean and stupid.
> They sometimes just *act* stupid and *that's* stupid!
> —GREGORY

Thus did Gregory emote about his peer problems when his parents brought him back for a second series of therapy visits. Compared to Marcia's "Dolly eat up a bottle" and "Give *me* a bottle!" his sentences were impressively formed to interlock with the linguistic expectations of the listener. When he began to approach the people world, he became ever more preoccupied with good and evil. I tried to tolerate his endless ruminations about his peers' "evil" and "bad" aspects. His mood changed dramatically when conversing about them: he became angry and sullen; his pacing and clapping increased. When discussing animals, he'd cheer considerably and I found myself wondering why he rarely, if ever, spoke of the "evil" or the "bad" in animals. He had read books about the bonobos, the apes recently studied by primatologist Franz de Waal and which are close to us genetically. Greg knew of their capability for empathy and their peaceful nature. Could he have concluded that bonobos behave more sensitively than humans?

I would watch respectfully as Gregory acted out one gory fantasy after another, like piercing a tiny male dollhouse doll in the groin with a "bad guy" weapon, a superhero's tiny knife or gun. I knew his passage from animals to humans was significant. I was determined to accord him the respect for his fantasies that he needed in order to maintain himself in the "people world." I thought if I listened attentively, I would, somehow, grasp why he was so intent on dichotomizing his surroundings into good and bad.

Once Gregory read my horrified face at some of his antics, and said mockingly, "This is going to be funny."

"To me what you are doing is not funny," I replied.

But Greg didn't appear to care in the least what I thought, and after many gorings and beatings of the tiny doll, I asked, "Why are you so into violence?" At this he jerked around to look at me and laughed wickedly. And there our brief conversation ended.

After weeks of listening and trying to talk to Greg, only rarely offering opinions and interpretations of the events he described or dramatized, I realized that my attentiveness to the way he saw things might have had unintended consequences. Because I had remained silent, he could have thought that I welcomed his every idea, opinion, and attitude uncritically. Since I tolerated (or tried to tolerate) his thoughts about violence, he may have assumed that I actually tolerated his violent behavior. It no longer seemed therapeutic to accept Greg and all his autistic ways in the hope that he would eventually respond to the social world more adaptively. I decided that the risk of listening to his every word was too great. His thoughts had become increasingly repetitive and were maintained with ever-vigilant rigidity. His behavior at school was deteriorating, and I once more became alarmed that he would be permanently suspended.

Even when Greg explained his violent acts in terms of what he knew about animals—"People are animals, you know," he'd declare in defense of his wild actions—my joining him in a discussion of the similarities between humans and other species only seemed to encourage more antisocial behavior. He didn't heed in the slightest my rejoinder, "The wild pigs you happen to be comparing yourself to are very smart." I had hoped to persuade him to consider animal qualities that would serve him in a social world.

Greg seemed unpersuaded by my logic, so I soon decided, against my personal inclination, that I must be firm with him and limit the wildness he so cavalierly indulged in. I had to be firm without appearing rejecting and uninterested in him.

After thinking about this therapeutic dilemma—a dilemma because I hardly wanted to jettison the work in which I had tried to convey to Greg that his ideas mattered—I made up my mind that there would be no more wild talk in my office. When Gregory came for his next visit, I heard him mutter under his breath, "Evil, evil, evil . . ."

I answered, "I'm very interested in you, Greg, but not at all interested in all the evil talk that I have heard so many times before."

Avoiding my gaze, Greg laughed a little. "I don't know what you are talking about," he said innocently.

"I heard you whisper 'evil,' and I heard a lot about that last time we met."

"No, you didn't," Greg replied, now defiant.

"It's time to do something different."

"Fine, then!" he exclaimed sarcastically. "No evil! I wasn't going to do 'evil' today, anyway."

Soon I got a note from his mother that not only was Gregory lambasting the other students verbally, but he was deliberately hitting them, not just bumping into them accidentally. She also wrote that Greg was once more refusing to turn in his homework. He'd insist on finishing it by himself; then he'd rip it up, probably to avoid didactic conversation with his parents, or he'd consent to take it to school where he refused to let his teacher see it, possibly fearing criticism and being marked wrong. Greg often thought his behavior and even his very self to be all wrong.

When next I met with Greg, I said, "Gregory, I have two things to say to you," as he was provocatively tossing some toys around the office, seeming to threaten me.

"Yes?" he answered in a surprisingly curious voice.

"You must not hit people, because it's not safe for you to do so.

And you must turn in your homework because you've gone to all the trouble of doing it. So why not get credit for it?"

Exasperated, Greg answered, "I keep forgetting to turn it in!"

"Then I'm going to write a note to your mom saying you need help remembering to give your homework to your teacher."

"But it's supposed to be *me* that decides whether to turn it in," Greg wailed as he admitted he knew precisely what was expected of him.

"Yes, I know that, but right now you need help so that you'll be able to get credit for your work."

Much sobered, Greg capitulated with a mild, "Okay."

Possibly Greg's change of heart came from his realization that in remonstrating him I had pointed out how he'd benefit from what I'd suggested: he'd be safer if he didn't lash out at others, and he'd receive credit for his work if only he'd turn it in.

As Greg was about to leave my office, I reminded him that it's not safe to start fights with people. He whirled around to face me and asked plaintively, "What *should* I do when people do mean things to me?"

Before, he'd characterized other students' actions as "evil"; now they were only "mean."

"Let's talk about that next week."

"I get very hyper in school," Greg admitted, thus showing he could be thoughtful about his behavior when he wished.

Yet Greg continued to cause a ruckus in class. He told me that he had recently "faked" an attack on his teacher and had been suspended. He said his parents were extremely upset by the suspension. His ongoing ferocity made me wonder whether my tactics with him were working. True, he'd begun to converse introspectively with me; he'd even confided how much he had upset his parents. Greg tried to reassure me by claiming he only "faked" his attack, much like Stacy, who tried to make her wild behavior more palatable by explaining its reasons. I was tempted to conclude, prematurely as it turned out, that because Greg's antisocial behavior continued and even worsened, my therapeutic plan was inadequate and, quite possibly, downright wrong.

For the moment, Greg was unable to sustain in school the resolve he'd achieved in therapy to cease his attacks and hand in his homework. I attempted a different approach as I said to him, "When you act up in school, it upsets your parents." This platitude, acknowledging his parents' importance for him, occasioned an eruption of self-blame from Greg, who imagined all sorts of disastrous, punitive consequences for his misdeeds. Now the proverbial pendulum had swung from his belief that he could finesse his uproars to imagining the worst of fates for his "evil" actions. He comforted himself briefly by playing Hangman, now his favorite pastime in my office, spelled the word "chihuahua," and suddenly disclosed, "I thought of that word because I tried to pet a dog in school, and its owner thought I was going to rip it to shreds."

"Were you?"

"No, and she didn't really think that. She just doesn't like me and doesn't want me to pet her dog."

Greg's disclosure, which revealed an accurate reading of his classmate, suggested that, all along, the purpose of his "evil" behavior was to wreak revenge on those who didn't like him. If so, this shows just how important the feelings and opinions of others were to Greg, and how hurt by them he'd become. Autists, like other people, defend themselves against adversity in any way they can. In Greg's case, he defended himself against the inevitable feeling that, because he was so conspicuously different from others, so "wrong," he would be rejected and forsaken.

Weeks later it dawned on me that Gregory had not talked about or acted out any gory, wild scenes since we'd discussed the fact that he had upset his parents by being suspended. His parents' concern reminded Greg that they cared deeply about him. He still liked to enact dramas that bordered on violence, but he often cloaked his thoughts with humor. Or he'd speak of the other children not as "evil" but as "mean" or "stupid." One day, after sprinting into my office like a gazelle, he blurted out, "Thank goodness the teacher moved that kid!" He was referring to a boy who sat next to him in school and who had taunted him mercilessly.

"What was he doing that he got moved away from you?"

"He was making faces and acting stupid."

"Is he stupid?"

"No, he just *acts* stupid and *that's* stupid!"

He went on to invent games with tiny dolls, examining them rigorously to test if they were "stupid," perhaps imagining a similar test of his peers at school. He assured me, "This is not an evil story; it's about stupidity." After many such dramas, I objected again, saying, "Let's do something different."

Laughing, Greg declared, "This *is* different. It's about a different stupidity!"

Then, eyeing my skeptical expression, he exclaimed, "I have a great idea!" He busied himself setting up the game of Hangman and suggested that the small dollhouse dolls would get knocked over for any wrong answer either of us gave. I was impressed by his suggestion to combine a structured activity with his fantasy and became amused by his plan. Encouraged, Greg began to write the most arcane animal names he could think of, anticipating I would make repeated errors, which meant he could knock over many dolls. Eventually, I thought his little game and its clever implication that I'd lent a hand to his assault on the dolls so funny that I began to laugh. Soon Greg started to laugh uproariously, too. It was one of the few times we genuinely and freely shared a great comic moment.

· · ·

I was never really sure what produced the change in Greg after he'd amused me with his comic antics. Was he heartened by our having shared humorous moments? Or had he simply realized that I appreciated him in an important way, a feeling he'd rarely experienced, except from his family. He'd gracefully cross the threshold of my office, saying "hi" audibly and warmly just as his foot touched the boundary between the outside and the interior. Why, I wondered for the umpteenth time, are thresholds so important to these children? He would broach current troubles spontaneously and earnestly. His teacher still had to remind him not to call other children names, but Greg was no longer threatened with suspension.

"You know what time-out is in school? It's a lot better than being suspended. I had that [time-out] yesterday for calling someone a name."

"Why'd you do that?"

"Because he kept chasing me around and wouldn't stop."

"Did he stop when you called him a name?"

"No, not really. And he's always getting into trouble for being disruptive and calling things out in class. I'm doing A-plus work in science now. We're studying the life process."

Greg went on to say that his father was impressed by his science grades, referring to the fact that they had often discussed Greg's interest in animals. From animals they had branched out to discuss science generally. Until recently, though, Greg had acted aloof, even bored, when his father attempted to enlarge upon Greg's store of knowledge. He needed time to process what he learned about biology from his father and from the science books his father gave him before he could claim as his own what he'd learned from both.

Continuing, he remarked upon his classmates' ignorance of biology but without the sarcastic edge of before. "Some kids thought there wasn't as much bacteria in prehistoric times as there is now. I think there was. It [what the kids said] must have been a joke." The reference to jokes reminded Greg of a riddle he'd heard recently. "Why does Santa Claus like to garden?"

"I don't know."

"Because he likes to ho, ho, ho!"

"Why did Comet stay home on Christmas Eve?" I contributed, laughing.

"Dunno."

"He was busy cleaning the sink."

"I don't really get that."

"You know, Comet, the cleanser?"

"Yeah, that's really stupid!"

"It's not as good as your riddle, right?"

"Right!"

How similar this was to the jillions of talks I've had over the years with other children his age. No kid, thought Greg, would think my riddle funny.

Greg's return to sociability came with progress in communicating. Furthermore, he'd established a niche for himself in class by acing science, which surprised and pleased his teacher. Greg even earned approval from some of his classmates. He had turned an "obsession," animal lore, into a topic of study that meshed with his school's curriculum. He began to attend his therapy meetings attractively clothed; his demeanor bespoke competence and enthusiasm as he bounded into my office like a fleet-footed, shy animal. He behaved less bizarrely and was ever more open to conversation. Most impressive was the ease with which he talked about his successes. Confident of my pleased reaction and looking straight at me, he told me, "You know, I was on a camping trip last week."

"How did it go?"

"I was the only one who won two merit badges."

He'd finished work on survival in the wilderness and a unit on animal species. The overnight camping trip provided ample opportunity for uproars and weirdness, but none materialized. I was once more impressed by how important the context is in working with these easy-to-identify and often very difficult youngsters. Gregory proved he could behave quite well when he was assured that the others liked and admired him, and the other campers had been impressed by Greg's achievements.

Despite all these gains, Greg, almost thirteen, would still lapse into disquieting fantasy at times. One day he drew some cartoon characters who, he said, were changing into "teenage mutants." In a bizarre, ominous voice, he spoke for the characters: "Oh no, what's going to happen to me?"

Could he be wondering, I speculated, what was going to happen to *him*, with all his personal "mutations"?

"What *is* happening to them?" I inquired.

"Here's a monster, scaring little children."

"Oh no," I thought. "Here we go again."

The monster Greg was drawing had claws with six fingers and long fingernails, as well as dinosaur-like feet with spikes.

"Do you enjoy scaring little children?"

"No, not really. I don't scare children," Greg answered soberly.

Maybe he's telling me, I thought, that all along it was he who was afraid of dinosaurs and monsters, the very subjects that had occupied his mind for so long. "I wonder, when you were young, if you were scared of monsters like this?"

"Yes, I thought there was a monster in my closet," Greg resonated instantly.

"Gee, I wonder why the closet of all places?"

"In the dark the shadows really do look like a monster. I could imagine it moving around, and I thought it was going to eat me."

Aha! Perhaps the beginnings of the gobbling, biting fantasy-making.

Then Greg volunteered, "You know, I used to live right across from the park? I could see red lights from my window, and I thought they were red monster eyes."

By now I understood that his use of "you know" signaled his feeling that we were communicating well. "Did you ever find out what those red lights were? Maybe they were the taillights of a car."

"They weren't moving so I couldn't tell . . ." Trailing off softly, Gregory seemed to ponder the problem further. Did he suddenly realize that because the red lights didn't move he could not determine, when he was young and impressionable, whether they belonged to a car or were monster eyes? If the lights had moved, he seemed to say, he would have known their source, since monsters, like animals, move fleet-of-foot, unlike cars.

Together, thirteen-year-old Greg and I tried to recast a past experience in which he'd been the scared child tormented by an imaginary ogre. Now, by identifying with an imaginary aggressor (the teenage mutant), he could poke fun at a young child's anxiety, as many children do when they struggle to cope with their irrational fears. Combating autism helped Greg understand not just how to cope with the here and now—he no longer instigated unspeakable turmoil in class—but also how better to understand his past.

The regularity of our weekly meetings sensitized Greg to time's passing, especially as it related to events happening to him. Time continuities seemed more vivid as he told me what had occurred recently and what was likely to occur in the future. He was less apt to avoid thoughts about his future, as he gradually came to believe that it held some promise. He could see that the events he had experienced were rather different from what he was experiencing now. Even though he didn't always talk directly but rather used an allegorical idiom, there was a beginning, middle, and end to his symbolic narratives. Gaining a better sense of who he was in the past, who he was now, and how he might be in the future helped him dissect his interactions with others. More importantly, he could imagine how relationships might improve, how they might actually solidify into real friendships. Unlike Greg, who first classified the world, then told tales about it, Nathan, whose story follows, had captivated others with his "ancient history" stories since he was a young child. His parents said he was inordinately fascinated by this topic to the exclusion of everything else. Because bookish Nathan was also interested in splitting words by syllables, perhaps he thought "history" really meant "his story." As it happened, he recounted a portion of his personal story just as his work with me was about to end.

To *him*, it's upsetting; to *me*, it's not.
Teasing's not emotional; I mean, it's not emotional to *me*!
—NATHAN

Ten-year-old Nathan was describing how he often got into trouble for teasing his younger brother. There was nothing wrong with teasing your sibling, Nate said, if what he said did not feel like a tease to *him*. In just a few months, his social perceptions began to include the perspectives and feelings of others more overtly. His view of himself and his optimism about his future had buoyed beyond the expectations of just about everyone who knew him. In Nate's case, learning about others did not appear to threaten his fragile hold on *self* but rather seemed to make him feel more expansive. He was elated when he shared with me his newly won—or perhaps newly consolidated— insight that two boys, his brother and himself, could have very different experiences of teasing.

At our first meeting, though, Nathan was despondent, despairing that he could not solve the host of problems he faced both at home and at school. He was doomed, he thought, because of his Asperger's condition. He was sure people didn't like him because he was odd and because he had academic and social difficulties such as persistent conflicts with his younger brother. He also had an unfounded fear that his peers would invariably reject him—unfounded because he'd lately made several friends in school who invited him over to play, even though Nathan would turn his back and act as if he didn't care when they mocked him about his odd ways. He staunchly maintained to himself that he did not "get emotional" about being ridiculed but worried inwardly, he confessed, that he appeared "weird" and that eventually his friends would discover that he was not at all like them. He reminded me of James, who became embarrassed, apprehensive, and even guilty at some of his atypical behaviors and who tried hard to camouflage them or to minimize their effect on others. So, too, did Nathan. Of all the autists I've known, Nathan seemed the most determined to overcome his autism, and precisely because of this investment he was exquisitely attuned to the reactions of others, quick to believe he had not measured up.

Greg, in his early years, didn't bother himself with social graces, but Nate had learned to compose himself even when he felt tense and intimidated. At first, he struck me as "hyperverbal" as he used his impressive vocabulary and polite, though somewhat stiff, manners to ease social situations. When he saw that his efforts were effective, he'd relax and bask in the affection others felt for him. These others were mainly adults—his parents, teachers, an older boy who'd take Nate under his wing—but also, increasingly, boys his own age.

Nathan felt inordinately compelled to tell the truth, which, he told me, was written down someplace, like in the Bible or in history texts. In conversation he was scrupulously conscientious. He'd tense up, though—I could see his shoulders stiffening—even when I remarked on the accuracy of his statements and the sincerity of his opinions. He'd rub his hands in the soft pile of the carpet on which we sat as we talked, trying to comfort himself by touching the plush fabric, much as a young child would cuddle a stuffed animal.

I soon noticed that he'd become nervous, fidgety, often withdrawn, even surly, when he thought the situation between us was adversarial.

If we were playing a board game, he would use military terms to describe his strategies. Slowly, he began to disclose an inner, fantasied sequence that accompanied his outward game tactics. Many of these thoughts nestled in a running, silent commentary, the details furnished, his parents told me, by his delving into any history book he could get his hands on. From Nathan's behavior, I guessed, retrospectively, that when James mimicked a television character while talking with me, he was revealing just how caught up he could be in two worlds simultaneously—ours and his. Nathan would become so overwhelmed by his inner world that he'd forget where he was, the name of the game we were playing, or whose turn it was. He was so mightily caught up in his intricate idea-system, common among young people with Asperger's syndrome, that he seemed, literally, to forget aspects of himself. Then he would jerk himself back to the reality of the game and become sheepish about his lapses.

I've witnessed many an autist get wrapped up in these self-generated imaginings, but I'd never talked with a young autist so excruciatingly aware as Nathan was of his own mental workings and of the implications for social discourse. Being ten, Nathan might have spontaneously developed just those mental abilities to assess himself self-consciously and comparatively. I saw the same self-evaluative process blossom in eleven- and twelve-year-old Gregory, but only after a great deal of struggle to put aside, for a moment, his egoistic interests and opinions. It would be interesting to discover whether other adept autists of ten or older show a similar progressive trend, one that can be seen in ordinary preadolescents.[4]

More than the average youth, Nate seemed accountable only to a certain idiosyncratic way of doing things and resisted the idea that some events might be beyond his control. Not being in control meant to him that he might have to change his preferred ways and habits. For example, he spoke enthusiastically about various game plans one could use against one's chess opponent. His face clouded and his voice dropped gloomily when he said that it wasn't good at all that he didn't always know which of the many strategies the other person would select. I was about to mention the probability of guessing plausibly when he brightened and remarked, "There are a limited number of possibilities, so I suppose you might be able to guess." Perhaps he despaired that—and then wondered if—the number of tactical possibilities is infinite, so there would be no way of guessing. Or better, maybe he silently wondered by what method one could determine whether the number is finite.

Speaking about his adversarial advances in chess and other games, Nathan admitted one day to his preoccupation with aggressive thoughts: "Maybe people who think all the time about aggression should be locked up in jail?"

He seemed doubtful, so a few minutes later I said, "If people went to jail because of their angry thoughts, practically everybody would *be* in jail!"

As was his custom, he anticipated my gist before I could finish the sentence and nodded his head ardently.

It occurred to me that Nathan had approached problems by pondering them immaturely at first, then shifted rather easily to more mature concepts. In conversation, he would first talk in a way characteristic of a younger child: there's no way to guess another game's strategy; there's no difference between thought and action; thoughts as well as acts could land you in jail. He would become elated by the more mature inquiry or insight—he understood he could make reasonable guesses about others' chess tactics, and he realized there's a difference between thinking and doing.

But why must he retrace less mature thought levels as he posed important questions? Perhaps he didn't trust abstract thought, so he felt he must ritualistically begin the cognitive step-by-step process anew with every advanced problem. I've seen kids who are not autistic quickly, accurately, and silently calculate the answer to a difficult math problem, yet resort to laborious basic math processes to confirm their solution. Possibly, then, Nate tried to confirm his social understanding by going over more familiar ground. Perhaps logical thought existed for him in a mental hodgepodge from which he could glean no obvious sense. In addition to being overstimulated by sounds, sights, and touch, maybe he also felt inundated by his own mental activity. What's more, logical thought might have rested in a kind of vacuum disconnected from sensory experience until he talked with someone about it. If so, game-playing gave him more than an opportunity to engage in his adversarial fantasies; it also provided him, conveniently and explicitly, with a forum for testing his ideas and his ways of arriving at conclusions against other people's.

And what better topic than human combat to test the viability of abstract thought? Talking freely, for example, of trying to "trick" or "trap" me, he'd exclaim gleefully, "If you think I'm going to move this piece, you're wrong! I could be bluffing, you know!" Thus, he knew that I knew he might be bluffing, a thinking process typical of ordinary children his age. Such thoughts are said to be beyond autistic children, even those with the less debilitating Asperger's syndrome.

Nathan's way of thinking—"I know that you know what I know"—even applied to conversations about his brother, who continuously irked Nate. He once told me that his brother was enamored of "childish" books, referring to the contemporary Goose Bumps series, chapter books containing ghost stories. I remarked that, of course, he and his brother had different opinions of books.

At first Nate responded compliantly, "Yes, that's true." Yet he brushed my comment aside with a flick of his wrist, adding, "But I still think I shouldn't do it."

"Tease your brother about being childish?"

"Yes, I should just stop it."

Then he began to clasp his hands together and pull them apart in rapid-fire movements, reminiscent of the hand-flapping I'd observed in less adapted autists. The feelings aroused by talking about his pesky brother seemed too much for Nate as he started slapping the chair repeatedly and rhythmically, eventually pulling his sweat jacket down over his arms to restrain them from this activity.

Yet a few weeks later he remarked that I was correct that his brother had a different opinion, contrasting his brother's interest in the Goose Bumps books with his own interest in history and science texts. Once more he had to retrace his steps from less mature to more refined thought patterns. And, like many a child, Nathan needed to check his thoughts with someone, a need that reflected his insecurity about being "different."

Since he had lately coped so well with his insecure feelings, had made friends, and had become a willing student, Nathan and I began to discuss that our work together might be coming to a close. His favorite board games became the forum within which to express his feelings about discontinuation. He invented a new way to play chess, saying he feared there would be "animosities" between us from now on, ostensibly referring to the game, but also reminding me of a time when he thought we were adversaries, not just in the game but in life. He linked our impending final separation to our final game battles. I commented that maybe he was upset and worried about our work ending. He sloughed this off with a wave of his hand, so I thought either I had misstated his feelings or he resented having his thoughts interrupted. Then Nate began to map out the "animosities"—the game battles—and commented matter-of-factly, "Soon we will have our final battle."

This time I kept quiet, but I did think he was referring metaphorically to our final session. Nate interrupted my thoughts by saying, "Our commanders [two chess pieces he so dubbed] should survive the final battle."

Instantly, I guessed he was talking about the two of us; he meant that we would survive the separation despite our varied feelings about it. I started to talk to him about our meetings, saying I'd become quite fond of him, but he was on a roll and wanted to talk about our "time problem." By this he meant we might not have time to finish our "skirmishes" before the final battle. A few minutes later he spoke of "time pressures." So I said, "Yes, Nate, we do have a time problem, and we are under time pressures." With a knowing, direct look and a widening grin, he replied, "Yeah, we *do* have a time problem, don't *we*? I'll miss you, too."

Hearing this, I felt exhilarated and loving toward Nathan, grateful not only for his stunning progress but also for our relationship. I wanted to give him a big hug and tell him how much I hoped for his future, but I confined myself to the suggestion that we might write to each other or speak on the phone if he wished. As he left my office, I watched him jauntily approach his mother. Arm in arm, they made their way to their car together. "The hazards of being a therapist," I mused. "What an adorably great kid, and I probably will never see him again."

Why had Nate connected separation with animosity? Maybe because he'd experienced so many animosities while relating to people. What other reason besides ill will between us could explain our parting? Nate's take on therapy's end reminded me of so many other autists I'd known, who assumed that any rift in a friendship meant a return to that insular, friendless life they'd led before. Yet I think Nathan sensed how much our meetings meant to me and he quite literally wondered whether I, too, would survive our separation. He couldn't have been so attuned to me, I thought, without having himself formed an attachment. Hence the great care he took to assure that our commanders endured the final battle, although previously he would capture, then "slaughter" my chess pieces with great relish. He had to invent his own new game to control the outcome of our work together so that we wouldn't merely survive the final battle in a physical way; surviving too would be the affectionate bond that had developed between us. He hoped, as before, to "capture" my game pieces, but the two surviving commanders represented his wish to retain his sense of self in tandem with his sense of the other.

Autistic children age ten or older differ from younger autists. They have accustomed themselves to their remote condition. Older autistic youth are likely to reckon with a mere portion of the social world, especially if they have yet to receive assistance; they require even more patience and tolerance from us than do their younger peers. They require at least as much respectful nurturing and ingenuity to fathom the meaning of their behavior and language, to broaden their perspectives and to dislodge some of their more persistently maladaptive behaviors.

Yet because of their predilection to look inwardly during our conversations, James, Gregory, Nathan, and even Stacy were like many an ordinary child who uses psychotherapy meetings to get to know himself and to better his relationships with others. This is yet another way in which young autists are like other children. By definition, "introspection" means knowing or trying to know one's own mind. In therapy, knowing one's mind often results from explaining oneself to another person, usually with the expectation that this special person, the therapist, will not only be interested but will also perceive the mind as making sense. It hardly seems necessary to add that theory of mind thinking occurs in the therapeutic dialogue. Autists like James, Gregory, Nathan, and Stacy are aided in their theory of mind capacities as they converse with their therapist about their place in the social world. And yet Bernard Rimland, long an authority on autism, adamantly advises parents in one of his newsletters, "Refuse psychotherapy."[5] In doing so, he attributes to all psychotherapies those excesses he believes typical of failed psychoanalytic attempts to treat young autists and their families. Quite simply, such a recommendation deprives young autists of the help they would receive should the psychotherapy be geared to their particular needs.

Psychotherapy's end has uncommon meanings for young autists, as well as outcomes specific to their condition. Since their bond to others is often tenuous and they have to struggle valiantly to begin and maintain human relationships, the threat of separation from a trusted other looms larger for them than for other youth. What's more, their sense of themselves, including their mind's capacity to function sensibly and responsively, is often unsteady. It doesn't always occur to them that they might, in the future, form another, different attachment once they have lost what they have worked so hard to attain. Likewise, they are not always aware that their thoughts will be appreciated and understood by a trusted other. Therapeutic measures that aim to assure young autists that they have the ability to relate to and interest others would moderate their social pessimism.

CHAPTER SIX

Theory of Mind Problems

[T]here is no self left to reason with.
—DONNA WILLIAMS

Magic tricks are not nice.
—GREGORY

These two statements, one made by Donna Williams in her book *Like Color to the Blind* and the other by eleven-year-old Gregory as we talked together about magic tricks, represent very different yet thoughtful reactions to situations requiring theory of mind acuity. Childhood autist Donna Williams writes of one of the many mesmerizing experiences she continued to have as an adult: being captivated by a pink streetlight and momentarily forgetting her friend, another childhood autist, who had accompanied her to a restaurant. She explains the disjunction between losing herself in the "puzzle of [pink] color" and her friend's attempts to call her back to sociability—the double stimulation of color and person overwhelmed her. She notes the sensorial "buzz" around her and views her retreat into oblivion a "compulsion," telling us that in this hypnotic state there is no self left to reason with. It might appear that Williams is admitting to no theory of mind. Yet to cogitate about an inability to think requires introspection, a highly developed and sensitive theory of mind thought process.

Gregory had been playing with magic tricks in my office and found the directions to one of them difficult and complicated. It wasn't that he didn't understand the reality–appearance confusion inherent in most magic tricks. For example, a bottle appears to cling to a rope as it's turned upside down when, in reality, a tiny ball fit in between the rope and the bottle's opening holds the rope in place. Greg commented eagerly and quickly that he knew how this trick worked, peering into the bottle's opening to check whether the ball was lodged there. The problem was that he had difficulty executing the trick with ease—his fingers and thumbs seemed to get in each other's way—which provoked him to declare that magic tricks are not nice. When I inquired what was not nice about them, he blurted out, "Magicians think they are soooo smart!" For Greg the irritant was not just the requisite physical dexterity but also the invidious comparison he made between himself and an imagined magician who, being smarter, would excel where Greg had not.

Whether autists can ever mount a mental feedback loop is discussed in cognitive psychologist Uta Frith's 1989 book, *Autism: Explaining the Enigma.*[1] Researchers interested in theory of mind want to know: Can autists locate mental causes and effects? Can they orient themselves to their own starting points, to the mind's own activity, and by logical extension or by empathy, to the activity of another's mind?

Reflecting on her experience, Donna Williams expends every ounce of her being to explain it to others: how flooded by pinkness she became; how difficult it was to emerge from social nowhereness to rejoin her friend, a "someone" whose words seemed intrusive and whose face she searched to make her feelings care enough "to turn from oblivion and clutch awareness."[2] And how exquisitely attuned she also appears to be to the anguished ambivalent state of her own mind! She is certainly aware of a kind of mental block: the press of a visual stimulus, then the sound and sight of her friend seem to barricade her mind like an unyielding curtain. And Greg's comparison of himself to a magician, contrasting his less smart mind with the magician's smart one, indicates his reverberation to the mind of at least an imagined other. Williams's ability to tell personal stories and Greg's understanding of trickery and his ability to draw interpersonal comparisons suggest robust theory of mind capacities for both autists. Researchers have linked the ability to trick others and the ability to tell stories to the theory of mind capability.[3] If autists can tell or understand stories or understand deception, writes psychologist Carol Feldman, and "[i]f such matters are evidence for anyone's having a 'theory of mind,' then [they] have a theory of mind."[4]

Autists, even articulate ones, may perhaps be "human oddities," as a 1998 *New York Times* article proclaims, adding that in the "gallery" of human variation, these individuals, conspicuously different from you and me are, "after all, human."[5] Yet you'd hardly draw this conclusion, even condescendingly, in reading the somber scientific works that profess evidence for their lack of theory of mind. Nor would you appreciate that much of this evidence arises from what psychologists call "false belief" or similar tests, many of which set up hypothetical situations among fictional people, requiring young autists to answer key questions designed to reveal their theory of mind functions—or lack thereof. Rarely is any other type of conversation reported, not even the children's reactions to the tests themselves.

A 1995 *Newsweek* article depicted one of these false belief exams, the famous "Sally–Anne" test, and reported that young autists do not predict as others do where a fictional character, Sally, will look for a hidden marble.[6] Nor do they appear to imagine the difference between Sally's perception of an event and the hypothetical actual situation. Not realizing that Sally's mind and their own possess different information, autists unwittingly reveal that they have no theory of Sally's mind as different from theirs. So young autists generally lack a theory of mind.

Or do they? The cartoon story shows Anne slipping Sally's marble into her own box after Sally has left the room. Perhaps autists realize that, in taking Sally's marble out of her basket and putting it in her own box, Anne may be attempting to "trick" Sally. Perhaps, then, they *do* perceive the Sally–Anne tests to be a kind of trickery. If encouraged to express their opinion, they might say, as Gregory did, "These tricks are not nice." The false belief tests may make autists feel as if they are being deceived, just as Sally is deceived by Anne. But there's no way of knowing because we are not told what the autistic children actually said in response to the questions they were asked.

Donna Williams's personal account provides a different, more complex interpretation of the apparent thinking lack. She thinks she has no self to reason with when bombarded unexpectedly by multiple stimuli. From Williams's writing and from my own work with autists, I infer that there may be a link between their social withdrawal and an apparent theory of mind deficiency. Similarly, Catherine Lord wonders whether the theory of mind deficiency drives other social behavior or whether it's simply correlated with social development (or not related at all).[7] I believe the social withdrawal of autists—sometimes accompanied by an utter dismissal of social stimuli, sometimes by their single-minded absorption in nonhuman stimuli—leads them to act *as if* they have no sense of mind. In other words, their hypersensitivity to human and other stimuli invites them to withdraw and pressures them to ignore the mind's social workings. This would explain the fact that when autists emerge from their private worlds, they often display a robust introspective idea of their own minds and a perceptive reading of the minds of others. The impact of the pink streetlight on Donna Williams was so powerful that she had to ask herself not only who *she* was but also who her *friend* was—that is, she had to ask of herself the most basic interpersonal questions. The pinkness of the stimulus, she says, had by then turned from a "sensory tickle" into an inevitable agony. That a sensation can be reflected upon as both hypnotically pleasant and agonizing, and that it can blot out the use of one's social mind, attests to the versatile complexity of minds like Williams's rather than to the absence of theory of mind.

Interpreting other minds is fraught with hazards, for it remains just that, interpretation, not certainty. Ordinarily these risky evaluations of the way other people think rest upon their spontaneous behavior and language, not on structured interviews or test outcomes. Second-guessing the other—say, an adversary—surely arose early in human history and most certainly conferred a greater chance for survival. There is nothing like the triumph of life over death to reveal how close to the mark one's deception, intended to gain advantage over one's adversary, had been. Since the use of deception for survival is a common human trait, we need to observe autists closely to discern if they lack what the rest of us possess. Even more urgent is the need to describe the precise and spontaneous language they use to speak, for it is their use of language that manifests a theory of mind. If we find that the lack of theory of mind thesis does not regularly apply to articulate autists, we ought to consider that it may not apply to mute autists either. The idea that they lack a theory of mind is pressingly germane—dangerously so—to those who have no linguistic forum to counter it.

Another group of researchers notes the same behavioral patterns in autists as do those who studied responses to false belief tests but advance a different interpretation of the alleged theory of mind lack in young autists. Psychologist James Russell and colleagues assert that it's not so much that a young autist's mind misses a theory of itself as it is that he cannot always act upon what he knows. It is the executive function that is impaired—the autist's control over action generally. "[I]t is still possible," Russell contends, "that the difficulty children with autism have with executive tasks is executive in nature. *They may have a theory of mind on which they cannot act*" (italics mine).[8] The self-reflective function may be available to autists, but, Russell hypothesizes, the capacity to discharge the full range of that function may be impaired. The receptive theory of mind function—an implicit understanding that one has a mind and others do, too—may be quite adequate, but not its expressive counterpart—the ability to act upon what one understands.

Russell suggests the animus for—and the pitfalls of—theory of mind research applied to autistic children: "[T]he failure of mental understanding to develop normally is not in itself evidence that there is an innate theory of mind module in human beings. Autism is not an existence proof of such a module."[9] It is a logical flaw to infer a capacity in normal children from its absence in autistic children. You cannot prove the existence of an innate ability in one human group by showing its absence in another. As far as young autists are concerned, our resources would be better spent if we focused on the autist's actual use of mind in everyday social situations.

The Sally-Anne Test

Cognitive psychologist Uta Frith marshals evidence from false belief testing and interviews of autists to support her theses.[10] For one experiment she subjects three groups of children to the Sally–Anne testing: autists, mentally retarded, and normal ("normal" by IQ metrics?—Frith does not say). Both the normal and the mentally retarded children tend to answer as expected. When asked, "Where will Sally look for her marble?" they say she will look for it where she put it. They do not volunteer, nor do they divulge, that they know Sally could imagine that Anne will take Sally's marble out of her basket in her absence and put it in Anne's box. Autistic children are found wanting because most of them answer that Sally will look for her marble where it actually is. Perhaps they think Sally is as smart as they are!

Some of the young autists may have wished to tell the bald truth at the expense of showing the interviewer that they knew what she expected. After all, the marble *is* in Anne's box, not in Sally's basket. The Sally–Anne narrative is depicted in cartoonlike drawings, which is all the more reason the children may have replied to one story with another. So the autists may have wanted to tell *their* story, one quite different from that of the normal and the mentally retarded children.

To turn this inquiry on its head, why didn't the others reply with a story similar to that of the autists? Why didn't it occur to the normal children that Sally may have anticipated Anne's deception so that Sally would look for her marble where it actually was? Doesn't it call for some explanation when the normal and the mentally retarded groups respond the same way, though the two groups are highly discrepant in other ways?

Mentally retarded children may not have the perspicacity to attribute mental maneuvers either to Sally or Anne, and so they simply answer that Sally will look for her marble in the basket where she left it. The normal group, possibly acting in line with what they sensed they were supposed to say, may have attributed less to Sally's mentality than they did to the tester's. Perhaps they wanted to please her by showing that they knew what she expected—and that's the story they told. How can we know for sure whose "mind" these normal children were reading? We would know about the underlying interesting differences in the children's responses if only Frith had asked them why they replied as they did.

Suppose the young autists were more likely to focus on Sally's mentality, ascribing to her a wily artfulness that permits them to infer that Anne, believing the marble to be some sort of treasure, took it and hid it while Sally was out of the room. If so, these children revealed that they were aware of what often happens in real life—that children are often tempted to or actually do take precious items that belong to others. (The normal children might have revealed this, too, had they been less centered on pleasing the examiner.) If anything, the test outcomes for autists may show that they *do* understand mental states, including deception, since they may have focused on Anne's trickery. They even may have thought Sally would figure it out as they did. While trying to confirm one alleged aspect of autistic mentality—that autists do not appreciate mental states—Frith may have inadvertently disconfirmed a related aspect of her own thesis—namely, that they do not understand trickery. The meaning of Frith's test results are not at all clear, and close, expert observation of autistic behavior and the autists' own statements might set aright what is quite possibly a misinterpretation. Oliver Sacks writes about the theory of mind that it "is only one hypothesis among many; no theory, as yet, encompasses the whole range of phenomena to be seen in autism." He concludes, intriguingly, "The ultimate understanding of autism may demand both technical advances and *conceptual* ones beyond anything we can now even dream of" (italics mine).[11]

Interviewing Autists

Uta Frith does report her observations when interviewing or otherwise conversing with speaking autists whom she characterizes as smart. Frith's reports of her conversations with autistic people allow for alternative speculations about their theory of mind processes. We are told that seventeen-year-old Ruth reads at almost a normal adult level. Yet Frith sees this as an isolated mental feat with little connection to Ruth's communication skills or wishes. In fact, for Frith, Ruth's struggles are typical of the autistic dilemma: how can one live in a peopled world without communicating deeply—that is, acknowledging others as individuals in their own right?

"Ruth does not talk much spontaneously, but answers questions willingly," Frith continues. "She has a rather grating voice and emphasizes final consonants of words. Her diction is oddly wooden, with little modulation, but her grammar is faultless."[12] Such incongruities, true of many other autists, may be one reason scholars wonder whether paradoxical autistic behavior reflects giftedness in some areas while showing alarming deficiencies in others. But autistic behavior may be more of a piece than we think. The apparent inconsistencies may be elements of a behavioral pattern that, though differing from our own in some ways, has an overriding social logic, especially to autists themselves.

Interviewing Ruth, Frith begins by assuring her that she's been helpful and kind, to which Ruth answers a stereotypical "yes-suh," stressing the last *s*. Her responses seem most stilted when she is required to participate in the polite, socially expected chitchat (Donna Williams calls it "gabble") that autists are memorable for ignoring. I witnessed the same labored speech while observing an autistic first-grader who was expected to contribute to a discussion on Earth Day. My impression was that this boy wasn't ignoring social expectations, but was doing his best to meet them. When it was his turn to contribute to circle time and his teacher called him affectionately by name, he stood up earnestly and replied deferentially, "Yesss, Yesss, Melissa," hissing his *s*'s to make the point, I thought, that she *had* gotten his attention, and by God, he was going to do the right thing, because he liked his teacher so much. Also noteworthy was this boy's speaking alliteratively, either practicing or playing with the *s* sound in the word *yes* and in his teacher's name. I checked these speculations with the boy's teacher and his principal, both of whom confirmed my hunches. Could Ruth, too, have been playing with sounds when she said "yes-suh" to Uta Frith, possibly to distract herself from being questioned or maybe even to get Frith to lighten up?

To me autistic behavior does not appear predictably "stereotypical." Labored, perhaps, but not unremittingly stereotypical. So I was interested in the times when Ruth did *not* answer "yes-suh" to Frith's questions. Praising Ruth's reading ability, which she may have prided herself on, Frith asks, "Have you *always* been such a good reader?"

"Yes, I have," Ruth replies with apparent conviction.

Frith continues, "Now you live in that lovely flat, upstairs?"

"Yes-suh."

The return of the stereotypy may have been the result of Frith's value judgment ("lovely flat"), which preempted Ruth's opportunity to make this judgment herself. Or maybe it was that Frith quite knew where Ruth lived, making her question to Ruth either redundant or just more chitchat. After all, Ruth freely answered a question when it touched upon her reading ability.

Ruth is asked whether she does some cooking in her flat, a question which is met with a normal-sounding "Yes, I do." But she quickly evades Frith's attempt to elicit exactly what she cooks. Continuing to probe for the requested information, Frith seems to treat Ruth the way many misguided therapists do when they assume that an evasive patient is behaving defensively when she simply views the ongoing probes as off-topic. Frith presses on and finally gets Ruth to admit that she cooks fish fingers.

One would expect Uta Frith to be delighted to obtain an answer at long last. Yet she returns to Ruth's cooking.

"And you cook them yourself?"

Ruth, enigmatically, "Nearly."

Perhaps Frith did not believe Ruth. She may have thought Ruth was for some reason telling an untruth about cooking, or about cooking fish fingers, or about cooking by herself. From Frith's account, Ruth appears quite defensive. But how could she be so without some semblance of a theory of mind? If indeed Ruth was dissimulating, how could she do so without understanding Frith's intent?

The conversation continues in the same vein until Ruth ends it by saying, "Work time now." It's hard to miss that the entire exchange seemed a test of whether Ruth could converse candidly and normally. Since this was hardly a reciprocal heart-to-heart talk, a good case could be made that Ruth's truncated speech was at least in part a response to the way she was questioned. Couldn't Ruth have sensed that she was being evaluated implicitly, unlike the first-grader, who seemed sure that his teacher was really interested in what he had to say about Earth Day? Frith's parenthetical summary on Ruth only deepened the queasy feeling I got upon reading Frith's report. "The characteristically abrupt ending of a conversation with an autistic individual is well illustrated. Ruth did *not* mean to be rude," writes Frith, "but the break was over and it was time to go back to work. Normally such a fact would be wrapped up in the language of politeness." And concluding Ruth's story, "Ruth does not present any wrappings, instead she gives bare information."[13]

Normally an individual is not subjected to this kind of *sub rosa* interviewing. When we are overly concentrated on proving what an autist lacks—such as social wrappings or the ability to reflect sensibly—we miss what might be an autist's personal reaction to the questions themselves. Frith seems casually disinterested in how *she* appears to Ruth. Why should Ruth converse candidly when her interviewer does not?

True, Ruth did not easily furnish Frith with the requested information, nor did she seem consistently interested in the conversation. Even if she had sensed that Frith was not probing for interesting information *per se* but for something more suspect, like cognitive style or social ineptitude, she nevertheless did not protest as another individual being covertly evaluated might have. This doesn't show an absence of social logic. On the contrary, it reveals Ruth to be quite consistent when she is spoken to. She could divulge her thoughts when the questions put to her seemed genuine. Thus she answered as expected when asked if she'd always been a good reader. What distinguishes autists, then, from ordinary individuals, is their reluctance to protest clandestine evaluations directly and vigorously. An autist may have a theory about what's going on but is somehow reluctant or unable to act upon it.

• • •

Another interesting exchange occurs between Frith and a twelve-year-old autistic boy, Milton, a subject in some of Frith's reading experiments. Milton read fluently and once gave a particularly suitable answer when tested for comprehension. We are not told what the answer was. This time Frith does ask the boy how he knew the answer, and he replied unexpectedly, "By telepathy." Frith contrasts his response with some imagined responses other twelve-year-olds might give: "My teacher told me"; "It's obvious, isn't it?"[14] Nothing more is made of Milton's intriguing reference to telepathy.

The *Oxford English Dictionary* defines "telepathy" as "the communication of impressions of any kind from *one mind to another*, independently of the recognized channels of sense" (italics mine).[15] Communication by inference, maybe? Since telepathic communication doesn't occur through the senses, it amounts to a hypothetical cerebral event. It's immaterial whether telepathic events actually occur—although many autists have told me they believe they can read my mind. Of interest is Milton's apparent view that he somehow gains knowledge from another person's mind. His answer scarcely confirms the theory that autists have no sense of mind. To be sure, we would have to inquire further, by asking Milton what he meant by telepathy. At the very least, we ought to consider why he chose this of all words as he answered Frith's queries. Even if Milton were said to be merely repeating something he had heard someone say, he could have chosen to repeat just about any word. Why telepathy?

Theory of Mind in Autists

That autistic individuals may lack theory of mind attributes has created a significant stir among several respected psychologists, doubtless evoked by the kind of cognitive studies just described. Presumably, because the theory explains the mental and behavioral mysteries of autism parsimoniously, many researchers not directly involved in theory of mind investigations have jumped the bandwagon in a way that may lead the unwary consumer to believe that this is a thesis proved. Psychologist Robin Dunbar, for example, author of an otherwise fascinating book on the evolution of language, marks the "two key deficits" of autism: the inability to pass false belief tests and the inability to play. Young autists "will not . . . run through the motions of a dollie's tea party," Dunbar confidently predicts. Evidently imagining how an autistic youngster might think, Dunbar continues, "[D]ollies are not living organisms, so how could they possibly do things people do?"[16]

Suppose, for the moment, that autistic children don't engage in imaginary play; they don't set up tea parties for the reason specified by Dunbar. If it's because the young autist does not take to imagining an inanimate dolly behaving as a real child, we can at least grant that she knows the difference between real and pretend. So it's not for lack of understanding this difference that these children shun make-believe.

Yet many autists *do* make up pretend games with dollies and other toys, as Marcia did when feeding her doll pretend tea, as Stacy did with mops and brooms representing people, as James did with elaborate make-believe scenarios with Legos, and as Greg did when he created farms, zoos, and jungles for toy animals. And isn't it possible that some autists are otherwise inclined, perhaps bored by imaginary events like tea parties or Lego set-ups, and so prefer to deal with the reality of, say, a quasi-scientific exploration? Stacy's questions to me about natural phenomena (described in Chapter 4), in which she inventively *played* with *ideas*, are a case in point, as are the investigations of Paul McDonnell, autistic son of Jane Taylor McDonnell. Because he didn't understand the world, Paul's mother writes, he set out to measure it and quantify it. He collected a vast number of electric lightbulbs in order to correlate wattage with brightness. Paul himself, in the afterword to McDonnell's book *News from the Border*, recounts how he played at creating pools of water and building dams in order to see how much water a pool he had made could hold before the dam burst. Noteworthy is Paul's friendship with other boys with whom he carried out these explorations.[17] Also noteworthy is that these playful and exploratory behaviors of Paul's childhood may have led him, as an adult, to ponder human behavior at the gambling table. After noting that gambling can be hazardous for people like him, he concludes, "They [autistic people] can easily get angry at losing and get very compulsive, or just have the mistaken notion that they can start making a slot machine pay out a lot of money by putting lots of money into it."[18] Does no one behave this way in Las Vegas? Does this sound like an individual who has no sense of his own or others' minds?

Yet, Dunbar asserts about young autists, "[T]here is no way to get through to them the deep emotional bases of normal human relationships."[19] Getting to the bottom of human relationships was explicitly the aim of both Marcia and Stacy as they spun their make-believe dramas. Marcia's tea parties for her doll enabled her to better understand and question the goings-on between her and her mother when Marcia was younger. Stacy invented imaginary people, represented by a host of inanimate objects, particularly human-sized items like mops and brooms, so that she might express to those who took care of her how she felt about life and family before the Orthogenic School. In fact, all the autists I've known who could or would speak engaged in play at one time or another, much of it imaginative as well as exploratory. Young autists may not always play as freely as ordinary children—hardly surprising, since their entire behavioral repertoire seems less "free" than that of other children. But play they will, when they are not frantically overstimulated or frightened. Psychologist Howard Gardner's uncritical generalization that autists are "unable *ever* to engage in normal human intercourse" because they block out much that is going on around them, besides being inaccurate, also discourages those who would help these children (italics mine).[20] Such statements give a false impression of their predilections and predicaments.

Gardner's overstatement unhappily contravenes another of his observations in which he compassionately and accurately imagines the effects of five consistent experiences a day for children valued by their parents and for those rejected by them. He concludes, of course, that the valued children would feel even more encouraged by consistently positive experiences and the rejected children would flounder, even become malnourished. When someone says or silently believes that a young autist will never be able to engage in normal human interaction, the inherent pessimism in such an attitude rejects the child. Normally resilient children are able to struggle against such pessimism, but autistic children are not. Test outcomes do not give a complete picture of anyone, least of all those who, throughout history, have been exceedingly difficult to understand.

A somewhat different tack is taken by researcher Janet Astington, who begins her interesting book, *The Child's Discovery of the Mind*, by anchoring it in everyday mental ruminations and conversations about mental events. We tell each other, she writes, why a person behaved a certain way ("She wanted to get such and so . . .") or why a person felt a certain way ("She was sad because . . ."). And Astington cautions mind researchers to look to commonsense psychology "in order to discover the mind."[21]

Ordinary children about the age of four begin to sense that they have minds, that their thinking is located somewhere. Earlier they indicate an intuitive awareness of mind when, for example, they follow their mother's pointing arm to the object it refers to or when they themselves point to a toy expecting their mother's eyes to follow their directives (called "joint attention" by psychologists). These early harbingers of the reflective mind are often lacking in autistic babies, giving credence to their missing or inadequate theory of mind, the ostensible cause of their anomalous performance on false belief tests. Yet failure to point or to follow a parent's pointing arm could result from an inability or inhibition of the executive function. Maybe the baby wants to point or wants to follow his mother's signals but, for some reason, his wishes are not easily acted upon. It's not difficult to imagine the frustration ensuing from such a situation, feelings that could subsequently lead to the baby's impassive response. If the infant is unable to act or if his messages are emitted in undetectably low doses, he may give up trying for lack of a social response. Felicitously citing the disappointments suffered by parents of autistic children, psychologists Marian Sigman and Lisa Capps write, "[W]hen another person does not provide the response we seek and expect, or any response at all, it not only affects our perception of that person but how we experience ourselves."[22] In this potentially intimate but ultimately frustrating context, it is difficult to imagine parent and baby resonating productively to each other's minds.

In regard to autists, Astington drops her premise that commonsense psychology is important to understanding the concept *mind*. So influenced is she by the *mind* studies and the interpretation of their outcomes that she fails to ask commonsense questions of the outcomes for autists. One reasonable inquiry would be how young autistic children can be expected to demonstrate theory of mind capacities when the social context in which these abilities ordinarily manifest is so unpredictably shaky.

Following other researchers, Astington believes that young autists are incapable of "metarepresentation"—those ideas that are abstracted from the concrete material world. When a young child pretends a stuffed animal is a person, she is imagining that one thing, the toy, represents the other, a person. A second level of representation, metarepresentation, occurs when a young child becomes aware that he or she is pretending, is aware of the difference between pretense and reality. Astington doesn't consider alternative explanations to the researchers' assertion that autists don't differentiate real and pretend; they will, for example, say an object both *looks* real and *is* real; and they don't use the words "think" and "pretend." Yet an object can both look and be real. The apple I see in the distance looks real, and as I approach it I find that it is real. It is also possible that some autists deliberately avoid such words as "think" and "pretend."

Astington herself concedes that fully one-fourth of the autists tested may have a theory of mind. Yet this statement is embedded in a text that stresses how deficient autists are in the theory of mind respect and that they never, ever fully discover the mind. Given their often oppositional, diffident, and uncooperative attitudes, that one-fourth of autists tested actually display a theory of mind is a startling finding. It should be emblazoned on the page in capital letters.

Could it be that some words have connotations and implications that young autists wish to avoid? What would these be? How to reconcile James Russell's thesis that autists employ the executive function only with great difficulty with my hypothesis that they actively avoid certain words, people, and aspects of reality?

I think that when a young autist finds herself in a responsive environment, a benign setting in which her words, acts, thoughts, and feelings are attended to with care and interest—no easy task because of the autist's likely aloof or even antisocial attitude—she becomes able to act more expressively and deliberately. In fact, Marcia did initially avoid such words as "think" and "pretend," although Stacy did not. Marcia even evaded uttering words referring to classes of objects, as though she was bound to stick to the here and now, the immediately tangible. While she would ask for her favorite foods, "Want cookie," or favorite toys, "Want tiger," in addition to avoiding the personal pronoun "I," she would not talk about the cookie as a snack or the tiger as a stuffed animal. When I began sentences without finishing them, I had no idea where it would lead beyond hopefully increasing her linguistic fluency. I would begin with "Tigers are . . . ," to which Marcia would reply, "Tigers." Sometimes her reply seemed to indicate ownership, as when she answered, "Marcia," to "Tigers are . . ." It wasn't clear if she meant to say, "Tigers are Marcia's," since she avoided the possessive. My rejoinder, "Your tiger is a stuffed animal, and Marcia is a person," only made her angry, probably because she knew that. Finally I hit upon, "Marcia likes her tiger and all the rest of her . . . ," to which she answered, after a very long pause, "stuffed animals." During the pause, she may have been considering whether she *did* like all of her stuffed animals.

Pleased that she had identified a superordinate class, I went on to assess whether she would or could talk about "pretend," since she was, at the time, setting up dolly tea parties. Just as playactor Stacy had done, Marcia created a neologism by substituting for the word "pretend" the made-up word "be-tend," the "be" ostensibly referring to the verb "to be," and thus giving a certain reality to the concept "pretend." I thought the issue for both girls was that their pretend games felt so real; the word *be* seemed to confer a validity to their emotional reality.

I explained to both girls that while their pretend games were very real to them, the dolls nonetheless weren't real people, although the girls might express some of their real feelings by playing with the dolls. Soon both Marcia and Stacy began to speak of "pretend" (not "be-tend") when they were playing with their dolls and stuffed animals.

Yet, I got the feeling that Marcia, in particular, did not want to generalize. The difficulty she and other autists have generalizing may be that doing so implies a shared criterial list qualifying an object for class membership. Young autists wish to avoid the implied consensus, which distracts them from their private worlds. Perhaps the attraction of their own solitary world lies in the fact that they can control it and thus imagine acting more freely in it.

Storytelling and Theory of Mind

Psychologist Jerome Bruner sounds a note of caution when he writes of autism and theory of mind that "understanding other minds is par excellence an interpretive process."[23] I might add that it's interpretive whether the exegesis is commonsensical or academic. Bruner's writing is nothing if not provocative. He spills ideas onto the page seemingly effortlessly, enticing his readers to think more deeply about problems both meaningful and urgent. He identifies as a "presumption of relevance" the value of a parent finding importance in what a small child does. This presumption is critical, I think, to the work with young autists.

A presumption of relevance is linked by Bruner to the importance of narrative in human social life. He worries, though, that without their being able to engage in and value the human love of spinning stories, young autists, even gifted ones, would be limited to "wooden algorithms and formulas in order to comprehend what people have on their minds or simply have in mind."[24] Hence autists' "stiff and unnatural demeanor." Bruner's concern is the link between the putative lack of theory of mind thinking in autists and their apparent disinterest in or inability to grasp the essence of storytelling. For Bruner, narrative is "one of the principal sources of knowledge about the human world . . . particularly relating to human desires, intentions, beliefs, and conflicts."[25]

This is an ingenious linkage between two seemingly disparate phenomena, the mind concept and the storytelling ability. In order to produce good stories, one must have not only a sense of what would appeal to the other but an intuition of the value of the story itself to humankind. Both realizations require a healthy, active, and self-conscious use of the mind. According to Bruner and his colleague, Carol Feldman, the young child must have the desire to "rework life experiences into narratives, beginning at a very young age, say two to three years, when most normal young children seem driven to encode their lives in story talk."[26]

Perhaps parents try to foster theory of mind processes through storytelling and thereby make sense of the charming, silly little things their children do and say—surely a presumption of relevance. Since their parents believe them to be sensible and smart, ordinary children are encouraged to ask what it is that makes them that way. What's more, they are led not only to question themselves—and in this process to refine their theory of mind capacities—but also to question their parents. What makes *them* think the way they do? How do *they* arrive at their judgments? These questions are the stuff of stories little children like to listen to and share.

Young autists, according to this view, have a weak or actually absent drive to engage in "story talk." And it seems hardly necessary to stress that presumed relevance and its benefits are essential to helping them cope with autism. Perhaps encouraging them to tell stories—better yet, to tell *their* story—would refine their theory of mind sensibilities and acquaint them with an important way to share human knowledge.

Remarkably, both Greg and Wendy did tell stories. Greg spun narrative after narrative in my office as he dramatized conflicts between himself and his peers, and Wendy typed or printed stories about girls being friends with one another or about mothers and daughters sharing good times. It might have appeared that neither autist had a narrative sense because they didn't share their stories easily. When I'd comment on Greg's "stories" and say that most people enjoy telling and listening to them, Greg would object strenuously that his dramatizations *were* stories. Yet this didn't stop him from continuing to elaborate them or from writing a lengthy fictive account for a school assignment. Wendy sometimes refused to let others read her stories, but stories she wrote, charming tales of both real and imaginary people. So my experience diverges from that of Bruner and Feldman, who write that the storytelling deficit in autists "continues into later life, manifesting itself even in high-functioning autistics as a difficulty in telling a story and difficulty in encoding everyday experience in story so as to give them a form that enters readily into everyday conversation."[27] Neither Greg nor Wendy were inhibited in spinning narrative; they were, however, reluctant to admit to it and to share it.

Stacy's pretend games with brooms and mops often conformed to narrative form, particularly as she spoke first for the broom, then for the mop, in an imaginary dialogue that had a beginning, middle, and end. Her stories, which she shared eagerly with anyone who would listen, told of her family. Her offbeat, comical, yet sometimes garbled dramas appeared eminently pertinent to me as I worked with her to sort out her past so that she might live more comfortably with it. We talked about the people she knew, how they behaved toward her, and how she'd reacted to them. Speaking with Stacy, though, was not always easy, and I wondered whether I had understood her play or her words correctly. I often found myself asking her whether I *had* understood her, sometimes rephrasing what I heard her say with "do you mean?" added. In these everyday conversations, young Stacy soon began asking me the very same question. She'd rephrase my question, tacking on "do you mean?" So the point wasn't just whether what she said was relevant and intelligible to me, it was also whether what I said was relevant and intelligible to her. In effect, Stacy and I practiced our presumptions of relevance together.

In the face of research suggesting an autistic inability to behave as we expect, it is all the more important for those who work with autists to sift through these results carefully and critically. We must remember that the lived-with and worked-with child is often different from the tested and theorized child. This is a distinction not often acknowledged by those committed to testing and theorizing.

Robin Dunbar reports on autistic children, chimps, and normal five-

and six-year-olds who were subjected to a "mechanical version of a false belief test which aimed to meet the standards of the Sally–Ann [sic] test used on children."[28] Dunbar allows that chimps might find the tests boring. Yet he makes no such allowance for autists in comparing them to either the chimps or the normal children. The only explanation he considers for them is their presumed theory of mind deficit. Isn't it possible, though, that autists find the tests boring, too? Isn't it axiomatic that one must get the attention of the subject for findings such as these to be meaningful?

About chimps, Jerome Bruner writes of another study, "The more a chimpanzee is exposed to human treatment, treated *as if* he were human, the more likely he is to act in a human-like way."[29] True of autists as well as chimps. The more we treat autistic children as if they feel human feelings and as if they can conceptualize the mind, the more they tend to act accordingly. It is important to lure them toward a protected social world so they can then experience the benefits and even the joys of being part of the "people world," of being treated as if they are human, which, of course, they are. Doing otherwise only saves our own egos from the seemingly inexorable autistic rejection.

A theory of mind deficit in autists, called a "hypothesis" by neuroscience researcher Terence Deacon, seems to explain why autists don't seem to notice us—a fact we find disturbing. "[T]hey tend to live their adult lives as relative loners," writes Deacon, leading researchers to "focus on their apparent lack of a 'theory of mind'" as an explanation for their diffident behavior. About the "primary social cognition deficit" and the "impairment of a 'theory of mind' module" theses, Deacon continues, "These suggestions are at best premature."[30] And what of the social consequences for autists of these premature theories?

Theory of Mind Manifestations

Experts doubt that autists, suspected of having a theory of mind impairment, can use higher mental functions like deceiving, analogizing, symbolizing, narrating, and joking. Yet, as Jerome Bruner notes, Old World monkeys deliberately trick each other to gain a social or food advantage, unlike normal three-year-old humans who apparently lack a tricking capacity. In grappling with this counterintuitive observation, Bruner remarks that young children *do* try to trick each other, but in spontaneous play. So they display a capacity in spontaneous activity that they do not in structured test situations. The difference in outcomes between a young child understanding deception in spontaneous play, writes Bruner, and lacking it when tested is that the young child's *intention* is activated in spontaneous play, whereas it is not in question-answering situations, when the child is "receptive"— that is, compliant with the tester's agenda.[31] I am suggesting that young autists, like ordinary children, have the wherewithal, when it suits them, to deceive spontaneously and to understand the implications of deceit for human interaction. Witness playactor Stacy's intentional trickery as she smoothed over her tossing paint to the ceiling to make her misdeed palatable to me. She tried to convince me that her wild behavior was okay if she explained her reasons for it. Or "little professor" Jamie's trying to "fool" me into answering his questions a certain way by asking me to match his Lego characters with Lego vehicles by some criterion known only to him. He had been trying to prove me wrong no matter what I guessed, and he cleverly changed his mind on the basis of what I said. When I joked with him (saying, "I asked you second," after he said, "I asked you first"), he put his hands on his hips, giggling as he gave me a look. Or consider Greg's ability to pun while enacting a made-up story of "Big Beasts versus Little Beasts," dubbing the largest donkey "Donkey Ho Ti" (Don Quixote).

Even Marcia displayed a sense of humor at times. When she was sixteen—to be sure, a little late to begin joking—she and some of her companions were playing musical chairs. Always sensitive to melodic line, Marcia could anticipate the interruption of a melody more quickly than could her peers. Time and again, she would slowly and deliberately deadpan her way to a free chair as those who played with her gaped in amazement or burst into laughter. When autists act on their own behalf, they exhibit capacities that they do not reveal in question-answering situations when they are "receptive" just as ordinary children are.

Stacy was once so enamored of the trickster idea that she called one of her pretend people "Tricky." This character would routinely say the opposite of what she really meant in order to deceive other pretend people. I have already quoted Greg as remarking. "Magic tricks are not nice," an observation that continued to intrigue me. When he played with magic tricks in my office, I'd try to interest him in telling me more about these detestable tricks. He was rereading the directions and eventually got discouraged about his ability to complete the "rope-in-bottle" trick described earlier. When I suggested we try to execute the trick together, Greg became angry, blurting out that I was the "magician" he'd been angry at before! All along he'd been comparing himself to me. He was angry that I seemed better able to trick him than he me. Again, it wasn't lack of understanding that thwarted Greg; it was his inability to perform magic tricks with ease that frustrated him. Scientist and childhood autist Temple Grandin writes explicitly how she uses visualization and logic to "work out how people will react," adding pithily, "[A]nd I have always understood deception."[32] She says she understood it as a *child*.

For many autistic people, symbolizing and analogizing—in essence, creating with a mind that reverberates to social experience—are well within their reach. Temple Grandin clearly would qualify for a robust theory of mind group. She analogizes to human ethics what she has carefully observed about cattle. Her consummate interest in animals apparently transferred to people in a way very like my protégé, Gregory, who for a time preferred to talk about chimps and dogs rather than humans and who eventually compared the chimp mind and the dog mind directly to the human mind. Theorizing about herself and searching for moral parallels between the animal condition and the human condition, Grandin told Oliver Sacks, who went to visit her at work in Colorado, "I find a very high correlation between the way animals are treated and the handicapped. . . . Georgia is a snake-pit—they treat [handicapped people] worse than animals. . . . Capital-punishment states are the worst animal states and the worst for the handicapped." Says Sacks of Grandin, "All this makes Temple passionately angry, and passionately concerned for humane reform: she wants to reform the treatment of the handicapped, especially the autistic, as she wants to reform the treatment of cattle in the meat industry."[33]

The passionate advocate for reform can sometimes be poetic. Take Grandin's statement to Sacks that she has no unconscious. "There are no files in my memory that are repressed. You have files that are blocked. I have none so painful that they're blocked. There are no secrets, no locked doors—nothing is hidden."[34] Need I say that Temple Grandin compares one mind to another—hers to Sacks'? And she likens the unconscious to a hidden, locked-up dossier, the very metaphorical image that some doubt autists can produce. Grandin's denial of blocked files might raise Freudian eyebrows, but her symbolic rendering of the unconscious enriches the concept.

While comparing animal and human intelligence, Greg once declaimed that dogs must be trained to be vicious and that this trait is not found in their genes. He went on to compare the brains of dogs to those of chimps, declaring that the chimps are intermediately positioned for smartness between dogs and humans. He was quoting a book he'd read on animal intelligence. Then he said of chimps and humans, "Chimps are smart but they don't *know* they are smart; people *know* they are!" He referred, of course, to the difference in consciousness levels among chimps and humans. How "mind-blind" is this?

Perhaps those of us fascinated by the autistic phenomenon get carried away by our prized conjectures. This is equally true of the authors of experimental studies and of observational and clinical reports. Yet the results for autists are presented as definitive and have been promoted by scholars not directly involved in the research. One cardinal rule of scientific investigation is to consider alternative hypotheses and explanations—a good reason to search the literature on observational and clinical studies.

If data are gathered objectively, a laudable event, we can nevertheless fool ourselves into thinking we've discovered something "out there" that exists in just the manifestation we've isolated. If we believe it's really "there," just waiting for us to discover, we tend not to look for alternative hypotheses or explanations, and certainly not to ourselves for reasons or motives for the investigation. We fail to examine the meaning of the research questions themselves, including the personal nature of our premises. And these premises affect the subject just as the interview questions do. They can be an important source of variation in the outcomes. We fail, then, to examine fully the tools we use to investigate. To quote physicist Freeman Dyson, who asserts that scientific advances usually arise from new tools rather than new doctrine, "the best way to understand [science] is to understand the individual human beings who practice it."[35] In addition to appreciating scientific outcomes, we must understand in which ways scientists choose to use their tools or concepts.

We should remember that we choose to attend to only a portion of what's out there. These choices are influenced by our psyches whether the investigation is experimental or observational. In the last analysis, we are all accountable for our conjectures no matter how they are tested or supported. When it comes to being responsible for what we think, science has yet to take us off the hook. "Science flourishes best," continues Dyson, "when it uses freely all the tools at hand, unconstrained by preconceived notions of what science ought to be. Every time we introduce a new tool, it always leads to new and unexpected discoveries, because Nature's imagination is richer than ours."[36]

Perhaps the inclination to divest the autist of the concept *mind* arises from the accurate observation that many autists refuse to acknowledge the existence of others. For how could solitary individuals overcome their egocentric perspective if they never shared the results of their personal investigations with anyone? Yet there is no reason to assume that young, intelligent autists would not be subject to the same coming-to-know processes as other children. Were they to bounce ideas off others they would find this an ultimately liberating experience that guards against the lonely, solipsistic dead ends many autists suffer, dead ends that not only stunt relationships but also impair thinking. I believe their sensitivity to human stimuli causes them to withdraw from the social world—autistic infants may very well sense that other humans are often responsible for the dreaded changes in their lives. Having withdrawn, young autists are loathe to check their ideas against those of others. They become inhibited in their discovery of mind. It's unlikely that you will discover and rediscover mind if you don't routinely compare what's on your mind with what occupies another's.

Working with young autists and reading personal accounts by former childhood autists has suggested to me that even if their knowledge acquisition is limited in their solitary world, they may attempt to explain what's on their minds and may even become open to new ideas when treated appreciatively. In everyday social encounters they discover—or rediscover—mind. Inviting autists to participate in whatever way they wish "in *the* world," as Donna Williams would say, is essential to our communion with them.

"*The* world" admittedly is a place apart from the private havens autists create for themselves. If we wish to convince them that *our* world is worth experiencing, we would do well to heed Williams's advice as we extend our invitations. Writing of her sensitive tactility, she counsels, "In order to receive pleasure from physical touch, it ought always to have been initiated by me and I ought, at the very least, to have been given a choice," thus alluding to the formative access, beginning in infancy, that one person has to another. She continues about very small autistic children that they "would need to be challenged to learn that they *can* choose" (italics mine).[37] Choice and action are the important ideas that enable these children to join our world more congenially.

CHAPTER SEVEN

Self-Revelations

Just as infants must develop, so must our theories about what
they experience and who they are.
—DANIEL STERN

My summer dream moon whispers, child born.
Upon my heart a baby cried far away.
—WENDY

Psychiatrist Daniel Stern writes on the difficulties in capturing actual infant experience, difficulties so entrenched in every observation, in every
clinical encounter, and in every infant study that we must be continuously open to recasting our take on who human infants really are.[1] And
ten-year-old Wendy imagines the details of a child's birth, as though she
were her mother, recounting them. Her splendid empathy with a
mother—quite likely her own—whose child has just been born helped
Wendy perceive herself in relation to her mother. Wendy's poem tells us
that she knew she was "far away" even as an infant, and she thought her
mother sensed it as she held her crying baby upon her heart.[2]

"Much of modern psychology seeks to know about others," writes
Bruno Bettelheim, "too much of it, in my opinion, without an equal
commitment to knowing the self."[3] Yet contemporary psychology has
shown that it is virtually impossible for a person to know the self
without knowing the other.[4] Stated differently, we'd be hard-pressed
to imagine the infant self emerging in a social vacuum. As Stern describes so eloquently in *The Interpersonal World of the Infant*, the
process by which the mother becomes acquainted with her baby attunes the baby to her mother.

Perhaps this is why many autists appear selfless and why Donna Williams asserts she has no self to reason with: without an "equal commitment" to knowing the other as they come to know themselves, autists are under a formidable handicap to recognize *self*. Resonances to the self from the other are the very grist for the self mill, especially in infancy. As Stern has shown, the advent of the infant self and her precious attunement to her mother are but two aspects of the same phenomenon: an intimate nexus in which the salience of self and other continually oscillates in the infant's mind and experience.

And how early in life this begins! "Between the seventh and ninth month of life," writes Stern, "infants gradually come upon the momentous realization that inner subjective experiences, the 'subject matter' of the mind, are potentially shareable with someone else."[5] Note that Stern refers to an infant's *realization*: a mental experience of self and other that presages the refined theories of mind children develop throughout childhood.

As it acquaints itself with the social world, the rudimentary infant self becomes marvelously sensitized to a mother who typically echoes her baby's behavior with amazing precision and appeal. An everyday example is a nine-month-old girl who reaches excitedly for a toy, bursting out with an enthusiastic "Aaaah!" as she does so, glancing at her mother. "Her mother looks back," observes Stern, "scrunches up her shoulders and performs a terrific shimmy with her upper body, like a go-go dancer. The shimmy lasts only about as long as her daughter's 'aaaah!' but is equally excited, joyful, and intense."[6] In so aptly reverberating to her daughter, this mother attunes herself not just to her child's overt behavior but also to her child's feelings. Being emotionally sensitive to one's baby creates an intense intersubjective experience that shapes the child's sense of who she is, which she retains throughout her life as she forms intimate bonds.

But what of the autistic infant? Fortunately, we do have a few accounts from parents of young wayward children describing how the soon-to-be autist seemed normally attuned before the age of about one year. Catherine Maurice describes in *Let Me Hear Your Voice* how her daughter Anne-Marie, although "serious," also looked lovingly at her mother, wrapping her legs around her, which many babies will do when they want to be carried.[7] The emotional attunement often manifests physically; as any mother of a small child knows, mother and infant adjust to each other's bodies, sometimes simultaneously, often automatically, so that the baby can be hoisted on the mother's hip or propped against her shoulder in the baby's most familiar, comfortable position.

Similarly, Jane Taylor McDonnell in *News from the Border* depicts her autistic son, Paul, engaging in a version of the childhood patting game. Eleven-month-old Paul had learned to climb the stairs and would pat the floor when he reached the top. When his mother reciprocated by patting back, Paul would pat even more loudly and energetically.[8] Little Paul tuned himself in to his mother in response to her emotional sensitivity to him. And Beth Kephart's not quite two-year-old Jeremy, portrayed in her charming *A Slant Of Sun*, implicitly expects that his mother will respond with compassionate understanding when one day he confidently asserts, "Hats." She bundles him into the car and off they go in search of a hat store, finding the wished-for item in chartreuse. Green, his mother tells us, is Jeremy's favorite color. He insists on wearing his hat despite the sometimes unfriendly attention it brings him.[9] Through the small child's overt behavior we often learn how firmly established his sense of self is and how responsive he is to his mother's attempts to adjust herself to him.

It must be devastating to the parents of young autists, who have initially shown an intersubjective sense, who have been encouraged to tune in to the social world by their responsive mothers, when they suddenly or gradually leave the world of others for their solitary existence. Wendy's poignant couplet catches the pathos suffered by these parents. It reveals her empathy with a mother whose newly born infant cries so far away upon her mother's heart. A measure of agony suffered by these parents also can be gleaned from their disbelieving relief when a therapeutic intervention works—and literally returns the child to her parent.

When she saw that her withdrawal deepened despite the best family efforts to stem its tide, Catherine Maurice provided a special tutorial program for her little girl. Barely two years, she would fall to the floor in a heap or simply walk out of the room when her behavioral tutor or speech therapist tried to work with her. Only a year later, after she'd begun to stay at her table and comply with some small request, Anne-Marie looked for her mother and called for her, finding her in another room. Other normally childish behaviors returned as well. In the office with two doctors, who were, like her parents, basking in the glories of Anne-Marie's recovery, Maurice told herself not to cry. "But the tears welled up anyway, spilled over. I reached out for her, my lost baby come home, my lamb. 'Anne-Marie,' I whispered as I buried my face in her hair. Her arms came around my neck. 'Mommy.'"10

Emotional attunement had been reestablished and Anne Marie's sense of self became more apparent. With some prodding by and practice with those who took care of her, she began to refer to herself as "I" or "me," notes Maurice, in such sentences as, "Do this for me, Mommy, I can't do it," or "Mommy, hold me."11

Safety in Closeness

Much has been made of the autist's apparent lack of self and even more of her conspicuous distaste for interpersonal relating. Even in the most socially obtuse autist we can see the rudiments of a lost self and, many times, evidence of a robust self, albeit one that is often at odds with our expectations. I've already described Marcia's varied musical repertoire and how she communicated through singing. She had also developed a small vocabulary in early childhood, so it's possible that before the age of one she played such childhood games as pat-a-cake or peekaboo, only to relinquish them as she advanced ever more intractably into psychical oblivion. By the time I knew Marcia, she was long past the age at which affect attunement games between mother and child are typically played. She was not quite eleven when she was admitted to the Orthogenic School, and although she rarely said anything, I thought the proper way to make contact with her was through language—to get her to talk somehow—not playing games like peekaboo or pat-a-cake.

Marcia showed me how wrong I was when her first attempts to engage with others took the form of chase games. She would deliberately hide behind playground equipment waiting eagerly and expectantly to be found, whereupon she'd squeal with delight and scamper to the next hiding place. In this game of now-you-see-me, now-you-don't, Marcia seemed to express her need to alternately present and withdraw her person. She certainly was expressing her ambivalence about being with others.

Bettelheim was impressed by Marcia's attempts to relate by way of being chased. He also made much of Marcia's journey toward a sense of self as she emerged from a *me/not-me* confusion, which he believed had arisen from her refusal to use the toilet and her parents' subsequent use of enemas to force her to defecate. Since she did not voluntarily thrust from her body those soon-to-be *not-me* parts, she was prevented or she prevented herself, Bettelheim thought, from learning the fundamental distinction between self and nonself. As she began to use the toilet spontaneously, she perceived that what was once part of her was no longer her. She'd tell her bowel movements "goodbye" as she tortuously but finally pushed them from herself into the toilet. Bettelheim believed that Marcia's now more normal toileting behavior formed the basis for her renewed (perhaps, her new) willingness to discriminate herself from other people, not just from body contents or things. Along the labyrinthine path to acknowledging her special self, she developed what Bettelheim called the "communal you." Since she perceived me as a safe caretaker, she appeared to merge her identity with mine so as to make an eventual individuation safe.[12]

I never felt, though, that young autists wish to merge, neither Marcia nor those with whom I now talk in my office. Bettelheim's theorizing, influenced to a significant degree by then-current psychoanalytic theory, can now be amended by more recent studies, such as those conducted by Daniel Stern. He observes infants directly, sometimes from the age of two months. The "observed infant" studies, so important to a theory of human development, are also useful in understanding the deviations taken by autistic babies. I believe Bettelheim's view of the Marcia–Karen "symbiosis" misstated Marcia's psychological status and her actual development as we worked together.

Certainly young James did not wish to merge. True, he'd step on my toes in an attempt to sit close to me as he perambulated around the room, or he'd grab hold of my foot as though it were an object, or he'd fondle my necklace as though I were not a person with feelings and opinions. Yet I never felt that his behavior signaled a need to regain his sense of himself by intruding upon my psychical being. Rather, I surmised that when he felt isolated from me, he wished to test whether I was still there. Once, when he was not quite three, he became so absorbed in playing with some tiny dolls that he forgot my presence. He suddenly jerked around to look for me, wailing my name loudly, as though he'd been forsaken forever.

Little James sometimes anticipated that I'd react personally when he'd step on my toes or abruptly grab my necklace. As he cuddled up next to me on a large chair, he expected that I would adapt to his body by adjusting mine. I think James felt reassured by my adjustments to him: they meant not only that I was there with him, but that I also respected his needs. Even more important in its implications for the autistic experience was his need to remind himself of my existence when he felt remote.

Likewise, I didn't think Marcia was trying to merge her body with mine or blend her psyche with my own. To Bettelheim, though, it must have seemed as if Marcia did try to blend with me when she determinedly backed up to me and studiously grabbed both my arms to wrap around her middle. She'd expend small, incremental amounts of pressure on her waist by wrapping my arms around it ever more tightly. The pressure she exerted, as I talked with the other children in her dormitory group, became a sort of interpersonal body wrap, much the way that, earlier, her legs propped in front of her as she sat akimbo represented a partial barrier between her and the rest of the world.

Years later, I read Temple Grandin's description of her ingenious "squeeze machine," which "hugged" her precisely according to her specifications. This enabled me to understand more fully Marcia's aim in wrapping herself with my arms. Marcia, too, had devised a clever and risk-free method of seeking bodily contact. In fact Grandin attributes her improved ability to socialize in college to a "breakthrough"—the direct result, she says, of the gentle yet controlled sensations she received from her invention. She went so far as to say that the machine's gentle effects taught *her* how to be gentle. "I was learning how to feel," she concludes.[13]

So, too, was Marcia. She was experimenting by relating to me without talking. I can't say whether Marcia, as an adult, would have had the technical wherewithal to invent a device like Grandin's, though I'm sure she would have appreciated its effects. She did realize how to gain the physical comfort, akin to cuddling, that she wanted from others by applying pressure from their arms wrapped around her.

In addition to having me hug her this way, Marcia would, at age thirteen, jump into my arms and enjoy being carried about for as long as I could manage it. Maybe this was her way of testing an intersubjectivity between us. Would I carry her around indefinitely as a sign of my affection? Staffers who saw me and Marcia this way asked, "Doesn't it feel odd carrying a teenager around all day?" In my mind, Marcia had shrunk to the size of a three- or four-year-old. Imagining Marcia to be much younger permitted me to enjoy carrying her. I was ecstatic that the girl who had once grimly eschewed human contact now could not get enough of it.

The hugging and carrying seemed to reflect how we felt about each other. If she felt affectionate toward me and sensed that I was hopeful about her, she'd wrap my arms all the more securely around her. If she felt ambivalent about me or sensed I was impatient or irritated at having to stand with her for so long, her touch was more tenuous, more like a question mark. I never thought, though, that Marcia wanted to *be* me or that she believed she *was* me. But to comfort and protect herself, she surely wanted to command my actions when we were together.

Language Usage and a Sense of Self

Bettelheim thought that for language development to occur or recur, young autists would have to distinguish between *me* and *not-me*. Marcia, he wrote, had not made a firm enough distinction between herself and others, and would therefore backslide into the "communal you" when she felt endangered. The "communal you" supposedly arose from the young autist's attempt to merge as she called herself "you" rather than "I." Since autists like Marcia and Stacy called both themselves and the other "you," their language usage seems to support Bettelheim's contention that on the route to selfhood the autist must blend into the other.

Since Stacy's language usage was flourishing, especially as she enacted her "pretend" dramas, I felt easy responding to Stacy's pronominal substitutions directly. When she referred to herself as "you," saying, for example, "You don't want to go to dinner" because the dining room was crowded and noisy, I'd answer, "Oh yes I do, because I'm hungry." Since she was verbally fluent and many years younger than Marcia, Stacy emboldened me to take more risks. To responses like these, Stacy looked puzzled and often jabbed frantically at her chest with her forefinger as she repeated earnestly, "You do *not* want to go to dinner!" "I do so," I'd respond. Staring at me, she would finally exclaim, "Little Stacy does *not* want to go to dinner!"

I never argued with her use of her own name; referring to herself as Stacy seemed closer to the affirming "I" than calling herself "you." When she talked about Stacy, I talked about Karen: "Karen *does* want to go to dinner, and maybe you'd like to come with me and sit close by." At this, she would sometimes accompany me to the clamorous dining room, albeit full of nervous, angry trepidation lest some imagined disaster befall her. The disaster to Stacy was, of course, the general pandemonium and noisy chaos of the roomful of children, which seemed to her like a personal affront.

Stacy gradually began to call herself "I." As I continued to take literally her use of "you," even though I knew she meant otherwise, she would become ever more fervent in rephrasing her statements. One day she said, "You *don't* want to . . . I *mean* Stacy . . ." Then realizing she'd said "I" to clarify what she meant, she burst forth with, "I mean *I* don't want to go to dinner!" And soon she announced boisterously, "I *want* dinner," and bounding off her bed, she grabbed my hand and bolted for the dining room.

Things went more slowly and perplexedly with Marcia. She was at once a small child in the way she related to me and a physiologically maturing adolescent. I often thought that what Marcia most needed was to extricate herself from the tight communion we seemed to have formed together. One day I began to enumerate her special qualities as distinct from mine. I talked about her beautiful blond hair and her musical sensibilities, stressing how adept she was at singing on pitch and switching octaves effortlessly. Summarizing, I said, "You are you and I am me." To this she replied, "You is you *is me is me!*"[14] Because she found speaking to anyone, even to me, arduous and distasteful, Marcia may have tried to simplify her language by avoiding verb changes, by refusing to conjugate as she used the verb "to be." She seemed to resist linguistic changes just as she did other changes. At the time, I was thrown back to the theory that she wished to remain unseparate, and momentarily overlooking her stress on *"is me is me,"* I replied, "You wish you and I were the same, but that is not so." "That is right!" Marcia answered heatedly, as though I'd told her the absurdly obvious. Plainly she was responding to the last part of my sentence, "but that is not so."

Despite her awkward use of language, Marcia tried to express, by twice stressing *is me*, that it was quite apparent she was her own person. Theory momentarily overran my ability to observe that Marcia typically responded to partial sentences. Theory is likely to distort observation, particularly when a young autist speaks inarticulately. And when theorizing distorts our impression of what the autist has said, her linguistic expression is even more likely to remain clumsy or bizarre. This is because she must attend to two aspects simultaneously: she must both speak to us *and* correct our misunderstandings, when she'd rather not talk at all.

It was tempting for me to attribute a theoretically based meaning to Marcia's statement: the sentence "You is you *is me is me*" might represent the preverbal ideation the infant purportedly has of merging with mother. Moreover, to say or imply, as Bettelheim did, that Marcia's statement reveals a residue of a normally enmeshed ("symbiotic") situation with a mother figure contradicts his own assertion that a sense of self appears before the beginnings of language. If Bettelheim were correct, how could Marcia-merged-with-me attempt to articulate the special nature of our relationship?

The abbreviated language of autists ought to be taken for what it is. Their linguistic disfluency is the best verbal expression they can muster at the time. Attending to what is actually said rather than reading meaning into it is, likewise, the best and safest tactic for us. At least the child feels understood when we struggle to get at what she means rather than at what we mean. And Marcia meant that she knew she was herself, even though she didn't have the linguistic facility to express it adroitly.

Not long after Marcia tried to assert her personhood by saying the equivalent of "I am me" ("me is me"), she began talking, not unreasonably, of her possessions and spoke of "my Karen." At the same time, she also disclaimed this ownership by saying, "Your own Karen." She seemed to reassure me that as much as she wished to own me, to control me, in reality I owned myself. But erring once again, we thought that in saying "your own Karen," she had returned to the enmeshed stance. We thought she meant that I was *her* own when she said I was *my* own Karen. We failed to recognize the progress she'd made in her use of pronouns by using "your" to refer to me appropriately.[15]

Taking her words literally, though, conveys an entirely different and more auspicious meaning. Reassuring me that she knew I owned myself shows a subtle social sensitivity: the recognition that people might not wish to be owned by others, like an object. So Marcia tried to convince me, again in truncated language, that she wished to avoid offending me. And taking care not to insult another person is a far more sophisticated, and kind, social gesture than is the baldly stated material wish to possess the other.

Thanks to Daniel Stern's work, Bettelheim's *me* versus *not-me* theory can be refined. Like Bettelheim, Stern posits a self-and-other scenario as he researches infant passages from the earliest weeks through the first language months. But Stern's thesis is more complex and precisely honed. He argues that normal two-through-six-month-old infants have two self–other experiences: along with "self *with* other" is a sense of "self *versus* other" (italics mine).[16]

The self-*versus*-other idea (in tandem with self *with* other) could have helped me with Marcia decades ago. Quite possibly Marcia's sense of who she was became threatened, because she sensed that I believed she was confused about her identity. I missed the impact of my own behavior on her by failing to attend to the impact of my theorizing. I thought she might still be immersed in an autist-merged-with-caretaker modality and wished to remain connected to me in some special way.

Though she probably did not guess the intricacies of my psychologizing, Marcia surely knew that I had high hopes for her recovery, which may have left her no room to be her shy self when she most wanted and needed to be, especially when she had become fatigued by being with me or because I had been tactless. I saw her retreats into isolation as proof that I was not a good enough therapist, rather than as a suggestion that the then-current psychological theory on autism didn't apply. Nor did I see her temporary withdrawal from me as a sign that she could comfort herself without my help!

The World of Pretend

Stacy's fiercely felt experience of self and other was the reason she smashed to smithereens anything within reach when she sensed affection emanating from her caretakers. In her early days at the Orthogenic School she seemed overwhelmed by intimacy expressed one day by two cryptic statements. She told her "pretend people," "You love me too much; don't cut me," and shortly thereafter, "True happiness will kill you." By these statements she meant, I believe, that she'd be hurt by too much love and that "true happiness" hurts people. It was not clear to me then whether her use of "you" in the phrase "will kill you" was colloquial, or whether she had reversed pronouns and referred only to herself as "you."

Playactor Stacy seemed particularly afraid of an intense relationship, as though the very strength of it would dissolve her sense of being Stacy. The fear of a self's demise is not the same as the absence of a feeling for self. I think it is the lack of ready opportunities to experience the other that renders the autistic self fragile. While Marcia would withdraw when threatened by interpersonal energy, Stacy would force others to back off from her by behaving obstreperously. In trying to protect themselves from one aspect of relating—its intensity—autists often deprive themselves of its overall benefits.

Yet, it's not true that autists live an empty existence because they are sometimes asocial, as implied by the title of Bettelheim's book *The Empty Fortress*. Rather, their special sensitivity to human stimuli leads them to act as though others don't exist, to shun human company, or to destroy items others value as retaliation for our "happy" or other feelings about them. When Stacy perceived that others did withdraw from her as the result of her wild behavior, which motivated her to continue her attacks on others, she would calm herself, assured that they would keep their distance as she played alone, silently rolling beach balls around the perimeter of her living quarters or sorting her possessions into piles of like items. Sometimes she panicked, fearing that her outrageous outbursts meant she would not be taken care of. She would then propel herself into an autistic fury the likes of which I had never seen before.

Stacy tried to solve the dilemmas that emerged from interacting with others by inventing intricate pretend games revolving around a make-believe family with whom she could be safely and emotionally connected. She chattered constantly about her made-up family scenarios. Everyone was inventively represented by toy mops and brooms. She even identified herself as being a toddler's push toy that she had brought from home, calling it "Little Rolly," the name inspired by the wooden balls that rolled around in a cagelike structure when she pushed the toy. "Little Rolly" easily equated in her mind to "Little Stacy." These props were held upright, the brooms' bristles, the mops' shaggy tops, and the push toy's wooden cage representing heads, in much the way a young child's first drawing of the human body consists of a vertical line for the body and a circle on top for the head—"lollipop people" or "balloon people." The prominent theme in Stacy's compelling enactments was that Little Rolly's misdeeds, always incited by the brooms and mops, needed to be rigidly contained, relentlessly punished.

Five years later, when we were alone together, Stacy told me she felt she was an incorrigible little brat whose behavior needed to be controlled at every turn. Her sense of self had been bound to her experience of being "bad." Similarly, Gregory, whose experience of self will be described shortly, thought he was "evil" or "mean" when others didn't appreciate him or when he would reciprocate their rejection of him. Or, if not evil and mean, he concluded that he must be "crazy" or "psycho" when he compared himself to others or registered their dismay at some of his antics. It was the intensity of feeling—essentially aroused by his being different—that caused Greg's deflated sense of self. Though these children didn't fault themselves explicitly for being autistic, Stacy, Greg, and Marcia felt overwhelmed in the company of others because of their autistic vulnerabilities—overcome by the intensity of affection in Stacy's case, by peer rejection in Greg's case, and by misinterpretations of her abridged communications in Marcia's case.

Today you would not expect to see complexity in an autistic child's behavior—the current professional literature is so often unidimensional in its focus on autistic deficits and dysfunctions. The conflict between Stacy's private world and the social world expressed in her make-believe dramas came to mind as, years later, I read Donna Williams's account, in which she opposed "*the* world" to "*my* world." In Stacy's world, she was "bad" and her behavior "abonible" (abominable), while in *the* world her caretakers often found her appealing and fascinating, albeit at times menacing.[17] Stacy tried to resolve the conflict between *the* world and *her* world by rejecting the affectionate overtures of others as she smashed toys or other objects to bits the minute she sensed how they felt about her. "I'm trying to break your feelings," she once told me. Her imaginary personalities seemed to act as a buffer between her experience of self and her experience of the real world, much like Williams's two imaginary characters, "Willie" and "Carol," generated early in her childhood, who seemed not just to traffic with the real world but also to keep Williams's real (autistic) self contained and, I might add, intact. As painful as the "bad" self was for Stacy, she hung onto it for dear life, much as anyone would prefer a genuine self to something alien.

For Williams, Willie appeared first, as a set of green eyes peering terrifyingly out at her; his primary emotion was anger, which he expressed by stamping, spitting, and looking at people fiercely, just as Stacy and her Little Rolly would do. Introspectively, Williams notes that the name "Willie" probably derived from her last name.[18]

Carol, who came later, was everything Williams thought a person needed to be to get on in the world, much like Stacy's mops and brooms, who, although they incited Little Rolly to act up at every juncture, also hilariously mouthed platitudes about how one should behave in polite society. Mimicking the sweet-talking tone of a caretaker, Stacy would admonish the toy representing herself: "Don't go and *do* those things, honey. You *know* you're not s'posed to break people's legs off. Now, don't go sayin' you're gonna shoot people dead, honey. You *know* you're not s'posed to! Be a sweet and nice little girl, honey." Williams's Carol also tried to smooth things over.

Carol's qualities were based on a real girl, someone Williams met once while swinging upside down from her favorite tree in the park. While hanging from the tree, her face painted with makeup she had taken from her mother, young Donna was approached by Carol and invited to her house. Carol's mother evidently found Williams unacceptable as a playmate for her daughter, cleaned her up after giving her a drink, and bade Carol to return young Donna to the park. Williams was devastated. "I glared [at Carol]—betrayed. The world was throwing me out . . . I wanted to live in Carol's world, in Carol's house." Then, the disheartening story of Williams's withdrawal: "I watched the person who had been Carol wave goodbye and say words. For many years, I wondered if she was real, for nobody had, till then, so totally held me with 'the world.'" Donna Williams continues, revealing how, if she couldn't *have* Carol, she would *become* her. "This stranger, who I only ever met once, was to change my life. . . . Later I became Carol."[19]

Perhaps Stacy tried to become the personalities represented by the mops and the brooms who seemed, at times, to act like the household help who took care of her just before she came to the Orthogenic School. Had she felt rejected by her family, I asked myself, when the maids took over her care and so tried to *be* the people who saw to her needs? What advantage would this confer?

In her book Williams refers directly to the self that was Carol. "If Willie waged war with 'the world,' Carol assumed she was part of it. Not knowing what a role was, Carol thought she was a self." Likewise Stacy had no idea of "role." Still her acted-out adult personae might have made her *feel* as though she had a self. If so, Stacy's dramas as well as Williams's statements challenge the supposition that autists have no inner feelings of self and, therefore, have no desire for commerce with the social world. The Carol "self" may have equipped Williams with the idea of selfhood and its interesting psychological nuances. About becoming ever more Donna, Williams writes, "It took this cheery, living facade [that was Carol] more than twenty years to learn that to 'function' was not to 'experience' and that to 'appear' was not to 'be.'"[20] Similarly, when Stacy toyed with what it was like to be an imaginary someone or to be with imaginary others, she played with the essence of selfhood. Like many young children who imagine they are mothers when they play at the dollhouse, or that they are firemen when they play with trucks and blocks, Stacy took on social roles when she enacted her pretend dramas. By playing, children define more clearly who they wish to be (perhaps their parents) and who they really are (wishing to be *like* their parents). Stacy had earlier enacted her wish to be like the household help who took care of her. Later, she wished to be like her counselors or her teacher. Thus her attempt to be someone else brought her closer to an actual self concept.

Many "Little Rolly" dramas later, Stacy startled me by articulating her problem with selfhood most cogently. While taking a warm bath and splashing water gently over her body, I heard her say softly to herself, "You're *real*. You're *real* Stacy. You're *not* pretend." By then she had been accustomed to calling herself "I," but when she considered the idea that she was thoroughly real, she had to phrase it as though the thought were coming from the outside, from someone else. Most probably the conscious idea of *self* was still alien, and she believed that only another trusted person could confirm her self as actual. Or, more simply, maybe her use of "you" instead of "I" was her eager wish to hear me say emphatically, "Stacy, *you* are *real*."

Stacy's language usage, like a toddler's, proliferated with incredible ingenuity, originality, and variety in her early years at the Orthogenic School, most notably her increased ability to articulate to others what her self-with-other and self-versus-other experiences felt like. But Stacy was six and seven years old, not two or three, the age when this development typically occurs. Yet the fact that language and other typical childhood developments occur in young autistic children should act as an antidote to pessimistic views of the condition that imply "once mute, always mute" or "once isolated, always isolated." The prescription, then, should be to identify autism as early as possible, ideally before the age of one year, so that tutorial and therapeutic interventions may aid early childhood development.

. . .

Perhaps Stacy's most inventive imaginary figure was a deep-voiced "he" who called himself "Doubleyou." Doubleyou appeared during one of my vacations, and I conjectured that she had created him to comfort herself in my absence. I was taken aback by the fact that this character sounded and behaved more like Stacy's male teacher than me. People who work with young autists can hardly avoid the narcissistic fantasy that only they are important to these children. It is not uncommon to find oneself jealously guarding one's perceived significance to them. I had thought, much as Robert Coles describes, that Stacy was waiting for the right person—me and only me—to rescue her from her condition. Since her isolation, her wild behavior, and her inveterate rejection of me were such severe blows to my equanimity, I sought to protect myself and to keep my focus on helping her. This I did by scanning her behavior for any sign indicating my personal importance to her, forgetting for the moment that her attachments to others augured well for her future.

Yet I was immensely taken with the extraordinary appellation, Doubleyou—a pun which seemed to me to have deep unconscious meaning. It could have symbolized Stacy's need for a "dual-unity," much like Marcia's alleged need for the "communal you." Since Stacy had earlier referred to herself as "you" instead of "I," the doubled yous might have stood for herself and me merged together. Yet this interpretation, in addition to returning her to a preoedipal stage when, the theory goes, the infant or young child has not clearly separated herself from her mother, did not do justice to Stacy's relationship with her teacher or to her play ingenuities. These suggested that Stacy had advanced, not regressed, when she invented her new character. The way Stacy played with Doubleyou—he was a piece of folded typing paper held vertically—and the way she talked about him suggested that she had not visualized him the way I had, as Doubleyou, but rather as "W." She'd begun to read prior to W's appearance, flipping through her storybooks searching for all the "w's" she could find. As though to make her meaning perfectly clear, she began to write his name, W, on the paper oblong that represented him, on which she had also drawn two eyes, a nose, and a smirking mouth. When she talked about W, she often enunciated his name precisely, elongating the vowels so as to stress both words, *double* and *you* ("duuuhbuul . . . yooo").

I realized then that W must be a double! To make her meaning plain, Stacy called out his name twice, "W. W.," and began to spell it this way. She sometimes would add a last name, "Okwells," which might have represented her new wish to be "OK" and "well." The "double" in W's name thus referred to her pretend figure, and "you" was the pronoun she used to designate her teacher. In thinking of W as a double for her teacher, Stacy seemed to have one foot in her pretend world and the other in reality.

Unlike some of Stacy's other characters, W did not incite her to act up. Quite the contrary: he would reprimand her, but always in a warm, soft voice. You might say W symbolized a kind daddy and a benign conscience wrapped in one. As he stood propped upright on a table facing Stacy, W also taught her math. She once cut a circle into the paper, which had been folded over three times so that it had four sections. Then she unfolded it, stared at the four holes, and exclaimed snappily, "One times four equals four!"

Stacy's creation was a bridge not just from pretend to real but also from autism to normalcy. Just as she had earlier recognized herself as real ("You're *real* Stacy"), now she became a real student to her teacher. Simultaneously, she had an imagined relationship with W, who kept her company when she was not in class with her teacher and who helped her show off what she had learned from him. As if this weren't enough, W's soft reprimands kept Stacy's impulse to act up under control when I was not with her. Although he wasn't represented by a mop or a broom, W's three-dimensionality made him vivid, quite the way a paper doll calls to mind a real person. Because he was created by Stacy herself, not tied to manufactured props like mops and brooms, W functioned, more than any other make-believe persona, as a template through which experiences with others could be perceived and evaluated. Stacy's W persona was based on her dealings, not with a parent, but with her beloved male teacher; it not only permitted adaptive behavior that was multiply caused, but it also encouraged her to analogize across experiences. She became capable of generalizing from one safe situation to another. It is thus not surprising that Stacy would fantasize not just about her teacher, whom she knew well, but occasionally about my husband, whom she hardly knew at all. They both represented her wish for a good father. Stacy appeared to be following the expected developmental sequence as she made her way out of autism. Her social circle had become an important oedipal triad: herself, me, and her teacher.

It may seem counterintuitive to claim that the *fantasy* life of a child will lead her to become more aware of *reality*. Inventing an entire cast of characters to meet her needs after forcefully rejecting the offers of real people to do so would seem to augur poorly for her ever relinquishing the solitary autistic stance. Wouldn't such intensely imagined personalities, as those in Donna Williams's experience or in Stacy's life, lead them even farther from the real world? Not if the imaginings of a gifted childhood autist reveal the lifelong wish to straddle two worlds against unimaginable odds: "This is the story of two battles," Donna Williams tells us in a note to her first autobiography, "a battle to keep out 'the world' and a battle to join in."[21] The sheer force of her determination, which pervades page after page, appears to have brought Williams to terms with at least those aspects of *self* in our world that she fervently wished to acknowledge. Those of us who took care of Stacy respected her world of make-believe enough to join in whenever she would let us, which led her to expand the drama. Williams adds that the truce she makes with the world must be on her terms. But isn't the truce any one of us makes with the world on our terms? Stacy seemed to feel that her terms had been met when we talked to W whenever he talked to us. If her dramas were important to us, then *she* must be important to us. She must be important, period.

Pretend worlds, I believe, may bridge not just fantasy and reality but also nonverbal and linguistic experience. Make-believe, both private and shared, originates as the child struggles to take in tolerable aspects of the environment and to make them over to suit her purposes. In communicating to others what a silently imagined world means, she must adapt to a social context to make her meaning clear. Whether or not Williams identified her imaginary selves to others in her life, she surely attempted in her memoirs to share her experience and her private world with her readers. When Stacy welcomed her caretakers into her dramas, she conceded that worlds *can* be shared. This gave her the feeling that her pretend world *was* real. It was real because those Stacy lived with took it seriously. If her world was real, so too was she.

Self-Narratives

Twelve-year-old Gregory had relaxed his autistic vigil somewhat and was sufficiently attuned to me to share events of the week without prodding from his parents or prompting from me. He was no longer ostracized in school for "bad" or "crazy" behavior. His play in my office spanned a broader range of activity: he explored adult puzzles, brainteasers, the Soma cube (seven differently shaped blocks that can be joined to form a cube)—toys that required just the cognitive and manipulative skills he had found so difficult when psychometrically tested a little more than a year before. He talked with me about computer games and his new interest in playing basketball; no longer content to merely *classify* animals, he now produced a series of animal *stories*, one of which he called "Awesome Pets." As we approached the end of our second year of meeting together, he would regale me with the latest riddles or jokes buzzing around his classroom. Most important, in his second and third year of therapy, he began to explore what kind of person he was and why he reacted to situations and people the way he did. He also wondered why I reacted or behaved the way I did and, more than incidentally, began to ask, curiously, why the other children with whom I met acted as they did. For example, he noticed toys or items out of place or inferred that they had been used creatively and would perplexedly wonder "why some kid" had acted a certain way. I think it not unlikely that Greg had begun to hone his intersubjective skills consistently and even happily as he sought to understand himself in a social context. The more he defined himself as a special sort of nice person, the more he used his mind's capability for introspection in a way benefitting interpersonal relationships. Observing Gregory's progress, I began to theorize that refined theory of mind aspects are intimately intertwined with self-development. A nuanced intersubjectivity might link the two.

Our conversations about *self* began in earnest when Greg spontaneously shared with me a homework assignment in which he had been asked to write a piece of fiction. He told a story about a nonhuman primate, begun during one of his therapy appointments, remarking offhandedly that the primate behaved as he did. He produced altogether a twenty-page manuscript in which the animal became socialized as he wandered from territory to territory, searching for primate friends. Greg's narrative, which amazed and thrilled his teacher, related how the primate taught himself the proper etiquette in his search for companions. He was rejected repeatedly until he perfected his befriending skills. The story's denouement depicts him integrated into a hospitable social group in which his fellow animals are each delighted to be his friend. Greg seemed to say that, by making friends, the generic nonhuman primate became human.

In his imagined alliance with an animal character, Gregory explored what it takes to form friendships and how it might feel. He told the story of a creature like himself entering a social world. Maybe he chose to begin the story of himself making friends in a meeting with me because he sensed that psychotherapy consists of telling one's story to another person. Interestingly, he enlarged upon our work to meet his teacher's assignment: he showed his completed story not only to his teacher but also to his classmates and to me, revealing that he was prepared to make it public. This was a major step forward for a boy who'd been reclusive for much of his life and who'd been too shy to acknowledge even the kindest, most gentle overtures.

Not long after Greg completed his story, he rushed into my office and, on a piece of typing paper, printed in minuscule, neatly formed letters the words, "Who am I?" He walked away from these words, which explicitly referred to his identity. When I took his question seriously, he brushed it off with a flick of his hand. "Aww," he said bashfully, "I was only thinking up a game. Never mind."

I got to thinking of Greg's cogent statement of a few months back when he told me that though apes and humans are both intelligent, humans are different from apes in that they are *aware* of their intelligence. At that moment, he realized he had to that point attended selectively to ape qualities: they were vicious and mean and run by their "instincts," he had said. So when he compared himself more propitiously to apes—he was smart *and* aware, even social—his feelings about *self* evolved in such a way as to make him more attractive to others. And he knew it—otherwise he couldn't have written of the primate's social transformation.

These new developments resembled those I had experienced working with Stacy when her make-believe characters, having been taken seriously by her caretakers, adopted more intricate and refined personalities. Living out auspicious dramas helped Stacy expand her view of herself in a real world. Likewise, as I responded with interest to Greg's primate story and when I took seriously his question "Who am I?," he could gather his courage to ponder explicitly the nature of his personality. His original story and his question to me and of himself improved his self-esteem and strengthened his self-image as someone who is smart, self-aware, friendly, and good. In effect, he could spin more auspicious stories of himself much the way Stacy enacted more felicitous dramas of herself with the advent of W. In the past, Stacy had thought of herself as a "brat" and Greg had thought of himself as "evil" or "crazy." Now both children entered a community of thinkers as they created *personal* narrative, "one of the principle sources of knowledge about the human world," which became as significant to them as it is to ordinary people, in which stories tell us about "human desires, intentions, beliefs, and conflicts."[22]

Yet I wasn't altogether convinced I could conduct the usual business of psychotherapy with Greg. Even though I was reasonably sure he felt strong enough being himself to withstand a more active psychological approach on my part, I remained wary of interpreting his behavior in a way that might lead him to conclude I was trying to control his mind. Bad enough, he might have thought, that "they" are trying to control my behavior; now "they" are trying to control my mind! Because of previous conversations with Greg, when he spoke of "evil" imaginary characters, those mentally omnipotent characters who could read others' minds and control their ideas, I feared that anything remotely suggestive of psychological tactlessness would throw Greg off and very possibly jeopardize our whole relationship.

One day he came for his meeting with me announcing, mischievously, "Something funny happened in English today." Is this not a good topic sentence for a personal story? But he immediately got up from where he was sitting to complete a favorite puzzle, of a country schoolhouse, apparently diverting himself from what he had, just minutes before, intended to say. He seemed to have associated a schoolhouse puzzle to his earlier statement about English class. Yet I debated silently whether his behavior was a sign of neurological misfiring—perhaps his mind got easily distracted when he was aroused or had too many things to focus on simultaneously. He once admitted, giggling nervously, that he'd gotten "mixed up inside" playing with a friend's Nintendo because it required "paying attention" to too many directions at once. Or could it simply be a case of a child's ambivalence about disclosing risky information? I responded as mildly as I could, "Yes, something funny happened in English."

Stumbling over his words as he spoke in fits and starts, Greg finally sputtered that in English class they played a story game in which one student was to begin by writing a few sentences. The students, Greg explained, were supposed to contribute sentences that were related in some way to the story's beginning. "One kid started writing about a little boy whose parents were getting divorced," Greg said, now laughing boisterously, "and I said that the little boy met up with a giant evil caterpillar." Greg stopped himself in his tracks and added, matter-of-factly, "The other kids knew I had written the part about the caterpillar because they saw me laughing." Since his contribution bore no obvious relationship to the story's beginning, Greg didn't accommodate, as instructed, to the story line and to the mind of the first storyteller. But he did acknowledge *mind* and how minds *work*. He acknowledged that the students could figure out his contribution by how he behaved. And, perhaps for reasons of humor, he did not wish to conform to the story's beginning; perhaps he hoped his classmates would laugh as he did about the sudden interpolation of a giant, evil caterpillar in the story of an innocent small boy.

As he saw that I had no conspicuously disapproving reaction to yet another weird fantasy, Greg soon set up another play scenario. In it, one of the superheroes was first to guard, then capture, a treasure that Greg nestled carefully in a wooden doll that comes apart at the middle, the largest of a Russian doll series. He specified that the treasure, a brightly colored marble, had been hidden in the "mother" doll; this tempted me to comment about a more promising fantasy, more promising because it quite obviously reckoned with a typical psychotherapeutic theme. Children sometimes feel their mother's power most poignantly when she whimsically declines to share her "treasures" with them. In expressing this, Greg was no different from any other child or adult in therapy who comes to terms with an archaic feeling of helplessness in the presence of an apparently arbitrary mother. Indeed, it was to Greg's credit that he brought forth this fantasy in therapy; it showed how normal he could be in identifying a core problem in relating to a parent. His fantasy was not evidence of having been raised by a "refrigerator mother"—quite the contrary. His conscientious, kindhearted, and reliable mother provided him with just the care he needed to invent such a fantasy. As a mother she was, in psychoanalyst Donald Winnicott's terms, "good enough."

Greg continued his enactment by having his superhero fail in his mission to get the "treasure" from the mother doll as he positioned an "evil" toy cat in the superhero's way. Greg seemed to fashion his fantasies to elicit my approval. I believed he knew just how interested I would be in his imagined attempts to procure a treasure from the mother doll and in his failed attempts to do so. Possibly, he felt a loyalty conflict: he was enough attuned to me to wonder whether his mother would resent our relationship or contrarily, whether I would resent his attachment to her. He acted out a compromise by narrating how important his mother's treasures were to him at the same time that he declined, for the moment, to enjoy them.

I decided not to comment about my speculations. Since an accurate statement resonates precisely and intensely with the listener, even a listener with an autistic condition, Greg might conclude that I wished to take over his mind entirely, in which case he would have good reason not to relate to me. The communication breakdown between autists and us may lie not in their simpatico understanding of our intent, but rather in what they make of this understanding—the motives they impute to us.

Continuing with his drama, which had the superhero doll finally capturing the desired treasure, Greg spun around to face me, exclaiming of the doll, "He turned evil." I still felt hopeful about Greg even as his toy hero "turned evil," and so I could inquire with some equanimity, "What caused him to change his mind?" With an equanimity matching mine, Gregory immediately replied, "Capturing that valuable jewel made him want all the power for himself."

Cogitating about Greg's alliance of himself with the "evil" superhero doll—evil because the doll had captured and hoarded the "mother" doll's treasure, I thought he meant that the superhero doll's actions were evil because he didn't share his treasure with anyone. Greg seemed to turn inward the import of the treasure symbol. If so, then Greg felt he was evil because he was autistic—because of his autistic tendency to barricade not just his possessions but also himself from others. Not sharing toy treasures may have stood for not sharing anything at all, which had for years been characteristic of his autistic stance. In fact, his parents had remonstrated him for not sharing his possessions, especially the ones his mother had given him, and for not sharing what happened in school.

Besides this, Greg may have meant to say of his autistic condition that he had all along wished to turn inward his mother's treasures—her power and, most of all, her nurturing. If so, here was a startling implication of Greg's self-narrative. It meant he was treatable in psychotherapy. He could trace to its roots his difficulties with people, including his mother, which were embodied in his belief that the sole use of a mother's significance, her caring and her power, is to bury it deep within a private fortress.

. . .

I watched silently as Gregory busied himself arranging some small toy dogs on my office rug, which he called a "pride of jackals." I was still occupied by Greg's narrative, which revealed how attuned to the psychotherapeutic process he'd become. Greg interrupted my thoughts to announce that one of the jackals had become injured and had signaled for help. I refocused as Greg, apparently aimlessly, drew deep lines in the rug's pile, uttering not a word. I suddenly realized that the toy jackal in Greg's hand was spelling the name "jackal." Possibly the injured jackal was signaling for my help by writing his name. When I said as much to Greg, he disclaimed, "Yeah, but he doesn't really know what he's writing. He's just writing lines." Not content to let him turn inward the significance of his interaction with me—he'd denied my meaning without clarifying his—I responded, "For someone who doesn't know what he's writing, he's spelling 'jackal' perfectly." Yet Greg paid no heed until I said of the jackal, "He wrote who he was!" At this, Greg's eyes lit up. He looked straight at me and called out enthusiastically, "Yes!"

He wrote who he was. Why had this particular sentence caught Greg's full attention? Perhaps my ongoing focus on his identity (I took seriously his written note, "Who am I?") was met by his drama of the jackal's self. From previous conversations I'd learned that taxonomic schemes were important to Greg as markers of one's identity. Rather than analyze Greg's feelings for his mother (as his superhero doll tried to get at the mother doll's treasure), I chose to concentrate on Greg's need in therapy to define *himself.* Apparently my persistent focus on Greg's own self prompted him, by way of the jackal, to signal for help. Maybe he didn't completely bury the notion of a nurturing other, since he shared with me his need for help. He continued to confide in me, risking that his ideas might be influenced or even altered by my responses to them. His private fortress had become accessible.

Exploring Greg's relationship with his mother seemed unduly perilous. If I had intimated that perhaps he felt his mother was withholding
something from him, Greg might have questioned his relatedness to
her, which he very much needed when he became ready to reach out
to others. I feared that if he concluded she wasn't the equivalent of a
good enough mother, he would then decide he couldn't relate to anyone. At some point in Greg's life he might benefit from evaluating his
mother–son relationship, but what he most needed now, in our delicate give-and-take, was to practice being himself.

Greg's situation reveals that autistic selves are not impoverished, nor
do they lack potential for growth. Rather, autists are accustomed to
their solitary selves. They are not familiar with a self in concert with another self. This is why one especially intense interpersonal setting—the
therapy hour—must seek to strengthen the autistic self in the heavy
presence of the other.

I said earlier that one way *self* and *mind* are linked is through the
child's intersubjective reactions. The infant realizes that his parent has
a self as he does. He later comes to conceptualize that others have
minds. The first realization is nonverbal and intuitive; the second can
be articulated and theorized. The infant reveals, by pointing to a distant, desired object, that she knows that her mother has a mindful
self. In later childhood, she tries to influence her mother's mind by all
sorts of devious maneuvers in an effort to have her childish way.

Was typically solitary Greg trying to convince me that his mind
wasn't working when he said of the jackal, "He doesn't really know
what he's writing"? Why would Greg try to influence me this way?
Most probably to protect his solitary self, to avoid being overwhelmed
by intersubjectivity and interpersonal relatedness. When I spoke to him
literally, saying that the jackal wrote who he was, Greg felt inspired
and sustained in his efforts to express a self who asked for help. For

once, he did not react as though I was invading his cherished, personal turf.

Though the dialogues Greg and I were having made more sense to me than ever before, and he evidently made sense to his peers for he now spoke of times spent with other boys—his remarks remained somewhat indirect and open to misunderstanding unless I sought to clarify with him what he meant. Greg now did not want to appear critical of others, despite his previous name-calling and provocative behavior. If he was unhappy about the way I treated plant life, for example, he did not say, as another child might, "Why did you prune back those trees?" Instead, he impassively inquired in a low moan, "Why are those trees without leaves?" Or, when he was upset with me because he caught my attention wandering as he related a fantastical story of a horse who used his tail as a paintbrush, he complained to me indirectly. Rather than say something like "Why don't you listen to me?," he asserted tensely, "I *said*, horses are painters!" His statements had the desired result, though. I did explain why the trees were pruned, and I apologized for not attending to his story. Only his style of communication remained reminiscent of autism; its intent and effect were ordinary.

It is sufficient for a young autist to overcome autism in some but not all ways. Sufficient, that is, if questioning the limits of his condition permits him to experience greater satisfaction being himself and being with others.

Greg continued to introspect about his problems, which eased his conflicts with peers and helped him open up more easily to his teachers. I noticed that his interest in animals had gradually shifted from the extinct dinosaurs to extinction in general. He focused especially on endangered species, explaining that if they weren't adequately protected they would vanish. I silently wondered if he referred metaphorically to himself and his condition. Would he survive if he weren't protected? Greg was determined to describe the large collection of volumes on endangered species that he'd amassed from bookstores and libraries.

He once brought a book on extinct animals to his therapy appointment. As I was perusing the title page, he instructed me not to read about the author. When he noted my surprise, he moaned dourly, "The author himself has become extinct." Greg had analogized species extinction to a person dying, yet he would not discuss the topic further. Perhaps he was anxious about a specific human death.

Greg was now almost fourteen. As the school year drew to a close, he and I began to discuss that we would soon end our work together. He'd achieved well in school and had made two friends. He was sharing more of himself at home, talking to his mother about his feelings and discussing science with his father. When his mother asked whether he would like to continue coming to therapy, he replied with more assurance than any of us expected, "I'll be okay without going."

As our last appointment drew near, Gregory again spoke of endangered species, confiding. "I think sometimes about extinct animals coming back. What I really like to do is make up stories about weird animals. I think I do it because many animals they thought were extinct have been sighted again. They came back."

"Are you saying that the animals people thought were extinct were just not sighted all those years?"

"Yeah, maybe, but three generations is a long time."

Struck by Greg's hypothesizing, I mused about what he'd just said. Had these "extinct" animals not been sighted for three generations, or could they have regenerated themselves in a kind of science-fiction scenario? He seemed drawn to the whimsical idea that environmental conditions might be just right somewhere for animals of the distant past to reemerge. Greg may have meant to say that, though his interest in scientific topics was satisfying, he was also preoccupied by his fantasies, a world of ideas that had held him protectively captivated for as long as he could remember.

It finally occurred to me that he may have broadened the extinction idea to include both classes of animals and psychological processes. He had previously likened human death to species extinction. Now he may have referred, metaphorically, to our relationship's end when he spoke about extinct animals being sighted or returning to the planet. Could he wonder whether it would be okay for him to return to therapy, again to be "sighted" by me?

I said that many people are interested in science and in other imaginative pursuits, like storytelling. Greg assented with a soft, "Yes, I know."

Then I suggested a connection between our impending separation and an extinction. "Maybe when we have our last appointment, it will seem like an extinction of something."

Greg shook his head and exclaimed ardently, "This is just like the time you made that joke about mother ships!"

He referred to a recent conversation in which he told me about a TV show on the function of mother ships in the fleet. He had repeated "mother" many times.

"Hmmm . . . mother ships," I had mused. "No father ships, huh?"

Annoyed, Greg had explained the reasons for calling a ship a mother. "It's because that's where the supplies are." He'd responded just like any youngster his age who wishes to be taken seriously and appreciated for the knowledge he has acquired, not brought up short by a remark that seems to discount his agenda, purporting to turn him toward a deeper understanding of his statements. Eyeing me knowingly, he had retorted, "Father ships? They don't exist. Anyway, they wouldn't be the same [as the mother ships]."

As he and I remembered this exchange, I said, "Yes, it is quite like that joke. I thought you might have been talking about our last visit. Of course, you could come back to see me again if you wish."

"Yes," Greg answered agreeably. "But that's not what I meant." Greg and I had come to understand one another despite our dissimilar orientations and the individual ways in which we used language. As before, he was content with his perspective. Now he could reckon more easily with mine.

Self-Awareness and Intimacy

By the time Wendy came to see me, I'd worked with quite a few children with Asperger's syndrome in weekly psychotherapy. In contrast to those with classical autism, children with Asperger's syndrome struck me as struggling more overtly than the others over *self*, if for no other reason than that they were generally more adapted to the social world. The autistic youth with whom I'd lived years before needed assistance with everyday living, not just with problems of self-awareness; many had sleeping, eating, and toileting problems, antisocial behaviors, learning problems, and attentional difficulties. The Asperger's syndrome youngsters with whom I worked in psychotherapy meetings had, by and large, adjusted well enough to home and school to forestall residential treatment. These autists reacted to the circumscribed therapy hour by bringing their feelings and fears about being autistic. They were similar to many nonautistic children who perceive psychotherapy as helping them with who they are and who they are becoming.

Wendy, who had been described by her parents and teachers as strange, given to prolonged tortuous angry outbursts and long bouts of social isolation, was determined from the beginning to work on her feelings about *self* in relation to me, the therapeutic other. Especially skilled in language usage and the arts, Wendy soon revealed that her interpersonal struggle was that of an intensely felt approach-avoidance conflict. She could readily escape others at home by going into another room. Although she would disappear in my office behind a screen that hid some shelves for toys and a sink with a mirror over it, the fact that she knew she must deal with me within the confines of my office, if she at all chose to do so, exacerbated her ambivalence about being in a give-and-take situation with another, potentially important person. Wendy would stop and start our relationship many times in mere minutes. I felt that her start–stop expressions of interest in me reflected her awareness of herself as peculiar. Would I recognize that she was in many ways unlike other children?

Of particular interest was the way Wendy used her eyes to signal the acute conflict she felt in being with me. She would look directly at me for an instant, then her eyes would wander casually about my office. Or she'd strenuously avert her head on some pretext, pretending to gaze at a toy, her feet, or the furniture. Sometimes her eyes seemed covered by a thin film. When she did stare at me for several seconds, I got the uneasy feeling that she wasn't really seeing me.

Wendy tried assiduously to mask her strange behavior. She attempted to blend asociability into a more pleasing, acceptable demeanor. She'd laugh congenially, if awkwardly, if she thought I was being politely social, or she'd flutter her eyelids to appear charming.

I soon began to wonder how this curious combination arises. How do autists like Wendy develop two modes of relating—one interactive, the other avoidant—which seem to exist side by side without ever becoming integrated? Does the forced social self represent an awareness of others' expectations only? Or is it a kind of playing with being affable, efforts that eventually blossom into genuinely felt social overtures? I puzzled over these thoughts as Wendy smiled graciously at something I had said but soon behaved as though she were smiling only to herself, or when she would politely invite me to join her at the dollhouse, only to cover her face completely with her hair, which appeared to enclose her face and thoughts within some inner, private and invisibly bounded space. She would sing lovingly to herself about a dollhouse doll, repeating endlessly the singsongy phrase, "Just like me."

Wendy's seemed a deliberately egocentric attitude. I say "deliberate" because, at other times, she showed that she quite knew that others have a perspective. For example, when playing the board game "Hangman," she became embarrassed when she realized that she'd spelled a word to be read from her perspective, not mine, and would hurriedly reverse the letters so that I could more easily read her word. It seemed to me that when she ignored my viewpoint—or that I had one—it was intentional.

Her mother accompanied her to her first appointment. Initially Wendy was friendly, yet talked in a loud, stagy voice, apparently trying on another's personality to measure its effect. She showed tactile sensitivity when complaining irritably about her wrinkled socks, yet she was drawn to other tactile experiences, expressing pleasure in rubbing her fingers against the terrycloth of a little doll's shirt. Alone with me during her second visit, Wendy did not relate to me at all. She said absolutely nothing for the whole hour and played by herself. On leaving, much to my surprise, she suddenly turned around to wave goodbye with a genuine smile. I guessed that I'd passed the silence test.

Wendy would try to arrange my office so as to reduce the stimulation emanating from the lure of toys and games. Though she was drawn to the dollhouse, she nonetheless began frantically to eliminate various items that didn't suit her. My attempts to unearth her reasons for doing so met with studied withdrawal. The silence hung around me like an unwanted guest. Finally, she turned slightly toward me, saying, "I'm rearranging everything."

"It's very crowded in that dollhouse, isn't it?"

"Yes!" she exclaimed with a relieved sigh.

It then occurred to me that Wendy had identified with the dollhouse girl, who was literally living in chaos. By creating a new environment for the doll, she tried to show me how she would like things to be arranged for her. From then on I saw to it that my office was tidy.

Wendy seemed to experiment with how much she could impact the empty space around her. It might not have seemed "empty" to her, since she imbued the air with such personal qualities as form and substance and the ability to answer back when she talked to it. Like James, who would slice menacing imaginary cartoon characters with his flinging arms, Wendy would thrust her arms as though punching or pushing the air; not only was she exercising her body, but she was also commanding the expanse around it. Similarly, Gregory tried to exert control over the space in my office by binding the area in which I sat as he paced around and around my chair, lecturing me on dinosaurs or animal taxonomy.

The more Wendy talked with me, the more mechanisms she produced to withdraw when her feelings became intense or when I misunderstood her. If I happened to be standing near her and she wished to avoid my questioning gaze, she would roll her eyes back into her head. I tried that myself with an object that loomed over me and found that while you can see the general outline of the thing, and so might feel confident about its whereabouts, you direct your vision away from that portion you wish to miss—in Wendy's case, the face.

Wendy would sometimes warn me of her struggle being with me and her wariness in getting too close. She once typed a short, pointed note, laid ceremoniously before me: "wach out" (watch out). Immediately after inviting me to join her in some activity, she would flip her fingers rapidly or incessantly repeat the same phrase in a fake voice while we were talking. Was she trying to discourage me from interacting with her? Or was she trying to discover how much I genuinely cared about her, how deep was my empathy for her autistic self?

Remembering the "silence test," I did nothing until she chose to return to our conversation. Then her behavior changed dramatically. She began talking to me again, with little, meaningful snatches to gauge their effect—not just on me, but also on her and her feelings about talking with me intimately—then trailed off vaguely lest she get too involved.

The same pattern prevailed when Wendy sat at a drawing table to write a story. The first sentences would be enticing and well-written, only to be interrupted abruptly in the middle. "Henrietta sat on a stool in her room writing," she began one day. "She heard her mother slip into the hall. When she got to . . ." And there it ended.

A few weeks later, Wendy explained her writing interruptions. She said that she did not want me or anyone to read what she had written, nor did she want me or anyone else to know, in any way, what the stories were about. "We can't talk about them, either." When she drew a picture, she would tell me not to look at it until she was absolutely ready to show it to me, which might be never. Possibly she didn't want me to see her spelling mistakes or what she considered inaccuracies in rendering her art, so she refused to let me see the finished product. Her behavior could not be solely the result of neurological misfirings, since it was so blatantly purposeful. I think she was mindful of others knowing her thoughts. She once asked me if I had ever written a story. When I answered yes, she asked, "How old were you?"

"About your age."

"What was it about?"

"A horse."

"Can you remember it? Could you write it down?"

I typed a few paragraphs, which she grabbed out of my hands as I was about to show them to her. Reading them, she burst out excitedly, "So this is what you thought about!" I supposed she meant that she had gotten a glimpse of what I remembered of my nine-year-old mind. And what better way, she may have reasoned, to find out how other people think than by examining their stories. In fact, I had exactly this motive in trying to get a peek at her stories.

Wendy soon chortled and boldly shouted, "You're *never* going to see what I've written," looking straight at me as she defied me. I took this stance as a sign that she felt safe asserting herself as she peered at me from behind her thick long eyelashes without the slightest qualm about the emotional reaction on my face. I guessed that, since I'd passed the silence test, she could be bold enough to take her interpersonal forays a little further, asserting herself in relation to me just at the exact moment she thought we were at odds with one another. Could she do so deliberately and joyously, not haphazardly and passively? Judging from her nonplussed delight at my obvious disappointment, I'd say I passed this test as well. I didn't retaliate. I cared a lot about her.

Being with Wendy made me wonder how she felt about her occasional attempts to relate. How did these figure against the backdrop of frequent socializing failures? Autistic isolation, whether deliberate or not, has exigent consequences for social development at the very time young children are typically refining their language and other social skills. Maybe Wendy impersonated the personalities of others because she was unsure of her self's survival in the company of others. Much like Marcia, Stacy, and Greg, she might have feared the demise of her self under the pressure of a too intense interaction. She may have had a firm sense of herself as a recluse, but not as a hobnobber. Rarely conversing with others over the course of her young life had deprived her of the ordinary social feedback accruing from one self to another. Quite possibly, the stability of her sense of self had not been embedded in her young psyche the way it normally is in babies and young children.

To put it another way, young autists are inexperienced in forming a social standard by which to evaluate the reactions, ideas, and behavior of other people. They have very little corrective experience for the notion, expressed by both Marcia and Greg, that just because a grown-up may appropriate a helpless child's favorite possessions, such an adult might also steal away anything that belongs to her, even her ideas. Since Wendy seemed to have presumed the truth of this concept, revealed by her secrecy about her stories, she had hardly ever tested the impact of her writings on others and as a result had very little idea about the probable reaction of these others. These phenomenona could occur no matter how dedicated, kind, and patient their parents. My point is that the youngster suffers the psychological effects of her own autistic condition. What psychologists call "prelogical" ideas fester in the young autist's mind, affecting social interchanges and future self-concepts. Since Marcia concretized words—perceived them as things—early on, she thought I would rob her of her ideas. Stacy and Greg believed I was determined to change their ideas. I was so eager to read her writing that Wendy may have thought I would take it and use it for my own purposes.

Like many an autist I've known, Wendy was not convinced by the results of one or even a few tests of her prelogic. Time and again, she had to prove her illogical presumptions doubtful or downright wrong before she could be with someone comfortably. When she thought no one was noticing, she would, much like Stacy, talk animatedly and uninhibitedly to herself, assured that telling herself her thoughts and fantasies was ultimately safer than revealing them to others. She looked quite bizarre during these moments and restricted this behavior to solitary times, unlike Stacy, who went on and on to herself about such things as flower petals, Victorian chimneys, swimming pools, and fancy drinking glasses, no matter who was with her. Then Stacy tested her ideas only against the imagined reactions of pretend people.

Neither Wendy nor Stacy would have reacted well to theory of mind testing. Since Wendy wished to prevent others from using her precious ideas to influence her in any way, conversations remotely suggestive of a genuine interest in them tended to turn her off talking. Stacy, too, came to realize that others were fascinated by what she said and believed they might try to influence her, either by changing some of her strange notions or by adding to them in ways she was not sure were safe. I imagine that in the face of theory of mind testing both girls would simply have clammed up, fearing that the more they revealed, the more hazardous their position in the world of people would become. If so, the theory of mind results for some autists reported by cognitive researchers may well reflect not a mental deficit but anxiety. For Wendy, Stacy, and, indeed, all the autists with whom I have worked, the fear of being influenced is grounded in psychotherapeutic reality. I do try to glean something of the child's own idea system in order to expand her view of the world so that she may adapt to it more vigorously.

Wendy helped me clarify what can be accomplished by conversing with a nervous, insecure young autist in psychotherapy meetings. When psychiatrists, psychologists, doctors, and parents believe psychotherapy to be inappropriate for young autists because the condition is not "curable"—that is, we cannot make it disappear or replace it with normalcy—they withhold a potentially restorative experience. After all, what we call "normalcy" is predisposed by our genes and our experience and so cannot be "cured" even if we would want it to be. And we often cannot "cure" such other conditions as a tendency to become overly anxious or to react to situations rigidly—we can't make them disappear or replace them with "normalcy." We can, though, ameliorate their noxious effects on peoples' lives. Why then do we use a basic autistic vulnerability to deny autists a psychological service? Freud proposed as the goal of psychoanalytic therapy the renewed ability to enjoy love and work.[23] I believe we can accomplish the same with young autists to varying degrees, depending on the child's age, the circumstances of her life and experience, and the motivations of all involved, particularly of the child and her parents. These goals and caveats are true for all young people in psychotherapy. Young autists are no different.

· · ·

Wendy became less content with solitude. She realized that she enjoyed being and talking with me. Her life became more textured and, insofar as I could observe, more enjoyable. Her mother told me that Wendy sought her out more at home and spent less time alone in her room. Since Wendy was the only daughter, her mother enjoyed the closeness that had developed between them. They shared "girl talk," went on nature hikes, and read storybooks together.

Soon Wendy sampled a variety of activities in my office and once read one of Maurice Sendak's books for children, *One Was Johnny*.[24] She'd begun the hour on a high note. She crossed my office's threshold with a warm and energetic "Hi!" Then she clamored, "Let's play cards!," soon followed by, "Let's draw together!"

In talking with Wendy about *One Was Johnny*, I realized yet again that she was signaling a need to be by herself for a while. This time, rather than just heading for the part of my office behind the screen where she could not be seen, she confided her wishes freely.

The story begins with a little boy, Johnny, sitting by himself happily reading a book, just as Wendy was doing. Various animals and a robber beset Johnny by barging into his tiny cozy room to bother and beleaguer him. The story's resolution shows Johnny all alone again, after his unwanted visitors have fled, absorbedly reading his book. Resonating to Johnny's love of solitude, Wendy came to the story's last line: "Johnny who lived by himself . . . LIKED IT LIKE THAT!" As Wendy sat very close to me on a sofa, she turned to me and confided softly, "I like it that way, too." Shy Wendy felt okay about admitting to me that she sometimes wanted to be alone.

She often sat next to me at a drawing table as I produced drawings according to her specifications. She told me that her own charming and explicit drawings were meant to illustrate her stories; she suggested that I, too, illustrate my stories! Checking whether my renditions were "realistic" enough, she would bashfully ask whether she could "copy" the way I had drawn trees and flowers. "I'm not really

copying you. I just think the way you draw trees is a really good idea."
Thus, she spontaneously differentiated mimicking and being inspired.
"Yes, there's a difference between mindless copying and getting ideas from other people," I responded. "Thanks!" she exulted gratefully. In an intersubjective moment she actually thanked me for appreciating her thoughts! She knew she wasn't trying to be me, yet she was inspired by me. At the same time she criticized my awkward attempts to portray people, she admired the way I drew plant life. This comparison gave her a more refined and immediate sense of who *she* was. What settled the matter was the different ways our minds worked in relation to depicting reality, which was, for Wendy, the crowning achievement in knowing two minds simultaneously.

Then more introspection: "One of my problems is that I'm always losing things," she said.

"Like what?"

"Like the favorite picture my mother drew for me. She's very good at art, too."

"But that doesn't mean you're copying her, right?"

"Right! I draw kids and she doesn't."

On a deeper level, Wendy realized that copying does not typify one of the most primary, profound attachments, that between a mother and a daughter. She recognized that one can share a trait with a mother without becoming a literal replica of her.

No wonder she could empathize so closely with her mother while she imagined herself crying so far away: she nonetheless imagined her infant self being very devoted to her mother. Now she could intimate, in a conversation with me, that she may have had to "lose" her mother's drawing in order to develop her unique drawing style more fully.

Probably because she felt helped by me, Wendy began to act as if she were my therapist. She once asked me, indulgently, about my drawing of a person, "Does that *really* look like a person's body?"

When I then had the idea of drawing a girl drawing plants, she saw right through my defensiveness and said with a laugh, "You're drawing that because of the plants which you draw so well, Karen!"

Ecstatic that she had addressed me by name for the first time, I thanked her for her praise and, implicitly, for her insight.

"You've really improved in your drawing of people, Karen!" she rejoiced reassuringly. Wendy was referring to my drawing of a group of children at a birthday party. I thought she was eager to critique my drawing of people, because her previously scornful or diffident attitude toward others may have seemed to her similar to my artistic clumsiness, my scorn or diffidence in depicting people. She prodded me, very like a therapist, into dealing with people more gracefully by assisting me in capturing their form on paper. To put this more psychologically, Wendy had restored her sense of autonomy not only in following through on her own ideas in her art, and in judging her work, but also by helping and judging the work of another person. Enthused by her independence, she could apply her energies to shaping the actions of others.

Wendy's sense of self had flourished during our ten months of working together. It has been said that self-awareness is the result of "owning" one's experience. "What lies at the heart of the present sense of 'self-awareness' is *ownership*—the ability to regard experiences as one's own"—meaning, according to James Russell, who writes of autistic potentialities, that young autists come to attribute to the self the activities of doing and thinking, of willing and knowing.[25] As these young people feel more certain of who they are and who they are becoming, they reassure themselves that being with others will not jeopardize what they've gained for themselves. They've become better prepared to anticipate a congenial, timely outcome when they seek to make friends.

CHAPTER EIGHT

Risking Friendships

In my high school diary, I wrote: "One should not always be a watcher—the cold impersonal observer—but instead should participate."

—TEMPLE GRANDIN

So much has been written about the social handicaps of young autists that you may well wonder why I devote an entire chapter to the ways in which they can and do make friends. How can they form friendships when they suffer a "disturbance of affective contact"—the inability to feel for and with another person? How can they, when they lack the ability to know or care what is on another's mind, when they often lack fluent language from which wondrous, engrossing, and confidential talks arise?

Sometimes naiveté works better. The principal of a public school, who knew of my interest in young autists, furnished me with anecdotes of the autistic children in her school who were integrated into regular classrooms. Remarking that children often make friends as they share newly won skills, she told me of a young boy who tried to teach his autistic classmate how to ride a bike. To the principal's perpetual amazement, the boy, about eleven, went about teaching bike-riding to the young autist exactly the way he would teach anybody. Our inexperienced young teacher "didn't *know* autistic children can't ride bikes," she exclaimed. "He didn't *know* autistic children won't or can't be taught by others," she continued zealously. "He just went ahead and taught the kid, and guess what? The kid learned!"

The same ingenuousness that our young teacher displayed permeated most everything I thought and did decades ago when I began to work with several autistic girls. I staunchly believed that if you truly cared about them, delicately but forthrightly charmed them out of their isolation, or deftly calmed their tortuous agonies and tumults, you could not only befriend them but also encourage them to befriend their peers. Some thirty years later I read avidly of the friendships gained—and sometimes lost—by authors who have written about their autistic childhoods. Their accounts confirmed what I had experienced in my work: autists sometimes want friends, although the passages to companionship are fraught with a profound inner skepticism and many an interpersonal hazard. Temple Grandin writes, "I wanted to participate, but I did not know how."[1]

I have described how the autists I knew told me that they thought they were "bad" or "crazy." In no small way, their feeling about self derived from their peers' responses to them, but the autist's own realization that he differs in many ways from other children often persuades him that he is "wacky," "psycho," "stupid," or "evil." It's not just that ordinary children tease and taunt autists—though this they surely do; it's also that the young autist, all the while behaving as if he does not notice others, carries on a running, invidious comparison with them. Thinking of one's self this way—Donna Williams refers to herself as a "nut," a "retard," or a "spastic," and Temple Grandin terms herself "bizarre," "dummie," and "weirdo"—hardly encourages the autist to initiate human contact much less to sustain it. In short, just when she wishes for friendship, she finds herself in the unexpected bind of desiring something she despairs she will never achieve.

All the young autists I knew, except for mute Paulie and runaway Burt, did make friends when one or two of their peers could somehow be conjoined with the autist's own particular, often peculiar, way of experiencing things. The successful friendships these autists maintained evolved only when they let the relationship expand beyond a closed, clandestine association, arbitrarily and mainly focused on the autist's own interests and preoccupations. Having experienced the benefits of being chummy with a prospective friend, the autist, loathe to lose his companion, sometimes adjusted to the interests and desires of the other. The strength of the relationship could be measured by the degree of this adaptation, essentially by the pleasure each friend took in it.

Early on, as he becomes more sensitive to *self* and desirous of engaging with others, the young autist is beset by anticipations of rejection, thinking "Who'd want to be friends with a dummie like me?" or "No one will want to be my friend because I'm wacky, I'm autistic." He often assesses accurately what his peers think of him—that indeed he is unusual, "weird." The feeling of being so different and the liabilities of being autistic are then etched in his mind ever more indelibly. The real and imagined rebuffs impede his search for consensual contacts and stultify his efforts to maintain a consistent and inspiring companionship.

His teachers and parents fervently hope (and pray!) that the young autist, especially one who is showing promise at school or at home, will seek a friend. They believe a friendship will provide the wished-for entrée to the social world, even if the youngster makes only one best friend. Often teachers and parents can create a propitious context for friend-making, even if it's only by suggesting that the autist and one of his buddies clean erasers together or take care of a classroom's pet gerbil, or by arranging a play date around the basic pleasures of sharing a favorite snack after school.

It is important for parents and teachers not to schedule an overly lengthy sharing activity. During the first encounters, the autist and his companion should maximize the enjoyment gained from a brief but significant time together, such as clapping chalk dust off erasers, feeding a gerbil, or sharing milk and cookies. They will remember the fun, not the length of time they were together. The new enjoyment they shared will motivate the autist and his friend to spend increasingly longer times with one another.

The hazard to the budding relationship is the autist's reckless determination to meld the other person into his own private world, no matter the interests or desires of the prospective friend, no matter his personal qualities. The risk, of course, is that the nonautistic other will soon conclude that his diffident companion is not really interested in the friendship; he appears disinterested in the other's qualities.

Some autists I have known—Wendy and Nate, for example—understood that they must appear attentive as they turned on the charm to keep their friends engaged. The motive was often to inveigle the other child into a strange fantasy scenario or thinking system that has likely occupied the autist for many years. The unsuspecting other, drawn into a complex web of often capricious or grotesque meaning and outlandish uses of factual knowledge, startles our insouciant autist by offering him a fresh, more commonsensical perspective on fantasy and fact. When this happens, he and his friend will benefit from each other's diverging viewpoints: the autist gets to know more intimately the commonplaces of typical social life; the friend is exposed to the workings of a curious and uncommon mind. Often an unexpected flight of fancy is given to the most ordinary of life's experiences, as when Temple Grandin commented inventively, aesthetically, on some of life's lessons, calling herself an "anthropologist on Mars." Speaking of her awkwardness in understanding complex emotion and the "games" people play with one another, she likened herself—wistfully, I thought—to an anthropologist studying others. Duly impressed by Grandin's insight, Oliver Sacks chose her metaphor for the title of his best-selling book.

Stacy gave a new twist to the commonplace distinction between people and things. She had forgotten, for the moment, if indeed she ever knew it, that other people understand this distinction. Yet her statement "People don't ruin in the laundry like socks" both amused and exhilarated her peers; they, too, began to talk of the dissimilarities between people and objects, contrasts they had assumed to be obvious and that now formed the basis for more mature, quasi-philosophical conversations. The debate went from people and things to animate and inanimate and finally to one criterial distinguishing characteristic. Of the fact that people, not things, generate movement, one of Stacy's companions shouted, "It's that people move, and things don't!"

When Stacy merged the meanings of two like-sounding words, "see" and "sea," her bemused dormmates helped her sort out the many meanings she had conflated into a tight significance web. In doing so, her companions learned not just how Stacy thought but also how *they* thought—about thinking processes generally. They had been enticed back to a time of their own freshly learned insights, which, inspired by a novel expression by Stacy, stood out like jewels in the tangle of tried-out thought patterns that had preceded them. In this important sense one can learn about oneself by communing with autists.[2]

Practicing for Friends

The autists I knew may have used our friendly interactions in therapy as a template to guide their tentative attempts at social contact. They felt that I had befriended them and that I had nearly always accepted them and what interested them. It seemed natural to expect a similar response from others, even if those others were children. My approach appeared to convince young autists that having friends would be fun. This was particularly true of those whose parents made every effort to adapt to their children's idiosyncrasies to ease the impact of the autistic condition and to gently encourage them to open up to their families. The efforts of their parents promoted the idea that being with people is enjoyable.

Respecting the autist's own perspective often does produce greater variety in his behavior. Feeling liked and even honored, he becomes bolder in trying new things. This preliminary nurturing, accepting context requires arduous work on the part of professionals and parents. Yet it is not enough to evoke in the autist genuine attempts to adjust sufficiently for friendships to blossom. These efforts must often be followed by outright coaching in the art of behaving reciprocally, including repeated requests for the autist to pay attention, not to give up, and to show an interest in others. "Some people have said that autistic people don't care about friendships," writes Paul McDonnell. "I just want to say that people mean more than anything to me. . . . However, I still need to work more on my social skills. They are not as good as a lot of people's."[3]

The need to coach twelve-year-old Gregory was abundantly apparent one day when he delayed leaving my office. Greg knew another child was waiting for his appointment, and he purposely, somewhat defiantly, prolonged his time with me, intending to deprive the other child. When I reminded him that someone was waiting, he shouted out, wearing his exasperating insouciance like an abrasive badge on his shoulder, "I don't *care* about anyone else waiting!" Quite irritated with him, I erupted, "Listen, Gregory, other people care about you, so you should care about them!"

His mother heard this exchange and began to nod her head vigorously, saying, "We tell him this all the time at home." Many weeks later, hindsight suggested that Greg had heeded my message and his parents' directives. He had become rather friendly, sometimes shyly inquiring how I was as he entered my office. He'd ask haltingly what the other children who came to see me played with and even spoke briefly about his and others' feelings toward each other.

Wendy and Nathan were able to relate to a select few, because these friends found their shy companions compatible enough and, once in their company, became captivated by some of their qualities. Scribe

Wendy's two friends admired her writing and delighted in her acted-out dramas and the stories she spun to accompany her amusing drawings. They reciprocated by teaching Wendy how to play card games, which she perfected in my office in order to challenge her friends more effectively. Scholarly Nathan's usually older friends shared and encouraged his intellectual interests and protected him when others taunted and teased him. Their protective behavior impressed Nate, and he responded with affection and a greater ease in being with people generally. The parents of these two rather well-adjusted autists told me that, along with increased confidence, their children unexpectedly— "magically"—found friends, seemingly overnight. I believe Wendy and Nathan felt that their parents and I had adjusted to them; they needed little coaching as they tried to behave toward others as others had behaved toward them. They just needed interpersonal practice; they could then approach their peers graciously and eagerly. No surprise, then, that their companions reciprocated and found in Wendy and Nate qualities to which they could relate.

Things were different for five-year-old James. His parents tried to persuade him to make friends, but "little professor" James, who visualized other children breaking or stealing his possessions, would walk away or cry the minute the others followed him, pestering him about his toys. James's parents were so upset by his attitude toward his peers that they accompanied him to our meetings, recounting their latest efforts to interest him in a neighborhood child or someone who sat next to him in class. They wondered whether I could talk to James, whether I could assure him that he'd have fun with friends, whether I could somehow "teach" him how to relate?

Eventually, James took up as his own his parents' mission to find him friends. He began to vociferate that other children wouldn't play with him. "Don't give up; try again," his parents would say. "Maybe that kid wouldn't play with you because he was already playing with someone else." These attempts to reassure Jamie, to help him pave the way for renewed friendly gestures, seemed doomed as he concluded pessimistically, "I'll never find a best friend."

One day, when he was fretting about friends, I asked, "You mean you don't know anyone your age in the whole world who's interested in emergency vehicles?" For the moment James was speechless and grabbed a cookie I had put out for him. "Maybe you could invite a friend over for snacks after school," I suggested, "and show him your emergency vehicles."

"Yes, the kids I know like my emergency vehicles, but I'm scared they will break them."

"But you wouldn't mind sharing cookies with them, would you?"

"Nope," Jamie answered, brightening. "Well, that's a beginning," said I, hopefully.

Shortly thereafter I visited Jamie's school to give a talk unrelated to autism. I happened to observe him interacting with another boy. At first he was playing alone with some blocks, pretending they were a police car and a fire truck. A classmate came over and asked Jamie what he was doing. "This block is the siren on top of my fire truck, and those blocks are the flashing lights on my police car," responded Jamie warily but proudly. The other child, an aggressive, noisy youngster, replied, "I'm going to bomb your fire truck now," grinning provocatively and watching for Jamie's reaction. Slowly, in an almost imperceptible way, Jamie began to move his blocks away from the boy. Finally, a gradual, cautious smile spread across his face. The boy began tossing his own blocks into the sandbox nearby, saying that he was bombing the dirt. At this, James turned to me and beamed from ear to ear as though to say, "See? I can do it! I *can* play with another kid. I can *survive* it!"

The next time I met with Jamie I told him how smart he'd been in school, how clever he'd been to move his fire truck slowly away when the other child threatened to destroy it. As though to mimic the boy's very aggression, Jamie startled me by grabbing a toy out of my hands and playing with it. Was he creating in me the intimidation he felt at school, even though, as it turned out, he'd finessed the other boy's threat? Possibly. He might have been fascinated by power just as he was frightened by it.

So I said of his grabbiness, "What do you think the other kids would do if you grabbed something from them like you just did with me?" Whereupon James bumped into me purposefully, saying, "I didn't grab it away. I just took your hands off it."

He just took my hands off it?! What an impertinent rejoinder! Did he wish to persuade me that he needn't attend to me personally, only to my hands, so therefore he hadn't really grabbed anything from *me?* He'd merely loosened my grip on the toy. This seemed a deliberately impersonal way of defending himself. As I was to learn some years later while visiting a school with several young autists in regular classes, these children can intentionally use their autistic behaviors for their own sweet reasons. For example, one nine-year-old, angry at his teacher, scooted away from her on the bench on which they sat as though to say, "Now I'm isolating myself from you big-time, because I'm mad at you." His teacher told me she had not given way that day to his brazen demands to do whatever he pleased.

James had been wary of offending me but also had wanted to assert himself. He compromised by seeming to return to his former stance of treating a person as a nonentity with only one body part that mattered, the hands. "What would the other kids say," I persisted, "if you said that to them?" Silence.

"I remember you played nicely with another boy in school last week," I reminded James. "So I know you can play well if you want to."

"Yes," Jamie answered testily, "but *you* are not a *kid*," now stressing that he would behave differently with me than with his peers. It was safe, he knew, to take advantage of me by snatching things out of my hands, but it was not safe to do so with his classmate. With him he had behaved as expected, if a little bashfully.

My efforts to coach Jamie in relating, to help him think out social situations in my office, seemed to evoke in him the thoughts and fears about socializing that often tripped him up in dealing with others. I knew Jamie was as worried about his own, often imagined, transgressions as he was about those of others, so I continued to talk with him when he acted unfriendly toward me.

He once pretended that his Lego policeman was hurt, so I got out the Lego doctor, suggesting his Lego man might get help from the doctor doll.

"You don't go to the doctor for having a knee scraped," he said scornfully, pushing the Lego doctor away firmly, as though to reject the idea of a "doctor" (me) helping him. "And anyway, these are *my* Legos so you have to do what *I* say."

"No, actually I don't, because this is *my* office so I don't have to do what you say."

Taking my retort quite seriously, Jamie countered, "Yes, this is *your* office, but you still have to do what *I* say if you play with *my* Legos!"

"No, I don't. I'm going to use *my* ideas, not yours."

Since James was less fragile than he had ever been, I thought he was tough enough to hold his own in a serious debate with me. He could not only assert himself bravely, but also tolerate, even welcome, my rejoinders. I felt as if we inhabited the trenches together, our sleeves rolled up and sweating, ready to work out one of the most basic interpersonal dilemmas autism presents.

In the past, Jamie had corrected not just my words but also my ideas. He now attempted to strike a deal with me. I could play with his Legos only if I let him influence my thoughts. In addition to being reluctant to share his possessions, he now was opposed to a mutually planned activity. Earlier he had done his utmost to control objects, but now he wanted to control people. Because he didn't want people to influence his prized ideas, he tried to control their every move.

His parents soon corroborated these impressions. They told me that Jamie would consent to invite other kids over, but only if they played as he wished. He dissolved into angry tears the minute he realized that other children had their own agendas or when his parents tried to persuade him that sharing could be fun. He brought his toys to my office so he'd be justified in bossing me around; yet I continued to say that it's more amusing to share play ideas. I advised his parents to talk to Jamie about sharing fun playtimes, but before his companion actually arrived. That way Jamie could prepare himself for the likelihood that his friend would interject his own ideas into the play.

Once, during one of these seemingly interminable conversations, he blurted out, "I like to play with Billy, but I'm afraid he'll take my toys away."

"Really? I don't think you'd do that, I don't think you'd take *my* toys away," I mused.

"That's because I'm not *interested* in your toys!" he snorted. "Anyway," Jamie continued, "Billy just said he would take my toys away, but he was only kidding."

"Yes, Billy was only joking, maybe to see what you would do. But even if he weren't, you and your parents wouldn't let him take your toys away, would you now?"

I realized later that Jamie wasn't so much centered on what people actually did, as he'd been before, nor was he interpreting what they said literally. Now he was curious about *mental possibilities*, those cerebral states underlying doing and talking. So I praised him for guessing what Billy's intent might have been and thought perhaps this was the end of the discussion as Jamie went on to do something else.

Soon he returned to our play, smiling a broad fake grin to hide *his* intent. "Can I take these Legos home?" he snickered. "I promise I'll bring them right back."

I told him he could play with the Legos any time he wanted to in my office, but that I couldn't let him borrow them, because they belonged here, "just like your toys belong to you and in your room at home." I hoped to model a firm but friendly stance that Jamie might adopt when other children tried to wheedle things out of him or have their way.

He had, I thought, recreated a situation he'd experienced many a time when other children tried to trick him into letting them borrow his toys on the false promise that they would return them. He'd learned that a child's overt behavior could mask other, more important, covert purposes. He had transcended the notorious autistic tendency to interpret things literally or to be naively trusting. Most important, he'd begun to act more like the others as he tried to trick me!

Perhaps to lighten the discussion with a joke, James remarked, "Did you know that dinosaurs have only three fingers? That's why they can only count to six!" Laughing, I wondered aloud whether he'd told this joke to his friend Billy. "No," Jamie answered breezily, "Billy told it to me."

Social Worries

Jamie soon befriended a second child, a boy who always got into trouble in school. He confided in our meetings that his friend "always gets time-outs" or check marks beside his name on the blackboard. Earnestly disclosing that *he* never got a "time-out" or *his* name on the blackboard, he fell silent, staring at his hands. He seemed as riveted on the acting up of other boys his age as he had been on shiny objects or toys that rotated. He seemed spellbound by precisely those behaviors that brought the reprimands. Unlike Nate and Wendy, who inveigled others to become part of their fantasy lives and whose friends often eagerly agreed to do so, James watched from the sidelines as his favorite classmates were rebuked time and again, evaluating the rights and wrongs of these situations without ever becoming involved himself. He inferred what would happen to him should he behave similarly.

Yet he said to me periodically, "I'm worried about getting into trouble in school."

"But you *don't* get into trouble!"

"But I don't *want* to get into trouble!"

"I know you don't. And your parents told me that when somebody in your group does do something wrong, the whole group gets into trouble. But that doesn't mean that you actually did something wrong, although it must make you very mad."

James lapsed into a thoughtful silence and finally muttered, "Yes, I *do* get mad!"

It wasn't simply that he preferred to sit disinterestedly on the sidelines as the others tended to their social business. He was afraid he could not control his emotions when reproached by his teacher unfairly. He cringed as he visualized his name on the blackboard and shrank from the imagined words, "Time out!" During these moments, his imaginings were so vivid and his feelings so strong that it was wellnigh impossible to convince him that this was only fantasy.

It wasn't until James was about eight that he allowed himself to make friends with children who shared his interests and who were proficient young scholars as he was, rather than troublemaking children prone to rebuke. He became less interested in "proving" his superiority over others and preferred the company of children who shared his values. His teacher remarked about this change in James, "He's become a team player!"

James nevertheless found it difficult to expand his social circle beyond the few, dependable boys he favored. Perhaps, as I had hoped, he had benefited from practicing how to behave with other kids in his meetings with me. Perhaps he had adapted to my attempts to recreate another child's reactions to his social intransigence, and I was heartened that he didn't withdraw when the going got rough. But if his parents tried to introduce him to an unfamiliar youngster or if he met a friend by chance, he'd stiffen into a nonresponsive demeanor until he adjusted to the newness of it all. Being a team player was nonetheless a great social coup for James. He genuinely enjoyed being with his friends, and these attachments presaged a more vital future.

Working Out Friendships

Try though he might, reclusive Greg, who was often absorbed with animals and their habits, couldn't quite be a team player. He played for years with only his siblings. And for years his brother and sister did most of the adapting. Greg's was an especially close-knit family; his parents eased his internal troubles and helped him surmount his tactlessness. Greg began to work out relating to others by befriending his sibs. Within the family haven he felt safe experimenting with his odd ways of being with people.

At school, he was altogether too tense and prone to hostile and vicious outbreaks to even think of befriending a child. He suffered enough, he told me once, when his brother and sister reacted to his autistic improprieties by teasing or avoiding him; yet he knew his parents would protect him and try to guide him toward more auspicious family interactions. Greg would essay a tentative, barely noticeable social gesture with another child outside the family, like a soft "hi," which, largely because of his academic successes in seventh and eighth grades, was sometimes met with a favorable nod from the others.

Earlier, Greg angrily withdrew from his classmates because they teased him unmercifully about having been suspended. He could see no alternative but to avoid them to inhibit retaliating ferociously, which would result in his being thrown out of school yet again. In a way, it's to his credit that he used his isolating tendencies to disrupt the vicious cycle. Seeking revenge for the taunts of others would only bring forth the very situation that had always instigated Greg's rage and his subsequent rejection by others.

Adolescent Greg soon realized that his siblings had become less content to endure his autism without commentary or protest. This actually motivated him to adapt more congenially. Now preadolescent, his brother and sister would say something like, "What's with you when you pace around like that?" or "Come off it, Greg, you're acting wacky!" Greg could process their remarks even though they were critical. He considered their reprovals, because they had earlier tolerated his eccentricities sensitively with a patience akin to Job's. Now it was time for Gregory to be forbearing and resilient. And he knew it.

Greg began to talk to me about his social life and even spoke of one or two classmates who, he said, had become his friends. He'd formed tight enough bonds with his brother and sister to suppose that he might befriend someone at school, but he approached only those youngsters who shared his abiding fascinations.

The idea the young autist has of himself as "evil," "wacky," "retarded," "spastic," impedes his socializing when his sense of his "bad self" too easily generalizes to a "bad" other person. Before, Greg had commingled his own feelings of worthlessness with the worthlessness he attributed to others—those very kids who seemed, by their teasing, to prove as wanting as Greg's autistic self. When Greg ceased feeling "evil," he allowed that, perhaps, others were not evil. Now viewing himself as "good" and "smart," he wondered if others might be similar to him in these ways, and he set out to confirm it.

An early friendliness, remarkable for its ordinary simplicity, was a gesture so common in others as to be hardly noteworthy; yet for Greg it was entirely out of character. He was helping me pick up some marbles he had strewn across my office floor, having pretended, with good aim, to fire them at some dollhouse dolls. I had tolerated his play because he was practicing a skill with dispatch. As always, when

I commented on his capability—I said, "Your aim is getting better and better"—he seemed lifted out of his usual humdrum things-are-always-the-same mood. After grabbing up a handful of marbles he casually approached me with them, handing them over, saying, "Here."

The following week he repeated this behavior. He rushed into my office and settled himself with some crackers, whereupon I asked him how he was. "Wait," was his terse reply. Then he slapped an envelope on the table in front of us. When I didn't react particularly, he picked up the envelope, which had his mother's psychotherapy payment in it, and announced yet again, "Here." Quite obviously, "here" stood for "Here are your marbles" or "Here is your check."

Autistic young people don't give things to others easily. They realize that to do so they must acknowledge the receiver. And they often do not want to admit to your existence. My thanks for the marbles and the check, casual but heartfelt, evoked, "I'm going to play with Legos for a while, and then I'm going to do something else, something totally different!"

"Great!" I realized he'd already done something different. For the first time, he'd given me the envelope holding payment for my help!

His "something different" turned out to be a request for advice on how to make friends. "What is a good thing to do when a person gets mad?" he began, talking in generalities. "What is a good thing to do when *I* get mad?" he continued, candidly focusing his important question on himself. Maybe he realized that others might get mad at him in response to his getting angry—that is, he might have referred to the endless irksome cycles described before.

"You mean the kids at school?"

"Uh-huh," came the curt reply.

Then Greg described the others' rude behavior toward him, impolite behavior he himself had often enjoyed. I thought it unwise, though, to zero in on Greg's own rude behavior, believing he would tune out any pointed remarks intended to persuade him to change.

And how could I know for sure that he hadn't changed? His behavior in school might have improved without my knowledge.

Instead, I talked with him about the others, hoping he would gain insight by analogy. "You could think to yourself that their rude behavior is really not your problem, even though it hurts your feelings. After all, *they're* the ones being rude."

With one final assaultive burst at the dollhouse dolls—his method of coping with *his* anger—he said reasonably, "Okay, uh-huh." But I wasn't convinced that he had really heard me.

The next time Greg and I met, he began talking specifically about two boys who had been annoying him. This time Greg named the boys as he described what they looked like and how they acted. "One kid used to be a lot worse to me; now he just doesn't want to be in my presence," Greg muttered laconically.

"So what do you do about it?"

"Mostly I laugh and then he gets mad—well, sometimes he gets angry but sometimes not."

"By laughing you're trying to join in with his joke?"

"I guess," said Greg thoughtfully.

"Any kids in school you like?"

"You mean *friends?*" Greg responded incredulously, then smirking. Again I got a vivid description of two boys' physical appearance as though they would, in this way, be brought to life for me as I visualized them.

"What do you like to do with your friends?"

"Oh, I don't know . . . act silly," came Greg's eager reply as he smiled ear to ear. Now energized, he suddenly began to pace my office. He also began to blush as he described his giddy antics with his friends. Never had I heard Greg talk so readily about other children his age nor had I seen him display such elation directly linked to *people.*

Attending to social cues had not come easily to Gregory as it doesn't to many autists. Childhood autist Temple Grandin notes that she didn't "read" people comfortably, if at all, but she does describe the psychological bonds that thrive between autists and others. Many commune, she writes, with their autistic soulmates or even marry them because of their shared experience being autistic. "The two partners," she says, "get together because they have similar interests, not because of physical attraction." Refining her point, she notes, "Friendships always revolved around what I *did* rather than who I *was*" (italics mine).[4]

Similarly, when Greg did make friends, he focused on their appearance and what they did together, not explicitly on who he was in relation to who they were. Yet there are those who would argue that who we are is determined by how we behave. "Our deeds determine us," writes novelist George Eliot, "as much as we determine our deeds."[5] And first impressions often center on physical appearances.

So just how different *was* Greg when, in conversation, he introduced me to his friends, people he knew I didn't know, by describing their appearance and behavior, to make their essence more vivid for me?

Eagerly he began to deliver a week-to-week commentary on the status of his relationships. Of his enemies he said, "Remember when I told you two weeks ago about those kids who bother me? Well, it's better."

"You mean those kids who are bigger than you?"

"Yeah, I mean those kids and it's a little better now." "It" referred to his being teased.

"Talking about it here helped?"

"Yeah, they're not my best friends," he added wistfully, "but it's better. They've stopped teasing me, and they're being nice."

He sighed deeply, happy and relaxed. Perhaps some of the silly stuff he'd indulged in with the dollhouse dolls had all along been a signal to me that he *had* formed friendships and that with friends he could act goofy—and normally—much the way any child would. But Greg was thirteen, not eight or nine, the age when most children I work with begin to converse earnestly and complexly about their friends and enemies.

Yet isn't a lesson learned later better than one not learned at all?

A Lonely Superhero World

Once he emerged from his isolation, Dirk, who was now seven, couldn't contain himself in the company of other children as easily as Greg could. Greg took his time entering the world of people and could more comfortably retire from it, thinking his favorite thoughts or being with his siblings. Dirk had become impossibly impetuous and vulnerable to social stimulation, often lashing out aggressively in a madcap way. Completely withdrawn when I first knew him, he surfaced in the social world about a year later and would become so flooded with emotion at acknowledging and interacting with people that his behavior resembled that of a frantic animal on a treadmill as he tried to keep up with the thoughts and feelings aroused by others. His mother had earlier spoken despairingly of Dirk's isolation, saying, "He's so *apart* from people!" And his older sister joined in, "Yes, he doesn't play with *any*body!" Now he was all over the playground, flitting from child to child, whispering bizarre inanities in their ears, and disrupting their childhood games during recess.

Like many autists with whom I had worked, he had readied himself for wished-for friends by befriending me. "You're my best friend," he'd say when he felt good about being with me. He straddled two worlds, his own inner space and the social world in which he had become inordinately interested, almost obsessed by. I often thought he was aware that he spanned two worlds, as though while occupying one he was teasing the other. He seemed to wonder, "Which world will win the battle? Which will claim me as its person?"

Dirk spun endless stories about good and bad people, the strong and the weak. He'd create mental binds for himself as he talked re-petitively about his fascination with Superman, trying to link good to strong, saying that Superman was both. Then he would counter his own assertion by saying that some *bad* people are strong. Typically, he'd turn to me for clarification. He seemed simply unable to escape his two-dimensional world to coordinate the two poles with each other (good-strong, bad-strong; good-weak, bad-weak). So how could he form lasting friendships when he realized that strong kids might not be "good," might not be nice to him?

He brought his dilemma into our interpersonal world. "You're good, aren't you? *Are* you good?" he'd asked urgently. Before I could answer, "But you get mad."

I'd say, "Yes, I'm a good person who likes you but who gets mad sometimes. How about you?"

"Noooo, I'm *not* good," he'd intone in his soft, musical voice, ever so slowly.

"What makes you think you're not good?" I'd inquire, hoping he understood that he could be good even if he got mad. Yet I'd never get an answer.

Once he came to his appointment sporting a Superman costume, wearing it proudly even though it wasn't Halloween.

"Now I see that you are really interested in Superman," I said.

"I *am* Superman," Dirk proclaimed pompously, annoyed that I'd suggested he was merely interested in Superman when he wished me to understand that he *was* Superman.

Did he think, therefore, that he could fly? "You won't be able to fly no matter how hard you try," I told him.

"But Superman rescues people and he *has* to fly to do it." A few minutes later, "Superman must be rescued, too. He might die."

"Does someone have to fly to rescue him?"

"Yes," answered Dirk tersely. "I do."

He seemed dead serious that not only could he fly with his costume on, but that he must. Worried that he might injure himself trying to fly, I told him he could make the Superman doll pretend to fly in my office but that real people can't fly.

"Except in planes?" asked a suddenly reasonable Dirk.

"Except in planes."

Often mute and confused, Dirk could reverse course in an instant. He could abruptly access sophisticated language: Superman "must" be rescued; he "might" die; and he could acknowledge reality: we fly in planes.

He enacted dramas of Superman being rescued by dolls and puppets he suspended on strings attached to the beams of my office ceiling, contorted efforts that suggested a dramatic last-minute save, only to fail dismally. "You see, Superman died again."

"Isn't there any way we can save the Superman doll?" I asked.

"No way at all," he answered, now speaking methodically, impersonally, routinely.

I remembered how his religious parents often spoke to him of going to heaven. They had tried to convince him that if he behaved himself as a child, he'd enjoy heaven when he died. I talked to his parents about his literal seven-year-old mind, that he had not matured enough to distinguish a literal from a spiritual interpretation of heaven; and how he might want to be there when he got upset and discouraged about his life here on earth. We devised a plan whereby we'd all stress that Dirk would never be able to fly to heaven as he imagined Superman doing and that we would all take very good care of him to keep him safe. We also assured him that his family and his friends on earth wanted him to be with us for a good long time and that we could have fun together, right here, right now.

Dirk began to struggle with the friendship concept, probably because we stressed live people on earth as potential friends. Torrents of emotion poured out of him as he bemoaned the fact that people hated him. "People hate me," he told me one day, "they don't know me and so they hate me."

"How can they hate you if they don't even know you?" I argued.

"They hate me *because* they don't know me."

Like Stacy, who often fused two unrelated ideas, Dirk blended *feeling hated* with the *stranger concept.* Dirk's fusing of these two ideas resulted in an inaccurate and tormenting causality association. Being just seven years old, he couldn't understand why strangers should be avoided. He concluded they must be bad, and if they were to be avoided because they were bad people, he was quite sure they must hate him.

Since they realized that Dirk had yet to treat people he knew differently from those he didn't know, his parents feared for his safety when he struck up droll, outlandish conversations with people in the supermarket, on the street, or at the park. Apparently heartened by the message that people he already knew could be his friends, Dirk began to pretend that the Superman and Batman dolls in my office were best friends. They were so friendly, he said, that they would even let each other dress up in their costumes (my superhero dolls wore removable clothing). Then giggling nervously, he tried to fool me into thinking that Batman was Superman and vice versa.

"You can't fool me," I teased. "I know Superman when I see him, and I know Batman when I see him. Everyone is themselves, your sister is your sister, your mom is your mom, and your dad is your dad." Dirk looked at me quizzically, so I finished by saying, "And you are you. You will always be you."

Seeming to be shocked by the obvious, Dirk protested loudly and vigorously.

"I'm *not* my own self. I don't *want* to be lonely. I don't *want* to be *by myself.*"

"I see," I responded, now fairly sure I could untangle his confused thought connections. "You don't want to *be* yourself because you don't want to be *by* yourself, and alone."

"Yes," came Dirk's whispered and anxious reply.

"Well, you can *be* yourself and still *not* be lonely," I interpreted.

"I like you," said Dirk immediately.

Brilliantly complex though it was, Dirk's insight was intuitive, thus only partially formed. He knew his failed attempts to form friendships had to do with how he felt about himself. He hated feeling lonely. He hated being by himself. In his precocious but overwhelmed mind, he deduced that it was a bad thing to be himself. His very avoidance of self in trying to be a superhero fatigued him and made him unresponsive to the overtures of others.

Years after reassuring Dirk that it was okay to be himself, that he need not be alone and lonely to be who he was, I read Donna Williams's account of her friendship with Ian in her book *Like Color to the Blind*. She recounts the ways in which she and Ian found themselves alike and different. They engaged in intense discussions to confirm and solidify their sense of who each was within the often quixotic relational nexus they'd developed with one another. Likewise, Dirk's relationships were often volatile. Their intensity seemed to turn him off relating at the very moment he dreaded feeling alone and lonely. Doubting that he really wanted friends because of the overbearing stimulation emanating from them, Dirk began to doubt himself—and his needs. It occurred to me that *we* doubt autists because *they* doubt themselves. Witnessing their tentative, sometimes awkward first social moves may convince us of their rock-bottom inability to relate to us, of their alleged inborn reclusion.

Williams's account shows why she learned more from Ian than she did from imaginary Carol and Willie. Ian responded in an authentic, continuous, and often unpredictable way, and so she was able to forge a truer identity from her reactions to him than she had when trapped in a made-up persona. For the first time ever, Williams heard herself speak in her dreams in her own voice.

That Williams had never experienced her own voice in her dreams suggests a dissociation in which the elusive depth of a person has been alienated from the basic feeling of "being me."[6] She had kept herself so distant from that person who was Donna that even in the looser, subconscious experience of dreaming, Williams failed to emerge as Donna. Yet her dissociation appears to have been undone by the success of her friendship with Ian.

To have a true, sensate experience of self, of feeling *real*, one must reckon with the emotional reactions to oneself of an attuned other. Otherwise the self remains underdeveloped; it might even feel "empty"—devoid of the numerous reminders of the particulars of one's social selfness emanating from a loved, trusted other. Ian's personal responses to Donna Williams, unpredictable though they may sometimes have been, nonetheless supported her sense of who she was when she trusted him enough to integrate what he said and did, and how he felt.[7]

When Dirk said he didn't want to be himself because he didn't want to be *by* himself—apart from others—he dichotomized being alone and being with people. He couldn't conceive of being truly himself in the company of others, so swamped was he by their impact on him. Being himself always meant he was alone, and lonely. By stressing the phrase *by myself*, Dirk may have meant that a part of himself stood off to his side, observing.

Temple Grandin experienced something similar. Taking a test in which a piece of classical music evoked images similar to those in others taking the test, she visualized these images only as an observer. She didn't visualize herself on a boat floating on the sparkling water as other people did. "All my life I have been an observer, and I have always felt like someone who watches from the outside."[8]

Dirk had doubtless experienced his loneliness before he tried to put his psychical puzzle pieces together and voiced his enigmatic but poignant complaint. Now his reconstruction of an archaic feeling got expressed in seven-year-old thought. He may have concretized his sense of self as he imagined himself standing off to the side, observing. As I sought to help him complete the puzzle by integrating the personal (being himself) and the social (he could be himself with me), he felt better and told me he liked me. In our conversation his very essence was confirmed, so he could turn outward and affectionately toward another person.

However lucid he could be sometimes, Dirk found it difficult to clear his thoughts when he was with children his own age. In my quiet office he could sift through the many ideas that bombarded his fatigued psyche in order to reject those that suddenly seemed wrong. In the height of emotion, when he'd try to persuade his classmates that either he or they were Superman, he simply could not contain himself and frequently got reprimanded by his teacher for misbehaving.

Dirk's interest in the others was unmistakable nonetheless. The first sign that he was ready for friendship came when he inquired whether the other children who came to see me played with the Superman and Batman dolls. If he saw some neighborhood boys pass by the office, he'd ask who they were and what they were interested in. He'd sort the information I gave him, classifying those children who were interested in superheroes and those who weren't. His teacher told me he was carrying out the same survey in school. He seemed genuinely eager to choose a small group of kids to play with who shared his superhero passion.

Invariably, he'd get into trouble at school because he tried to beguile some boys with his wild and vivid fantasies, tempting them to act aggressively toward those boys relegated by Dirk to the alien group. These were the boys, Dirk decided, who wanted to kill Superman.

Sometimes Dirk's teacher was able to convince him that he didn't have to play with kids who weren't his friends, who were "alien." For a time, Dirk dropped his aggressive stance toward these children. When he realized the implication of his teacher's suggestion, that he could no longer divide his peers into "friends" and "aliens," Dirk's befriending attempts took a turn for the worse. He could not restrain himself from acting like Superman, now toward his friends, as he attacked them, trying, in his view, to save Superman, who was himself.

Dirk's parents became distraught by their son's antisocial behavior and began to despair that he couldn't or wouldn't relinquish his private world for the social world. Yet Dirk would talk to me about his "friends," concentrating on one boy in particular, calling him by name, Travis, telling me how much he liked him.

"I hit Travis today."

"Why'd you do that? Isn't he your friend?"

"I don't know why I did it," he replied. Then switching to a high-pitched, sweet voice, "He's such a cute and nice little boy." Once relentlessly echolalic, Dirk now mimicked his mother, and probably his sister, with a comical flair when it suited him. His willful use of mimicry infuriated Dirk's mother but amused his sister. His mother became angry and frustrated when her son would *deliberately act autistic*, a reaction I've seen in other parents of young autists I've known.

Yet, isn't an intentional use of what was formerly a "symptom" a sign of progress? At the very least, the child no longer feels the helpless victim of his condition, no longer thinks he's hopelessly and irrevocably hemmed in by his autism. He may relish the fact that sometimes he can control it, turning it off and on at will.

Talking with Dirk about the school's rules only evoked more frustrated, wordy bursts: "I don't know; I don't know why I do it [hit Travis]. I just love Travis, and he calls me 'sweetie.'"

"People don't usually hit others if they really like them," I answered warily, wondering whether Dirk actually liked Travis.

To this Dirk erupted, "All the kids call me stupid in school! Travis calls me dumb and stupid! I hate that!"

"So you love Travis but not when he calls you 'stupid'?"

"Yes!"

In contrast to Gregory, who was more composed and who gave himself time-outs when his friends and acquaintances rejected him, often avoiding these youngsters for days, Dirk was much more driven. He would fixate on making his play scenarios turn out just the way he wanted. He'd seek to orchestrate an interaction the way he wished and expected, often oblivious to the desires and plans of the others. Although he was doing well academically, his peer conflicts at school escalated. In his frenzy to enlist the children as his accomplices in a fantasy world, he'd neglect to grasp and respect their perspectives and wishes. He even tuned out his teacher, who attempted to contain his aggression and to teach him more congenial ways of being with others.

Sadly, Dirk was asked to leave his school and eventually was enrolled in a day program for handicapped youth. He was aware of his failed attempts to adjust to his classmates. The overwhelming stimulation he experienced when with them often made him feel powerless in his struggle to adapt to social situations. He was reluctant to moderate his Superman fantasies, believing that getting along in the world of real people would mean abandoning his exciting world of fantasy. Since he, like his parents, had become pessimistic about his future, he stubbornly clung to his wild thoughts lest he be left with nothing.

Dirk resonated painfully to his parents' disappointment in him. Yet living with and teaching him made it imperative for those who knew him best to contain his aggression so that he might cope better in school. Dirk created so many emergencies, so many impasses between himself and others, that it was difficult to consider his talents.

I do believe, though, that too few people in his life recognized Dirk's startling use of intelligence. His parents doubted he was smart, because he seemed incapable of solving his social problems. Eventually Dirk's teacher concurred in this opinion. Tragically, what Dirk most wanted to hear from others was not how "stupidly" he sometimes acted but how smart he could be.

Attractions of the Social World

In her private world Marcia, who sang to signal her feelings, imagined no "social selves" so far as I knew or imaginary companions. She hadn't the equivalent of Donna Williams's "Carol," nor did she speak with a made-up personality as Stacy had done with "Little Rolly" and the paper doll "W." With few exceptions, she did not befriend her dormmates. Possibly the very idea of "friend" was foreign to her, unlike Stacy who used the term freely and would invent both friends and enemies ("bad people") with her all-too-fertile imagination. One exception for Marcia was an adept girl, Elsa, several years Marcia's junior, who was appalled by the mechanistic, unfeeling, and inhumane way Marcia treated her favorite doll.

Marcia permitted Elsa entry into her life because of Elsa's intense, genuine concentration on Marcia's doll play and the fervent determination she adopted to teach Marcia the correct way to feed a baby doll. Neglected as a child, Elsa sought to correct her own experience by playing with Marcia and turning her robotic ministrations into healthy, humane ones, even if these were given only to a doll. This single event, feeding a baby doll, exemplified both girls' feelings about their past: Marcia seemed to relinquish hope for humanity as she, in early childhood, turned away from people; and Elsa clung to hope's last vestiges, wishing that her future would be better despite the neglect she had suffered. Properly feeding a baby doll came to represent for both girls the nurturance they needed to sustain a human relationship.

Together they would sit side by side, teacher and student, as Elsa firmly but gently wrapped Marcia's arms around the doll and rocked

Marcia and her doll to demonstrate how a baby ought to be cradled, cradling Marcia so that by her own experience she would know how to be affectionate to others. When Marcia would stiffly insert the toy baby bottle into her doll's mouth, Elsa, protesting vigorously, would exclaim, outraged, *"That is no way to treat a baby!"* Then she would grab the toy bottle and, once more, show Marcia how to cradle the doll while holding the bottle gently in the doll's open mouth.

For a time Elsa was the only one among Marcia's peers to whom she'd speak regularly. Others might have tried to befriend her had she shown any sustained interest in them or had they not been resentful of the attention she garnered from the Orthogenic School staff. Marcia was one of those beautiful, dreamy-eyed, mysteriously compelling autistic children, vigilantly watchful but so far away, whose ethereal presence captivated her primary caretakers.

Yet Elsa soon chose to move out of Marcia's dormitory because of the impact relating to Marcia had on her. Trying so hard to lure her out of her dreamy solitude and guide her toward a less indifferent sociability, Elsa saw only too clearly just how entrenched Marcia was in her asocial ways. Despite all the benefits her relationship to Marcia might have had for both girls, Elsa needed more sympathetic and stimulating companions who would react to her more fully as a person. Part of the hardship autists have in making friends is the relentlessly forbidding effect they sometimes have on others who would be their friends. However possible it is that a young autist, motivated to find a friend, will exert some effort toward this goal, there is often the lingering feeling in the friend that the whole interpersonal edifice might topple at any moment.

Although she often created friends in her imagination, Stacy could not maintain a friendly attitude toward people for very long. To be sure, her imaginary friends did not act in Stacy's best interest as they bullied or provoked her. When she acted out the commands her pretend people gave, it seemed as if she were creating a folie à deux, make-believe though it was. Simultaneously she would blend her imaginary dramas with real conflicts. Sometimes they arose from her habit of checking her image in other people's eyes. Since the shadow of her very being could be seen in the eyes of another, that other seemed, to Stacy, to own her. Small wonder that she often engaged in power-of-the-will battles and attacked those who seemed to possess the precious "I" she lacked.

She'd roam two worlds simultaneously, speaking first to a bossy, even tyrannical imaginary person, and then to a real person she'd antagonized by her obstreperous behavior. Her imaginary enactments were so vivid, seemed so real, that I frequently found myself beseeching her pretend people to let Stacy be or to be nicer to her. Some of Stacy's peers reacted this way, too. Probably because they "defended" her against her imaginary demons, she felt protected by her companions, and this sentiment readied her for socializing. Her very first ventures, though, often degenerated into behavior reminiscent of her imaginary dramas. She seemed determined to recreate in real relationships the bullying, cajoling, and provoking psychological deal-making that she had heretofore realized only in her make-believe world.

As she recognized that she had evoked anger in the other girls, Stacy would either retreat from the social scene or attempt to retaliate for their rebuffs. Fortunately, her make-believe personae took on more varied and developed personalities, as if Stacy were practicing a different kind of relating. As a result, her overtures toward others became more attuned to their precise qualities, and thus held more promise. When Stacy tried to integrate another girl into her fantasies, she even used the girl's actual personality traits or life situations, having selected her because she truly fit the drama. If she were anxious about getting sick or hurting herself, and one of her dormmates also was sick or hurt, Stacy would enact a drama about the illness or injury, sometimes inventing imaginary disasters, sometimes concluding with a happy ending. Her prospective friend, in turn, would be variously amused, offended, involved, or remote, depending on whether Stacy's plans were benign, mischievous, consensual, or grotesque. Stacy counted as successes some of her interactions with others, which encouraged her to leave her fantasy world for the pleasures of the real.

Noticing other children mainly when they were sick or hurt did not endear her to them, nor did it always augur well for future liaisons. At first Stacy wasn't so much interested in making friends as she was in protecting herself from the tortuous anxieties she suffered about her own body's functioning. She tried to control her fears by learning as much as she could about the misfortunes of others. She wanted to know the causes of the mumps or the flu, of sores and scabs. She was frantic to know the nostrums, magical or otherwise, that might affect people's sufferings.

These efforts to protect herself by searching for the cause of every little bump and scratch, every ache and pain, both in herself and others, were met with disdain, anxiety, or downright rejection by the other children. They grimaced with disgust and fear when Stacy stared impertinently at the injury or badgered a child with a million questions.

Even these misdirected and invariably aborted attempts to interact with others served Stacy better than did the implacable aloneness of a child like Marcia. What's more, Stacy's pesky behavior allowed me to counsel her on how to approach other children as if she really wanted to be their friend. Why not, I thought, impute a "social" motive to Stacy since the seeds of wishing for friends had appeared in her make-believe dramas? I had had good results expecting that she'd make sense of my answers to her questions about the weather and refrigeration; so why not imagine a beneficial outcome to her struggles to be with her peers? An overly guarded, doubting attitude seemed cruel to me. Had I excised my hopes for this girl, I might have brought about the very result I feared, her return to a chimerical world in which she communed only with ghosts. I hoped that by imagining a social circle for Stacy, she, too, would consider the idea.

I praised Stacy for trying to find out how her peers were doing at the same time that I limited her verbal assaults. We had many talks about what actually caused the illness or injuries and what really remedied them. The conversations bound Stacy's fears at the same time that they taught her about aspects of the world.

The other children would sometimes participate in these talks, adding what, to them, were reasonable palliatives for what ailed them. The discussion often turned to psychological ills. Stacy heard time and again their various pep talks: "If you want to get better [psychologically], you have to try." Or, if Stacy bumped herself and lashed out at whoever was nearby, blaming a child for her suffering, they'd declare, "Stacy, nobody *made* you bump your knee. You just didn't see the chair," thus detoxifying one of Stacy's stubbornly rooted beliefs, that someone had deliberately caused her misery. She was so stimulus-sensitive that she was apt to blame the world from which the sensations appeared to emanate.

Once the notion sunk in that she could make things better for herself, she became fiercely competitive. Though competing at board games or learning to read brought her into greater contact with others, a boon to her socializing attempts, her cutthroat attitude menaced possible friendships as she determined to excel and overtake others. Her companions often concluded that she didn't care about their feelings, only how often she could best them. She was caught repeatedly between her achieving and affiliative needs, a not uncommon childhood dilemma. Children often agonize over their desire to excel and their need for friends.

Stacy and Marie

Young Stacy nevertheless became friends with two girls. Since she seemed capable of mastering just about anything, Samantha, who was several years older, became Stacy's inspiring mentor. Samantha read prolifically, was a whiz at checkers, excelled at arts and crafts, and had several lasting friendships among the teen cohort.

Stacy's other reliable friend, Marie, was about Stacy's age. Though not as bright as Stacy, Marie exuded an unruffled competence and her composed demeanor often infuriated Stacy. How could Marie maintain her aplomb, Stacy wondered, when who knew when the next thunderstorm would descend? Marie's personal differences aroused Stacy's curiosity and tended to stabilize both girls' attempts to secure their friendship.

Stacy and Marie initially joined one another as they tried to decide whether to play fantasy games or board games. Each held fast to the intractable stance that she should be the one to choose the first game. They jockeyed for the right to choose first and learned to negotiate with one another. Particularly Stacy, who'd never squared with anyone, gained from settling with Marie. Stacy always wanted to play "house" or "counselor" while Marie would choose simple board games, like Candyland, Chutes and Ladders, or Bridge-It.

In the sweetest voice she could muster, Stacy would tell Marie, "First we'll play 'counselor' and then we'll play Bridge-It." Stacy loved the game of "counselor," because if she were the "kid" she could act up without consequence since it was only a game—and anyway, Marie took the edge off Stacy's stunts by raising her voice authoritatively. Soon Stacy wanted to be the counselor and overly compliant Marie took great pleasure in strutting her stuff. For once, Stacy enjoyed being "good" as she playfully and noisily scolded Marie for throwing her stuffed animals around. One day, much to Stacy's delight, Marie became serious about acting up, heaving chairs as Stacy used to do and marking the walls with crayon. Stacy tattled on Marie self-righteously just as Marie had told on Stacy. Both girls were immensely pleased with themselves, toying with one another's typical behaviors. Soon they formed an easier rapport in which Stacy agreed, restlessly sometimes, to play board games with Marie.

Stacy had learned to play Marie's favorite game, Bridge-It, with me. Easy game though it was, I was still astonished at how quickly she grasped it. She not only learned the logic of this game but also began to question game logic generally. As she arranged her game pieces strategically to form part of a bridge to my side of the board, she asked, a little nervously, "What does 'win' mean? Does it mean to stop the game?" For her, winning a game was inextricably tied to a separation from her opponent—in this case, me. In fact, Stacy resisted the very idea of being an opponent; she wanted to be with me without the threat of a rift. She didn't really want to win the game, because then I might go on to something else. I might actually get angry and leave her, once and for all.

I assured Stacy that if she won the game we could always play another or do something else. She was surprised by the idea, because she thought the end to anything—even to a seemingly innocuous childhood pastime—meant the end of being with people. In a way, it was more liberating for her to play games with Marie, because she wasn't as invested in her relationship with Marie as with me, her primary caretaker. Also, Marie's sanguine flexibility about beginnings and endings and her unflappability seemed to reassure Stacy.

She'd invariably try to persuade Marie to play Bridge-It to Stacy's own advantage. When a direct request to do so had no effect, she tried to intimidate Marie by chanting, magically, "You'll stop blocking me; you'll *stop!*" This delighted Marie who, naturally, continued playing to her own advantage. When I would say something like, "Of course you both want to win; you're both kids," Stacy, to her credit, maintained herself in the game, although testily.

As much as Stacy resisted knowing that Marie would act in her own best interest, I still hoped to sensitize Stacy to the shared aspect of her experiences with Marie. Games with Marie, both real and pretend, had become important enough to Stacy for her to reconsider her earlier, tenaciously held notion that she could manipulate people just as she could objects. She realized that playing and talking with Marie were wholly different from dictating to "W," the oblong piece of paper whose affection and companionship she had imagined herself so earnestly coveting.

Still formidably insecure, Stacy thoroughly believed that real people, unlike her pretend people, could not like her. This was not an idle insecurity, since she often alienated others by her irksome antics and her outrageous instigations. She once remarked candidly, "I can be bad with pretend people, because they don't get mad." When she decided it was more enjoyable to be with real people, she began to ask incessantly of them, "Do you like me?" No amount of sincere assurance that we did seemed to matter, even if we addressed her likable qualities. Even when I would give her a hug, she would, releasing herself from my arms, stand off at a distance and invariably probe, "Do you like me?" "Why else would I give you a hug?" I'd reply, knowing the same question would be repeated many times over before the day was done.

Stacy wished to control aspects of my affection for her. Although she didn't try to regulate the pressure of my arms around her as Marcia had, she did feel compelled to calibrate the quality of my stated feeling for her. Words, especially *like*, were not to be believed facilely. They had to be accompanied by the true happy face and sensate emotion.

Stacy's good times with Marie nuanced her feelings toward me. Attending to Marie meant she must attune herself to Marie's attachment to me, since I was often invited to enter their play or settle their disputes. Once, following one of Stacy's outbursts, I said, "Maybe you think I like Marie better than I like you." I knew I was treading on thin psychological ice since there was not the merest suggestion from Stacy that she'd take to any insinuation at all that I also liked Marie.

"Go to hell, deep dark hell," Stacy intoned murkily.

"I didn't *say* I like Marie better. I said maybe you are *afraid* I will like her better than I like you."

"Oh."

Strange, I thought, that this brilliant, linguistically gifted charge of mine would so easily confuse an intimation of what might be true with what is actually true.

Stacy soon widened her social circle to include another girl about a year older, Julie. Stacy would approach Samantha almost affectionately, asking the older girl if she would teach her how to play checkers. Sometimes bossy Stacy even asked to join Marie and Julie in a game already in progress. If they happened to be making tents out of chairs and blankets, Stacy would beg to participate. Then the three girls would hide in their tents and giggle until someone found them. Stacy had always loved playing hide-and-seek but played the game of "getting lost" only with me, trusting me enough, I supposed, to "find" her, because I seemed to want to be with her. Now she risked being "lost" when it would be other children who found her. She trusted that they liked her enough to want to be with her.

Once the game took an unusual turn when Stacy began to elaborate on it by pretending she and her friends were camping and building a campfire outside the tent. Then she became frightened by the idea of fire. She also assumed that the others would be equally frightened, and possibly offended, by her introduction of this scary notion. Instead of leaving the scene in a panic or acting so obnoxiously that the others would refuse to play, she introduced one of her dolls to the girls as "Karen" and had the doll protect them from the imaginary campfire.

Much like ordinary children, Stacy could finally put aside her fears and find enjoyment in the kind of childhood games that lead to general learning. By mastering real games and by elaborating dramas that more nearly fit actual experiences or that appealed to her companions, Stacy prepared herself for more extended commerce with the world.

Stacy and Samantha

Stacy's friend Samantha was fond of watching the younger girls' inventive antics, particularly Stacy's, and often listened to the conversations I had with them. Once, much amused, Samantha told me she'd witnessed Stacy engineer a game of Duck, Duck, Goose with Marie and Julie in such a way as to deliberately catch the older girl's attention. In this circle game the child who is "it" runs around the perimeter of the circle the children have formed, reciting, "Duck, duck," finally tapping one child on the shoulder, crying, "Goose." This child chases the person who is "it," who rushes to her place in the circle so as not to be caught, else she is "it" again.

Roguishly transforming real friends into make-believe personae, instead of saying "goose" Stacy began to chant the names of her favorite pretend characters. "Duck, duck, W!" she shouted gleefully. Then, for Samantha's benefit, she switched to famous pop singers to make this rather repetitive game interesting for herself and her friends, especially Samantha, who was thrilled to hear Stacy call out, "Duck, duck, Elvis Presley!" On hearing Presley's name, adolescent Samantha—much to everyone's delight—could no longer resist joining in this prosaic pastime. The girls enjoyed Stacy's vivacious clowning immensely, so much so that she became ecstatically giddy. Yet for once she remained sufficiently composed to continue playing.

Soon Samantha invited Stacy to play hide-and-seek. At first, Stacy wanted to be "it" so that she could find Samantha. The older girl eventually persuaded Stacy that it was her turn to hide. Stacy hid her eyes as many younger children do, believing for the moment that because she could not see, she herself could not be seen. Giggling, Samantha exclaimed, "Just because you can't see me doesn't mean I can't see you!" At this Stacy instantly uncovered her eyes and found a hiding place for her whole self. When it was again Samantha's turn to hide, Stacy shut her eyes, then unabashedly but quietly opened them and, with a smirk, calmly observed as Samantha went off to hide. At first, the other girls, who were watching, didn't notice that Stacy was cheating, but her witty behavior started me laughing. Now really hamming it up, she began to prop her eyes wide open with her fingers lest anyone miss the comedy, which sent the girls into gales of laughter.

By way of original, often funny, variations on games intended to delight and amuse others, Stacy better understood that her friends had their own perspectives. During the game of hide-and-seek, Samantha could "teach" this to Stacy, because she'd admired Samantha for so long.

In her absorbing book, *The Scientist in the Crib*, psychologist Alison Gopnik describes something similar. In an experiment with young children, she found that they initially clung to a "false belief"; they insisted that they had always thought pencils were in a candy box instead of the candy they expected to see. They changed their minds about what they initially believed after an adult gave them systematic evidence to the contrary. The children were told outright that they had said candy was in the box. They experienced a "big, sweeping change, a sort of theoretical revolution." They also became open to counter-evidence generally.[9]

In much the same way, Stacy reacted propitiously to "contrary data"—which arose from a different perspective in the hide-and-seek game—presented to her by an older, trusted person. The child's living context and that of a psychology lab produced an analogous result!

So when Samantha offered to help Stacy's teacher and me instruct Stacy in the basics of reading and spelling, she responded willingly, even eagerly. Who wouldn't want to be taught by an idolized mentor from whom one had already learned such valuable lessons and had fun in the bargain?

Probably because she, too, had once been a confused, sometimes unwilling student, believing she was not quite up to tackling school subjects, Samantha sympathized with Stacy's learning insecurities and could imagine the younger girl's reasons for becoming fiercely competitive, since Samantha's own successes were based on an intense need to excel. Determined that Stacy, too, would learn to read, Samantha sat for hours reading books to her, discussing the pictures and story themes.

When Samantha would read with Stacy, I'd use educator Sylvia Ashton-Warner's teaching method in my work with Marcia, hoping to supplement the learning experiences she had in class.[10] Samantha noticed that I wrote single words of Marcia's choosing on separate pieces of paper for her to arrange in sentences if she would. Marcia and I often didn't get beyond her intoning her chosen words methodically, sometimes angrily, when she would avert her gaze, refusing to string the words together to form a sentence. But Samantha and Stacy were fascinated by the idea.

Samantha soon asked Stacy what words she'd like to read. Then Stacy supplied words that represented her pet topics: names of her pretend people, her teacher's and her counselors' names, the address of the Orthogenic School, names of her favorite foods, and Samantha's own name. Eventually the girls had collected about fifty words. Samantha then added prepositions and conjunctions, words with little meaning for Stacy as they weren't as vivid in her mind as those that named people and places, actions, and a few descriptors. "Good" and "bad" were quickly added to the pile.

Stacy, like many children learning to read, became angry and frustrated when she couldn't recognize a word instantly. Everyone watching would suddenly, tensely, fall silent, fearing that Stacy would blow it and ruin the lesson by having a temper outburst. Much to everyone's relief, she stuck with it, her efforts to sustain herself in the lesson praised and appreciated by Samantha. One day when Stacy was tempted to erupt with an angry invective, she put her finger to her lips and whispered to herself, "Shhh!" A few minutes later she read the word correctly.

Much like the Maori children Ashton-Warner taught, Stacy sometimes intruded her feelings into the reading lesson. She had previously acted upon her feeling that she was "bad" by attacking others, making messes, screaming obscenities, and being hopelessly provocative. Now she *spoke* her reasons for acting up. "I came to the [Orthogenic] School very, very bad," she moaned dourly. She took this feeling of self to the reading lesson with Samantha, writing, "Bad Stacy." I objected vehemently to her statement, whereupon she hid the word *bad* behind her back. Then Samantha protested Stacy's characterization of self. With an appreciative, knowing grin, Stacy dropped the word *bad* and brought forth the word *good* to write, "Good Stacy."

When she was with Samantha, Stacy read and spelled more easily than she did in class, probably because she realized that she lagged behind some of the other students, especially one proficient reader who was younger than she. She caused a ruckus in the classroom so that, as she told me angrily and vengefully, the others could not concentrate on their work. When I asked, "Why not concentrate on your work instead of theirs?" she answered wistfully, "To catch up, you mean?," a doubtful look flooding her face.

The more Stacy tried to master the language basics with Samantha, the more vulnerable she felt about herself as a person. She was desperate to know that she was "good" at reading and that people liked her. She was proud that she could read better than Marie, but she still thought I'd like Marie better, especially if Marie were to learn to read as well as she. "Do you like me or just Marie?" she'd ask pointedly, perceiving her comparison a zero-sum game. She'd soon continue, "Is just Marie good or is just Stacy good?" When I explained that she and Marie were good in their own distinct ways or when I'd say for the umpteenth time how much I liked *her*, she'd counter, "Even when I do bad stuff?" Something was missing from my attempts to reassure her.

So I tried again. "Here at the School there are no just bad or just good children. Everyone has bad feelings sometimes. You are not bad, Stacy, because of bad feelings."

"Do you like me?" came her rapid response.

"Yes, I like you very much."

"Even when I act up and throw chairs?"

"When you act up and throw chairs, I get mad and upset," I told her, "but deep down I always like you."

Still skeptical, she gazed at me for a long time, lest some flicker of ambivalence cloud my face. Poised to intercept an angry, violent outburst that Stacy might produce just to prove, once more, she was bad, I stood my ground until she stopped staring at me and went off to play counselor with Marie.[11]

As she became ever more involved in her lessons with Samantha, Stacy projected onto them some of her deepest concerns. In an attempt to make "that world out there" safe, she fused it with her familiar but inner, private world. The way she talked about her reading lessons with Samantha revealed how deeply absorbed Stacy had become in the ideas generated by what she read. The reading discussions thus had the same imaginative quality that her conversations with "W" had had.

Perhaps the reason for the figurative quality in the language of linguistically gifted autists is their tendency to relate to the real world through their often rosy-colored, personal lenses. One had only to gaze upon Stacy's joyous, beaming face when she was talking to her paper doll to realize how exuberant she felt merging her real teacher with

the imaginary "W." Just as poets seek to express themselves by probing the depths of their inner experience, some autists are equally attuned to that precious inner self, which they live out, voicing it ever
so cryptically.

Donna Williams's writing is poetically evocative. Referring to the
conflict she felt about subjecting herself to society by publishing her
first book, she contrasts the child within her with the adult. "Was it
the want of my heart or had it been the compulsion of my fear to
burn the manuscript of *Nobody Nowhere* after coming out of the
closet to just one person who would read it? . . . Or was it," she continues, "the want of my child heart?" Likening the child within to a
prisoner and the adult to someone on the outside, she combines both
"wants" splendidly: "Perhaps my adult heart had a want that went
beyond this, cradled in the arms of a sense of humanity and morality
that evaded my child-heart, like the view on the other side of the walls
of a prison that evades the prisoner contained within them."[12]

No stranger to metaphor, Williams allusively defines her social distance. Using the number *one* to signify a person, she remarks that, to
her, one plus one always equaled one. This personal equation referred
to her unrelatedness to anyone. She remained within herself, the only
one. Until her friendship with Ian, she did not easily "compute" with
others.

Since Stacy's use of language was similarly evocative, her alluring
metaphors naturally transferred from spoken language to the reading
of simple words and sentences. One day when Samantha was shuf-
fling through Stacy's word stack, her favorites called out from memory ("swimming pool . . . Samantha! . . . cherry soda . . . *The Honey
Hunt* . . . Marie!"), Samantha couldn't locate some of them. One elusive word was *yes*. Realizing that her friend was searching for a "lost
yes" threw Stacy into a despondent frenzy. "What happens," she
wailed, "if the 'yes' gets lost?"

For years Stacy had avoided even saying the word *yes*. *Yes* appeared either to have no meaning for her or was so noxious that she side-stepped the word entirely. Maybe she didn't want to say *yes*, because she feared it would negate her old reliable standby, *no*. Now, missing the printed word *yes*, she agonized over whether she could, or would, somehow return to that insulated, non-yes state when she was unable to welcome the invitations, ideas, and sentiments of others. The "lost yes" meant to Stacy the disavowal of the social affirmative. This because she so completely, so emotionally, identified the paper on which the word was printed with its referent, so tenuous was her understanding that, however intimately related, a word is distinct from that to which it refers. Yet we call it poetic license if an artist willfully exploits the suggestive nuances of a concept like the lost yes. "We make out of the quarrel with others, rhetoric," William Butler Yeats counsels, "but out of the quarrel with ourselves, poetry."[13] Stacy turned her rhetoric into a poetic: before she tried to convince others of the worth of her thoughts, feelings, and actions—of the worth of herself, really—and now she quarreled with herself over becoming a person who says yes.

"But we can always find the 'yes,'" I implored, wishing to reassure her and to respond sensitively to the poetry in her language. "And even if we can't find it we can always write 'yes' again and again." At that moment Samantha found the *yes* paper, and the two girls continued working on Stacy's sentences without further ado. The implicit *yes* in their continuing to be together and to read almost brought me to tears.

Young Stacy was almost ten but was neither capable of writing poetry, even though she spoke metaphorically, nor was she the age at which children generally begin to master reading and writing. Youngsters typically begin to coordinate the relationship between the spoken and written word and the ways in which literal meaning differs from story meaning in third or fourth grade, ordinarily before the age of ten, the age at which Stacy reacted imaginatively to the lost word, *yes*.

Yet Stacy's autism may have helped her find poetry in her reading lessons, late bloomer that she was. Perhaps she brought artistry to learning precisely because she was a late-developing reader. Some of her immaturities, including her emotional reaction to the printed word as if it were its referent, may have allowed, even encouraged her to create a poetic symbol, the lost yes. "[I]t is perhaps best to think of the mind of the five-year-old as a curious blend of strengths and weaknesses, powers and limitations," writes Howard Gardner in *The Unschooled Mind*. "[I]n its artistic endeavors, it can be creative and imaginative."[14] Though Stacy's mind had advanced in many ways beyond that of a five-year-old, her gifts and her immaturities stood side by side as she entered a communicating world. Very like a five-year-old, she showed strengths and powers in her artistic creations. Could she have learned, I now wonder, to arrange words to form poems even if she wasn't yet a fluent reader or a legible writer?

Could the mysterious, inspiring, audacious combination of unexpected pockets of talent, readiness, context, and dedication characteristic of Stacy's experience be found in that of other intelligent young autists?

Despite the trials entailed in friend-making between an autist and his companion, difficulties can be overcome when the two potential friends find themselves in auspicious circumstances. One of these potentially liberating situations is the regular classroom. There the young autist is not surrounded by children who suffer the same social malaise as he does but is tempted, despite his insecurities and his invidious comparisons, to join in the learning and the fun with inquisitive and energetic classmates. If the ordinary private or public school is able to modify its curriculum and its procedures to accommodate a few young autists, regular classrooms offer these children the benefits of an engaging course of study and the opportunity to participate with other students in a give-and-take exchange of ideas. For those who can manage its demands, there is probably no better forum to draw young autists out of their private worlds than a regular classroom headed by an enthusiastic teacher. One such public school setting is the topic of the next chapter.

CHAPTER NINE

School Days

About the autistic kids I'd tell my teachers, "They're not going
to be responsive right away. You're going to have to look
closely to see what's happening. Helping them is really
a matter of liking them."
—PUBLIC SCHOOL PRINCIPAL

In spring of 1996 I was invited to visit a regular first-grade classroom of a public school in which there were six children with special needs. Before the visit I'd had many talks with the principal about the efforts of her teachers to engage personally with the children and to teach them. Five of the six had been provisionally or firmly diagnosed as autistic or as exhibiting behaviors typical of the autistic spectrum. The sixth child was hearing-impaired. I had begun working on this book by then and from it I prepared a short talk to interested faculty and the parents of the autistic students. Utterly fascinated by what I'd observed in the class, I arranged for three more visits in subsequent years to monitor the effect of the teachers' efforts and the appeal the school's curriculum had for the children. My last visit, in the spring of 1999, happened to be the principal's final year, an anticipated event that the autistic boys had been dealing with since her announcement earlier that year.

Four boys in the autistic group were seven years old; the fifth was eight. They'd been enrolled in the same class a year earlier, when the special program for these children was designed. That year, the principal told me, was the first time the school—for that matter, any school in the town—had developed a classroom to accommodate the particular needs of young autists. Before this, there had been a separate class to mainstream children with special needs, or mainstreaming had consisted of atypical children, for example, Down's syndrome children in addition to autistic children, enrolled in a regular class but with a substantially different curriculum. In 1995 the town's special education department asked the kindergarten teacher to include in her class a small group of young autists and provided the classroom with two aides and auxiliary teachers, specifically an occupational therapist, a speech therapist, a gym teacher to help the autistic kids adapt to the same curriculum offered to the others. This team approach, so critical to integrating these youngsters in a regular classroom, was headed by the enthusiastic kindergarten teacher and was such a success that she was asked to take the young autists to first and second grades. For three years, this teacher coordinated the efforts not just of the aides and the other teachers who helped out but also of the boys' parents and any psychotherapeutic or other mental health professionals involved with these children.

The autistic boys, so far as I could observe, felt a part of this small classroom of eighteen children. (One of the autists moved out of the area the year after my first visit, so I had little opportunity to observe him.) They engaged with their teachers, sometimes enthusiastically, and they responded personally, sometimes affectionately, to their main teacher. Each in his own way related to her, sought comfort from her during tense moments about his ability to fit in with what I soon began to think of as the classroom's exceptionally enticing ambience.

The Public School

This particular school was in many ways like no other I'd seen in my years of visiting public and private schools for talks, consultations, or meetings on how to advance a child's learning. There were many lovely touches in the way the learning spaces were arranged. Parts of it were built up on levels, giving the impression of a school without walls. On every level there were open spaces where kids could gather in small groups. Gazing at levels above and below me I often wondered how children felt about being elevated or netherward, protected, to be sure, by obstructions such as railings and bookcases. Kids can look up at or down on various classroom activities and be soothed by or get curious about the low hum of voices speaking of schoolwork and friendships, of home life the previous weekend, of recess or lunch to come. Much that's happening is potentially visible but doesn't seem to detract from the children's ability to concentrate on what they're doing. From top to bottom, interesting curricular materials are on display: for example, an array of math puzzles, or a terrific mural done by some older children, a brightly hued assembly of tiles representing people of various ethnicities in colorful outfits. Roaming the premises with its vermilion stairwells was a visual pleasure right down to the lowest level where even a dank hallway was lightened by another gorgeous mural, this time hand-painted. I imagined the children walking through, uplifted as they viewed the painting's design and dazzling color. The library, likewise, was an open space, yet distinct from the others. Children attended art, music, and gym in spaces appropriately furnished and equipped. I felt lucky to be able to visit these special rooms to familiarize myself with the ways in which these subjects were taught to the autistic students and the impact the curriculum had on them.

On my first visit I was ushered by the principal into the first grade class and introduced to its teacher, who greeted me warmly. Experienced, cheerful, and energetic, she approached her class with didactic care. Rather than merely direct children or modify their behavior according to a fixed agenda, she'd alter, on the spot, the situation facing the child in order to refocus or interest him in what he was required to do. She'd approach a young autist who was dreamily gazing at the ceiling, flipping and dropping his pencil, take hold of his hand so as to help him grip the pencil more firmly, or give him a rubdown on his back, only then to instruct, "You'll need to focus now." She had enticed him away from the isolating, solipsistic state he'd been in and had created a psychological space in which he might learn. She later told me she'd read Temple Grandin's *Thinking in Pictures* and, in fact, had this very book in her classroom. She had even attended one of Grandin's lectures. The author's descriptions of her squeeze machine and its relaxing effects prompted the teacher to rub the shoulders and back of a tense young autist.

The teacher directed me toward a chair marked "visitor," an implicit welcome and a signal to the children that, while I was not their teacher or an aide, I might nevertheless be interested in what they were doing. As I looked around, I was struck by the spaciousness of the setting. There were four discernible sections to the large room, delineated by the furniture and equipment but open for all to observe the ongoing activities. The main section was larger than the other three and consisted of tables and chairs at which children grouped themselves for reading, science, or math. Adjacent was the section where the children first gathered in the morning to go over the day's schedule and to share ideas and discuss topics of interest. The third section was a roomy play area, almost as large as the main portion of the classroom, the most notable item in it being a large yellow bouncing ball to which one of the autistic boys would retreat when nervous or overwrought or simply to have fun. The fourth section, smaller than the others, was where children often worked on their language arts workbooks. The kids could work in two of the spaces, talk in another, and play in yet another.

An ongoing science project occupied the largest classroom space. There were numerous displays scattered around it and nature posters on the board showing how seeds grow into plants. The overall theme of these displays was the continuity of living things. Some of the posters consisted of artistic renditions of butterfly larvae, the insect stages laid out for the children to observe. Another showed how flowers grow and reseed themselves. Information was readily available on how our feeding and caring for plants help them grow. There were many living plants in the room, including some beautiful African violets. One decorative flower, a three-dimensional pastiche made by the children, was an interesting mélange of color, charming but not sanitized, thank goodness, lacking that fake perfection characterizing the art in so many classrooms.

A winsome poem, printed in bold, dark handwriting, tacked to an easel in the middle of the room, made it easy for children to read or to follow when their teacher read it to them. Titled "Polly's Butterfly," it was about the metamorphosed insect flying around, finally landing on Polly's nose.

The Autistic Boys

The autistic boy who first caught my attention was an alert youngster who was not immediately conspicuous as different. After some minutes, I did notice that he would dart his head first in one direction, then in another, in what initially seemed to be an effort to avert his gaze from his teacher's face. Soon I realized that he'd briefly scan the face not just of his main teacher but also that of the American Sign Language (ASL) teacher who was signing to the hearing-impaired girl. Then he'd jerk his head around to watch her reactions. This boy wasn't so much looking *away* from someone as he was looking *toward* the main object of interest, the adult who was attending primarily to another special needs kid. What a wrong conclusion I'd drawn in thinking this boy was avoiding eye contact with his main teacher!

After class his teacher told me that he'd been fascinated by sign language and had actually begun to learn some of the signs while watching the ASL teacher communicate with his classmate. He'd observe the signing and then propel his head around to observe the girl's reaction, then abruptly turn his head toward the teacher again. He was obviously following a gestured, silent conversation between the two. I had the impression he did not want to miss a thing that was going on between the hearing-impaired child and her special teacher.

Soon I noticed another autistic boy, a year older than the others. I picked up on this boy's unusual behavior and on his teacher's approach to him, which differed from how she dealt with the others. She was extra-clear in her remarks, trying to make sure he heard and understood what he was asked to do. Both boys spoke intelligibly, but the one who'd learned sign language spoke in short staccato bursts while the other spoke so softly it was difficult to hear him. As long as he was the focus of the teacher's attention, he appeared to follow the conversation, which was about Earth Day, and softly answered his teacher's questions monosyllabically or with a few words. As soon as the children dispersed for language arts, this attractive, rather babyish looking eight-year-old ran to the play area where he began to bounce enthusiastically on the yellow rubber ball, his eyes rolling, catching sight of distant objects in a strange, excited fashion. He appeared to smile at nothingness, presumably fantasizing. Until, as I rather sheepishly realized, he seemed to be playing a sort of peekaboo with his teacher and his classmates, who were working at the language arts table in a part of the main room slightly more elevated than the play area. I got up from where I'd been sitting to observe him better, and sure enough, he'd catch sight of his teacher and the others, whom he eyed perkily on the up bounce, then block them from view on the down bounce. Wondering why I hadn't originally spotted his antics, I noticed he looked at me once or twice in a kind of bounce-up-and-see-people, bounce-down-and-not-see-people game. So even this autistic boy, who had a much harder time focusing on his schoolwork than did the others, showed he was not totally rejecting of people. Rather, he had mixed feelings about observing them. He wanted to control when he saw them and when he didn't.

Later he repeatedly isolated himself, tempting the others to pursue, even chase him, to be brought back with a smirk to join in the day's activities. He enjoyed the influence he exerted over being with people: he did exactly what he knew would get the others to go after him. His teacher didn't say, "You must come back and sit down and do your work." When he got up from his seat to bounce on the rubber ball, she said instead, "Remember you need to tell me where you are going." Perhaps, I thought, she was just as interested in socializing this boy as she was in teaching him. She'd created a situation in which he'd have to take responsibility for his actions: he must inform his teacher if he chose to isolate himself, something he readily complied with.

It had also been impressed upon him repeatedly that his decision to leave was followed by being pursued and brought back to the world of people. I hoped he'd gotten some inkling of his responsibility for this part of the bargain. And indeed he was brought back to the language arts table by one of the aides. He hadn't just taken strategic advantage of the break between chat time and work time to sneak in a bit of exciting bouncing and amusing fantasy; he had also practiced a bit of socializing: now you see me, now you don't; now I run away, now I get chased.

A third boy, quiet and retiring, avoided looking straight at people. He seemed shy, dreamy, and almost fragile. Although his speech was more forthcoming and audible, more natural sounding than that of the other two autists, this child was noticeably out of it. He'd sequester himself next to a bookcase whenever he could, flipping pages of several books, seeming to read some of them. He'd been described as "hyperlexic" by his teacher who, during lunch break, related compassionately how withdrawn he'd been the previous year. She was not sure he comprehended what he read, and she described how he had refused to enter the classroom and how he'd head for the nearest secluded area he could find. He'd read absorbedly for a while, but at other times I'd see him nervously turning the book's pages, smiling subtly to himself. Perhaps he meandered through the text rather than concentrating fully on it. Some three years later, his teacher told me that he'd begun a chapter book series, often carrying one of the books in his pocket, opening it up during scheduled free times to resume reading absorbedly.

Suddenly I was distracted by one of the boys blurting out, "Where is the clock?" It was the boy who'd been bouncing on the yellow ball just minutes before. So he wasn't merely gazing randomly as he scanned the environment. He was searching for an important classroom item that was missing from its rightful place. He first looked up at the ceiling, though, as if he weren't doing anything in particular, then searched for the missing clock, dropping his pencil noisily, becoming quite disorganized as he strenuously avoided his teacher's directions, until she was able to focus him once more on his workbook pages. Even then it took a lot of doing to hold his attention. She gave him his pencil and took his hand to hold it on the line he was supposed to be reading. Interspersed with his mostly accurate reading, he obsessed about the page number because the handmade work pages were out of order. As his teacher explained that a page was misnumbered, he refocused briefly, only to start smiling to himself as he searched, yet again, for the missing clock.

I wondered how his teacher could maintain her steady composure with all the implied rejections of her teaching. She even realized there might be a psychological reason for his deliberate avoidance of the work she'd laid out for him, an aversion that took the form of arguing about page numbers or remarking on classroom lapses (the missing clock). There was a sentence to which he was expected to supply the correct word from several choices. It was clear to me that he understood what he was reading, because when he came to the correct choice, he put his hands to his face, palms to his eyes and nose, then pushed the paper away as he reared back in his seat a bit and made a face. His teacher took the cue and said, "Yes, you don't like to read about fire."

This empathic observation seemed to make him even more desperately inattentive. His teacher immediately suggested that he skip the troublesome exercise and go on to the next. Then and only then did he complete the last two correctly. In order to bring this boy back to the lesson, his teacher had to help him evade a noxious stimulus, the word *fire*, and move around the table close to him so that her stated aim to help him concentrate better would more easily sink in. Again, she rubbed down his back and arms, which he seemed to like, as a young child likes to be cuddled. Then he finished his work. He wrote his name legibly and drew a circle around the correct answers.

Because he'd been absent, I didn't get to meet the fourth autistic boy until the next day. Diagnosed as having an autistic spectrum disorder, he could be dreamy like the others, but I soon noticed that he was more direct and forceful than they were in rejecting parts of his assigned work or some of his teacher's suggestions. His classmate, our shy autist with whom this boy could be friendly yet fiercely competitive, would retire inconspicuously into his own world or else act like nothing of interest was happening around him. His more assertive peer, a late reader, would strenuously avert his face when he was given something to read, or turn himself away from the work when it didn't please him. Yet he'd be openly curious about certain other portions of the lesson. His teacher told me that, even though he wrote illegibly, he'd suddenly begun to draw and showed an interesting artistic gift. Earlier he had only consented to scribble a few marks on the page, but now he drew recognizable animals, centered aesthetically and surrounded by attractively arranged flora. His relationships with his peers, while not easy, were maintained by his hamming it up with the other boys to gain their approval, perhaps to become one of them.

The School's Culture

Piecing together my impressions, I realized that the teachers of the young autists had adapted the curriculum and the pedagogy to their needs without forfeiting the educational values of the school as a whole. The teachers would inaugurate their autistic students to school procedures and policies, as well as to important facets of the curriculum, so as to promote cohesion not just among the autistic cohort but also between the autists and the rest of the class.

I soon grasped that the key to integrating young autists in this regular classroom was the school's people-oriented style. For example, the school's "three R's" consisted of respect for self, respect for others, and respect for property. The faculty was committed to integrating socializing and learning and to acknowledging the children's feelings about learning. This was true whether the comfortable being-together occurred during the lesson or in the kids' interactions or as they listened to their teachers' thoughts and feelings, freely expressed, about their workday—their personal reactions to the benefits and pitfalls of their lessons. The teachers' style was neither sentimental touchy-feeliness nor an alien and arbitrary imposition of "social adjustment" protocol. Rather, what people felt about each other could, and did, influence the teaching and learning experience naturally, including when things went wrong.

Teachers shared with one another an easy, companionable camaraderie that must have suggested to their students that it was okay for them, too, to express themselves, and that it might even be helpful for them to do so when events didn't turn out as they wished. Teachers frequently commented to the children and to each other about their own state of mind. Yet this was done in an entirely respectful, sometimes humorous way. Once, during music class, the teachers conferred openly about the schedule for the remainder of the school year. They joked when none of them could remember exactly when school let out and commiserated with one another about the hardships of teaching. The students, including the autists, listened attentively, some smiling indulgently, as if sharing feelings is to be expected. The students might have felt just as strongly as their teachers that the school year had had its hardships. I thought it just fine that teachers felt free to express how hard it is to teach. Then the children might concede that it is indeed hard to learn, true to fact, and a boon to their self-esteem when they experienced setbacks.

When I remarked to the principal on the respect the teachers showed the children and the freedom with which they spoke in front of them, on the "we're-all-in-this-together" feeling I had about the school, she replied, "That's the thing I like about our open spaces— we're obliged to respect one another." Continuing emphatically, "You know what chaos would reign—are you kidding me?—if we didn't treat each other respectfully?"

If a teacher, concerned about her students' well-being, could share the children's frustrations about a work page not having been printed clearly or the classroom's being hot and humid—two classroom commonplaces—then the children, even the autists, might feel free to express themselves when things didn't work out as expected. Especially the young autists, typically behind the others in learning or tending to make it something private and personal, might be reassured by the effects of genuine conversation. Even if they never actually availed themselves of the opportunity to complain or protest, the humanization of learning in their school setting, I thought, could hardly fail to serve them—even to impress them. The classroom's atmosphere communicated to the children, particularly to the autists, that it's perfectly normal to express oneself.

Respecting others' feelings inheres in this school's social climate. "The kids understand that the respect is there, day in and day out, that they will be kind, try to get along, work together to solve problems, be accepting and warm to others," the principal explained. "I don't ask the kids to be friends necessarily. I say to them, 'Maybe you don't want to be on the same ball team, and that's okay. But if you *are* on the same team, you ought to play respectfully with one another.'" The primary gift this school provides its autists may be its social influence. As much as the children learned academically, their everyday learning seemed part and parcel of the curriculum's socializing benefits that taught about being a person.

Lessons

A significant aspect of the school, one which pervaded the curriculum and was especially helpful to the young autists, was its teachers' sensitivity to slight changes in the kids' ability to adapt, to a bit of enhanced productivity in them, often traceable to their teachers' pedagogic efforts. I had arrived for my first school visit the week before summer break. Each of the teachers was summarizing the year, attending to the ways in which the children had grown since September. In art class, the day's agenda had the children review their art work since the year's beginning, to assemble it into their folders. They were to attach the piece of art they liked best to the outside of the folder and explain to the class why it was their favorite.

One young autist stood out from the rest as he sifted through his amazing pencil drawings of dinosaurs, one of which had a very small American flag in the center of the page, the animals on the periphery, arranged carefully into a pleasing configuration. Might the artist have imagined the animals saluting the flag? The aesthetic effect of juxtaposing the prehistoric dinosaur with a modern flag struck me as unusual. His teacher, nodding in agreement, showed me this boy's earlier art work. He'd progressed from erratic scribbling to an ingenious pictorial rendition.

One of his autistic classmates, about the same age, remained at the scribbling stage and, in fact, did not progress much beyond this until two years later, when he created a colorful collage at the same time he used a journal assignment to trace his progress in reading and writing. This year, he'd jerk his head around in art class to remind himself what to do next by observing the others assiduously drawing, only to flip his pencil between his fingers or drop crayons noisily.

It wasn't until he was almost nine that he would create a colorful collage of reds, oranges, pinks, and blacks; it made me feel bombarded by exciting stimuli, as he himself may have felt. The same year he wrote in his journal about learning to read. When his teacher asked him to write about his school memories, he wrote that he couldn't read in second grade, that he could only read little words, like "the" and "big." He described how he would ask his friends when he didn't understand a word. He wrote that he'd ask his teacher for help sometimes. He had used the computer to compose his story, and there was one misspelling and some punctuation errors. He also wrote that he would ask for help if he didn't know how to pronounce—to say—a word. About asking for help with pronunciation, he seemed to reminisce that he was assisted not just with reading but also with talking. Maybe, I thought, that's why he'd been so fascinated by the ASL signing in first grade. The gestural language could have bridged his mute moments with his struggles to talk. He ended his little story by writing, "Now I'm in fourth grade and I can read hard books."

An autistic classmate also scribbled at the beginning of his first grade year. Though he didn't appear to be graced with a striking artistic bent, his self-portraits in the spring had become quite personal. When asked to select his favorite art, he sighed audibly, "But I like *all* of it!" He'd divided the page into four sections and had put a stick figure of a boy with glasses into each with a prominent head and the eyes bearing glasses even more so. The figure representing himself was drawn consistently across renditions, revealing that he had a graphic schematic sense. His self-concept appeared predictable and had become stable at the expected age of about seven years. I'm suggesting that attributing an artistic schema to this boy's drawing is a more accurate description of its development than to ascribe it to autistic perseveration.[1]

Another drawing his teacher showed me consisted of four faces, all with different emotional expressions. They reminded me of Stacy's cartoonish drawings, the people having obvious smiles, upside-down grins denoting sadness, exaggerated wide-eyed looks to suggest surprise, or a straight horizontal line symbolizing seriousness. Were these two young autists, who showed a distinct predilection for portraying human emotion, also mocking the very feelings they so capriciously pictured? Doesn't mockery of emotion reveal an implicit understanding of it?

The oldest autist of the group I'd been observing drew a serious family portrait. Each person was represented by a fleshed-out human figure with shapes approximating body limbs, hands and fingers, and torso. He had conspicuously omitted two sense organs—the eyes and the ears. I wondered whether he attempted to communicate in this way that these bodily organs offended him, because he himself had frequently felt inundated by sights and sounds, especially if more than one sensory modality had been activated simultaneously. He seemed quite satisfied, even complacent, with his portrait and its omissions. In class he'd control sensory input by trying to take charge not just of the clock, as described before, but also of the electric lights. Turning them on or off seemed to make their stimulation more tolerable. At least they were under his purview.

One day his classroom was unbearably hot. His teacher, noting the children's lethargy and their audible sighs and yawns, remarked about the heat and how hard it must be for the children to concentrate. As soon as his teacher said that the children might be getting tired, our young autist appeared to anticipate that she'd suggest the overhead light be turned off to reduce the heat. As she started to speak, he got up from his seat with a great sense of purpose and marched across the room to flick the light switch. A few students called out his name exasperatedly as though he'd diverted their attention from their work. Instantly, his teacher emerged from her seat to talk to the children who were complaining, and said she'd asked him to turn off the lights to reduce the heat so the children could concentrate better. Our young autist stood nearby, listening attentively, as his teacher continued to explain in a friendly, matter-of-fact way that he'd understood just what she wanted done and that perhaps the others hadn't heard her request.

A little later, it was time for music class, and the young autist headed for the play area instead of standing in line with the other children. Another child went to fetch him and tapped him on the shoulder to remind him about lining up for music. Our young autist wriggled away irritatedly and started back in the direction of the yellow bouncing ball. Then their teacher advocated for both boys: she thanked the autist's classmate for helping his companion get ready for music and explained to our autist that the others wished him to join them. At this, he veered away in the direction of the others but mischievously just missed joining them, as though to entice the teacher to pursue him. Pursue him she did, whereupon he went off to music with the rest of the class.

In fact, his teacher had formed such an empathic bond with this young boy that when he avoided drawing eyes and ears on the people in his family portrait she felt free to urge him: "I want you to put eyes and ears on your people." As soon as he complied, he got up from his seat and began to pace nervously and agitatedly, moving away from his art only to return perturbedly again. It seemed that he wanted to adapt to the art lesson but the sight of eyes and ears on the four people of his drawing was too much for him, and he could barely look at it for more than a second or two.

There was little doubt that his perturbed state was due, in part, to his efforts to adjust to his trusted teacher's expectations. Quite possibly his teacher knew this. This gifted, dedicated, sensitive teacher could not help feeling discouraged and disconsolate when her ingenious efforts appeared to flounder. "Sometimes I just don't know *what* to do with these kids!" she exclaimed to me later when we shared some thoughts over lunch break. Confronted by a seemingly Sisyphean task, perhaps she could not imagine pushing the legendary rock up the mountain yet again. "A face that toils so close to stones is already stone itself," writes Albert Camus.[2] Far from shutting down her remarkable expressivity, she once more undertook to reach her student, head now bent over his workbook pages, as class resumed after lunch.

Why would the teacher's tactics not accomplish her objectives with this autistic boy? It was as though her compassionate expertise mirrored his supersensitivity: both teacher and student thought they'd fallen short when, in fact, they could not have done better. They had achieved the optimal outcome in their educational endeavor even if it wasn't exactly what either wished. The teacher had communicated to her autistic student that in school one must use one's eyes and ears, and the boy, in turn, had not only complied with his teacher's request, he'd expressed by his behavior the nature of his difficulty in doing so. It was excruciating for him always to have to watch and listen, to focus, to read and write, especially when the stimulation of the classroom became too much to bear.

The Teachers

The teachers who worked with these stimulus-sensitive young autists were among the most proficient in the school. If the school didn't invite its best teachers to the program and it faltered, it would be difficult to ascertain whether this was because the teachers were inexperienced or whether the program was in need of fine-tuning. If even a dedicated, seasoned, and attuned teacher could become perplexed, distraught, and dissatisfied with the program's efficacy, it wasn't for lack of inspiration or planning. It might be that the needs of the young autists required the program to adjust in some small but significant way.

I shared these thoughts with the principal during one of our many conversations. "You don't know what to expect of them," she explained one day. "These kids go through their own growth processes, they react in many different ways, so it's hard to predict what they'll do. You always feel that you're in a survival mode with them." This resonated to my own experience when I'd worry whether a therapeutic plan would have an effect, then worry whether its effect would last. "The frustration mainly comes from the teacher's own expectations," she continued. "They figure the school system allowed these children to be in their classes. The system provided the aides and the ancillary teachers, and so there's this anticipation that they're going to get to a certain reasonable point with the kid by the end of the year. And then they ask themselves, 'How in hell am I going to get there?'"

She went on to explain that the teachers of the young autists understood, intellectually, that autistic development is different from what they're used to seeing in their other students. When a young autist begins to stumble, seems unreachable, "In their heart of hearts they believe it's their fault, and they blame themselves." These teachers, the principal persisted, often needed to review the day's happenings with other faculty to convince themselves that it was *not* their fault that an autistic student seemed stuck or had withdrawn from his teacher's efforts. Invariably they would look inside themselves to identify what they could have done better. "Maybe I'm not doing enough," one teacher told me. "Maybe it's my personality." Or they avoided blaming the youngster by referring to him as a "high-maintenance" kid, implying that something different must be done with such a student if the program is to function properly.

"Why not measure the progress of the young autists against themselves and not against the progress of the others?" I asked. "Yes," said the principal, "but that's a very hard concept for a good teacher to accept. Your job is defined by one set of kid behaviors, and then you've got to adjust to very different kinds of responses from the autists, and you get precious few rewards for doing so. With a regular kid you can see they're responding to what you've done. They solve a problem, they read a book, they learn how to write. With the autistic students, you have to look so hard to see what's really happening. And you don't know as much about these kids as you do about ordinary kids. We've got a vast amount of knowledge about regular kids so it's easier for us to interpret what's going on."

"So what can you do to help?" I inquired.

"One thing I do," she replied, "is to remind my teachers that they've forgotten that they have two different measuring tools. They sometimes leave the autistic measuring tool around the classroom someplace and they've lapsed into using the one they had before which was the regular measuring tool for regular kids. They aren't going to see themselves as successful when they review the progress of the autists with the regular measure."

Gym Class

The curricular niceties that the faculty devised to help young autists impressed me once more as I trooped with them down to the gymnasium for the special "prep" gym class. It was prep, their main teacher explained, because in the small class of only four boys they could be acquainted with the procedures and exercises of the larger regular gym class. Their bodies could be strengthened, and their coordination improved. In this small group setting the autists were better able to get to know each other and the gym instructor.

On the way to the gym, the autistic students hugged the walls as they propelled themselves, somewhat reluctantly, away from their main classroom. As soon as we reached the gym the teacher reminded the children of their schedule, but the autistic boys evidently remembered on their own, because they instantly took their places on the floor, sitting or standing in individual squares that had been drawn to form a larger square. Given the evasive behavior of the boy who resisted the reading lesson because of the word *fire*, I was amazed at how eagerly he participated in the warm-up exercises and even in some rather complex games with the others, when he became downright enthusiastic. He did not have to be brought back to the gym activity the way he had in the reading lesson. He seemed, like the other boys, to delight in the release that physical activity provided and this time, unlike when he was bouncing by himself on the yellow rubber ball, he outright basked in the company of others. Although a little clumsy, he knew precisely what he was expected to do, and he did it, pushing himself up while on his back and then off his tummy. In fact, all the boys began to socialize with one another because they were enjoying their activities so much.

Next on the agenda was an exercise in which the boys raced about six steps up to a ramp on which they ran to six descending steps. A boisterous to-do ensued between two boys who had been friendly with each other during the warm-up. They suddenly became competitive about who was to race first, as if this had happened many times before. When one of them was chosen by their teacher, his erstwhile friendly peer became upset. The gym teacher tried to console as well as guide him by saying, "You may try to get ahead of him but don't push him." The boy who was second in the lineup found it difficult to heed his teacher's guidance. Perhaps the combination of two instructions, one geared to his competitive strivings and the other warning him of a possible mishap, was confusing. He began to cry in earnest, possibly because a two-pronged directive was unpleasant or difficult to follow. Staring angrily at his rival, he began to make faces and hissing noises. As the teacher urged him to join the race, he did so, trying hard to catch up to his classmate, who not only ran faster but proudly announced he'd won. A few minutes later, the two boys resumed their friendship, miraculously it seemed, and played ball together.

Meanwhile the gym teacher sat the boys down to discuss what had happened during the racing game. In this way, she gave both boys time to think about her guidance: run fast, but respect your friend. After explaining this once more, she said to the young autist who'd been upset about not winning the race, "I have spoken to your friend about his bragging, and he understands that bragging is rubbing it in. And so now I want *you* to let go of this." Daring to bring up the incident once more—and risking that he'd become distraught again— she waited for a few seconds before she said any more. With an angry face, he subsided, and in a few minutes joined in the ball game with his companion.

Now concentrating on a simplified baseball game and having a fabulously organized plan for the boys, the gym teacher oriented them to the idea of bases. She assigned them each to a base and directed them to stand on it. Then she prepared the boys for what was to happen next, asking each one in turn what would happen if one of them ran to first base, to second, and so on. Then each boy got a turn at bat. They chose which ball they'd try to hit, one boy choosing a larger ball so as to maximize the probability of hitting it. Three of the boys were rather awkward standing at bat, so the teacher again structured the game by reminding them how to place their feet by home plate. She also urged them to take a practice swing. By the time she pitched the ball—she would toss it within their easy reach—they'd miss it by only a hair's breadth. After two or three tries they would actually hit the ball, first to the cheers of their gym teacher and then to the shouts of their peers! One of the young autists, the boy who'd been upset about the missing clock, hit a home run to the other side of the gym, and everyone whooped loudly, much to his obvious delight.

The children, now somewhat fatigued, not just because of the physical workout but also, I thought, because of their robust socializing, were divided up into individual activities. Their teacher negotiated with them about who would be the one to choose these activities. She removed some splendid pieces of gymnastic equipment from a cabinet, among them a rowing machine. There was also a trampoline in front of a mirror on which the boys jumped while observing themselves. In fact, the teacher asked the young autists to watch themselves in the mirror as they jumped. Surprisingly, the boy who'd bounced so hard on the yellow ball in class did not become inwardly preoccupied when, following his teacher's direction, he observed himself while using the trampoline, which he did with a little, proud smile. Another dreamy boy had to be reminded to watch himself. I was amazed that the teacher dared ask this shy child to risk watching his somewhat awkward self. Yet he complied with his teacher's request, and his jumping became a bit more coordinated, surely the object of the lesson.

The boys came together again to play catch. The same two who'd been rivals in the racing game seemed reluctant to adapt to the movement of the ball as they passed it back and forth. They reminded me of Marcia some forty years earlier when she resisted moving her body according to the ball's trajectory. It didn't appear to occur to her or to these two boys to anticipate where the ball would land. Though when Marcia was twiddling—engaging in those rapid and repetitive finger and hand movements she would use with objects—she'd adapt her body perfectly and complexly to what she was twiddling. Perhaps autists adapt in this situation because it is they who've initiated the activity, not a peer of whom they might be wary. Initiating one's own activity might render it safe, which suggests that, however sensitively attuned and compassionate the other person might be and however nicely structured the situation, the autist will feel most protected when his world revolves solely around his own actions.

• • •

As the gym lesson drew to a close, one boy began to ask urgent questions of his gym teacher. He wished to know when he'd be seeing her again. Since there was only one week of school left before summer break, he might have been anxious about the impending vacation and the temporary loss of his teacher. She asked him when he'd be returning to gym class, and the boy answered truthfully. This didn't satisfy him, and he continued to ask the same question; perhaps he needed reassurance about something else. "I told you that we're not going to talk about this anymore, because you know the right answer." But he repeated his question yet again, much like a younger child who is told to stop something he's doing and then tries it one more time to bring his own closure to ceasing an activity somebody else prohibited. Or so I thought.

It wasn't clear when this boy first sensed his school's program was not working for him. During my visit the following year, I realized that the school would not be able to keep him in the program. He'd been assigned a full-time aide in class so the main teacher would not have to spend as much of her time adapting class procedures to reach him. Hindsight suggested to me that he'd understood the faculty was reacting to him differently. When he persisted in asking the gym teacher a question he knew the answer to, I wondered if he wished to be reassured that he was making progress, that he was really *liked*, and that, indeed, he would see his teacher again. After all, his teacher did like him, as did his regular teacher, who had spent hours adapting her teaching to his needs. His gym teacher told me much later how much she loved working with autistic kids, saying, "I feel very lucky to be able to connect with them." So in his way this boy *had* formed attachments to at least these two teachers and naturally wished to know whether he would see them again soon.

The faculty, the principal told me, had many discussions about his progress, how to develop the program to meet his special needs more effectively. She again referred to the structure of the program and the structure of the class. In describing how the young autist's main teacher had lately been diverted from the rest of her students as she tried earnestly and tirelessly to continue working with this student, the principal remarked that if a teacher is unable to teach her whole class, something has gone awry with the structure.

That was the whole point of the school's philosophy: the focus ought not to be on what's wrong with the kids, but on what's wrong with the structure. This was why, I realized, the first-grade teacher had altered the situation for the autistic boys before expecting them to attend to the curriculum. The program's structure had provided this boy with the wherewithal to learn basic skills, but only up to a point.

Predictably, his teacher clung to her hopes for her student for most of his third year at the school. She conferred with the principal, proposing alternative techniques for helping him. She'd say fiercely, "We can do it! I know we can!"

The principal thought another plan for the young autist more viable and during faculty meetings would say something like: "Look, this boy's behavior is his language. He's trying to tell us something. We've tried a lot of things with him and he knows it. He responds initially, because he sees that there's been an effort to help him. So he gets hopeful, he responds, he tries. And then he realizes he can't do it. He gets disappointed in us, he gets disappointed in himself, he knows we're not making it with him. And so he withdraws, rebels, acts silly or strangely." Yes, I thought, thinking of similar experiences with autists I'd had, this boy *is* saying something by his behavior.

He might have thought, though, something like, "I'm not doing well because I'm not trying. I'm not doing well because I'm being silly." If so, he may have tried to save face as he became inattentive to learning and preoccupied by his own thoughts. It wasn't that he *couldn't* make it at school; it was that he *wasn't* making it.

Nevertheless I thought it extremely important for people who try to help autistic children to realize when they've reached the end of what they think they can do in their setting. Accepting one's own and one's school's limitations could pave the way for a sensible, acceptable new plan, one equally sensitive to the child's needs.

For the time being, the teacher and the child must go through the painful, arduous process of accepting that their work is coming to a close, that separating is inevitable, and that the child must move on to an educational setting structured differently enough to make a difference. "How do we know," I tried to comfort the principal and, by extension, his teacher, "that his relationship with his teachers, the ones who worked so diligently and so caringly with him—how do we know that the enjoyment he did get from their instruction, from being supported when he helped his teacher by turning off the light on a hot day, from the fun he'd had in gym class—didn't act as a kind of template for what he might expect of his future teachers?" We couldn't be sure, I thought, that this boy wouldn't approach his new school setting with a more positive attitude than he would have had he not been exposed to the special program designed for him in kindergarten.

School Relationships

Just as the young autists gained from specific classroom alterations made for their benefit, they also profited from being exposed to the values of the entire school. The primary socializing message, communicated to all children, ran something like this: we are not only tolerant of diversity, we welcome it; we must be kind to one another and respectful. Such an attitude surely arose many decades before as the school struggled to integrate its ethnically mixed population.

Children throughout the school were taught that ethnic differences were inherently interesting and to be received gladly; social class differences were to be honored. It may have seemed like a short step for teachers to welcome children whose differences were individually anomalous.

If a student found himself face-to-face with a young autist acting weirdly, it seemed natural when he'd eye the young autist a little skeptically, then venture a social gesture, and eventually play with his offbeat friend, sometimes enthusiastically. The gradual warming to autists took place during a reading or math lesson; on the way to gym, art, or music; on the playground; at lunch. In turn, the autists, however awkward or withdrawn their behavior, however unusual their ideas, behaved as though they expected their peers to be interested in them. Curiously, they sometimes seemed not to have the slightest doubt that their classmates would respond in a receptive way. I noticed that transition times often offered the relaxed, companionable setting in which autists seemed particularly open to friendly interactions.

Once I observed our shy autist, who, apparently uncomfortable about relating to others in a large group, had that day retired from formalized learning. He enticingly invited another boy to play while the children were waiting in line for music class. Recorder in hand, he stealthily approached the other boy and, with a subtle, mischievous smile, challenged him to a recorder duel. The two boys brandished their recorders, jabbing at each other playfully without uttering a single sound, as if by some silent pact they'd agreed to share this exciting activity by themselves so the others would not interfere. Then it was time to head off for music, and the two fell into line together, the autist's friend now giddily chatting with another boy, our young autist watching, somewhat at a distance.

His teacher had actually paired our retiring student with this other boy, knowing of the autist's interest in the classroom pet, a gerbil. The two boys were to feed it and clean its cage. A semblance of friendship developed between them, and the teacher encouraged it by assigning them joint projects in math, for instance.

One day, the teacher gave the children some geometric shapes of various sizes. They were to calculate how many of these small shapes were needed to fit into a larger one she'd drawn on a piece of paper. She called on a pair of vivacious, talkative girls, who seemed to have already aced the assignment. The whole class cheered them on to success—except our shy autist who appeared to daydream throughout. I noticed that every so often he'd glance at the girls sideways, feigning only the mildest interest. Perhaps he was reacting enviously to the girls' showing off; or perhaps, yet again, he became inhibited in joining in the larger classroom group.

When the kids paired up to do more problems with shapes, the autist and his partner went to work in earnest. His partner started adding out loud, coaching his shy friend, turning to him urgently, and asking, "What's nine and nine?" Then he'd wait, smiling encouragingly and breaking into a wide grin when his friend came up with the answer, "Eighteen," loud enough for all to hear. Now convinced that his partner could manipulate numbers, the boy prodded him again, this time loudly, for everyone's benefit. "What's twelve and twelve?" "Twenty-four!" was the noisy, energetic answer.

Then his partner handed the entire project over to his autistic friend, who attentively finished it, head bent over his work, utterly absorbed. He worked slowly but methodically. When he finished, to my surprise, he gave no indication to his partner that he'd completed the lesson but sat stock still, waiting for the other boy to notice. After a while, his partner did scan it, counted the shapes that his friend had arranged, whereupon they both stood tall and yelled in unison, "We were right!" At that, the young autist appeared to anticipate his partner readying for high fives; each slapped the other's outstretched palms, our shy student shouting triumphantly, "Yes!" How normal he could be in this friendly situation; how competent his demeanor!

. . .

When the autist struggles to follow the lesson, momentarily fending off the allure of his inner life, the teacher can liberate in him an accommodation to the curriculum. The autist often gets bogged down with his feelings about routines already begun or about to be set in motion, so that he can't attend also to those stimuli that emerge from the lesson. By remarking in simple, pointed sentences on his temptation to daydream or his momentary confusion, which often prompts him to leave our world for his own familiarly ordered one, our shy autist's teacher was able to get through to him, to show that she understood his dilemma in focusing, to clarify his confusion, and to promote the hope in him that he could pay attention, could do the work, just like the other kids. Once, during a group math lesson, when he was lost in thought and appeared not to know what to do next, his teacher said softly but firmly, "You're only thinking of where you should sit, not the lesson."

Again paired with the boy with whom he'd shared high fives, he seemed reluctant to sit down next to him. His teacher's statement showed him that she understood, but she didn't go too far with the explication. She waited for the boy to mull over what she'd said; she let him consider what to do next; perhaps he'd even conclude that he had a choice about where to sit. These clear but truncated communications from teacher to autist act like a psychological signal that says, "I understand, and it's okay."

His teacher could have interpreted to him that he might not want to sit next to his partner, because this boy had a visible black bruise under one eye after bumping into another child. The shy student, like Stacy, could be chary of physical injury yet fascinated by it and the aggression inherent in roughhousing or in the other ways children risk hurting themselves. To speak of this, even if statements were to be framed accurately, bombards the autist once more with too many stimuli. The teacher let her autistic student deduce from her statement whatever he would, to draw whatever conclusions he might hazard if, to *him*, it was *safe* in the school setting to do so.

Suddenly the shy young autist's friend, his autistic buddy, chirped loudly, "Come sit over here," gesturing toward a spot near him. Our retiring autist abruptly "came to," sighed deeply, and gratefully took the proffered seat.

Several minutes later, the partners who'd shared high fives were again working math problems together. Both boys had been all ears during the math presentation, our shy student now seemingly comfortable sitting next to his friend with the bruised eye. When it was their turn to present their math solution, his partner did all the talking so their teacher said to her autistic student, "Your friend is doing all the work. You'll have to do some, too." Again, a short, firm, gentle statement, one which directly referred to the autist's *friend*. Soon the bashful partner began calling out the answers he'd worked out, shyly at first, not looking at anyone in particular, then turning with a proud smile to his partner.

Talking to me about his breakthroughs in math and in relating to his partner, his teacher said of her autistic students, "It's time to stop worrying about their fragile egos!" Nothing like solid progress, I thought, to convince teachers that these kids need not be coddled. Yet she cautioned, and rightly, that simply including autistic kids in regular classrooms would not make them "normal." This did not mean that the educational and social expectations would routinely overwhelm them. Hard work would be rewarded by significant gains, even in recalcitrant students. In fact, many times the autistic kids seemed invigorated by the demands made on them.

A Class Skit

Two years later this retiring youngster, who had graduated to fourth grade, was willing and able to reveal more of himself. When his teacher called him by name to get his attention, he'd abruptly jump to it, leaving his daydreams behind, and proceed with his work. His rivalrous attitude toward the other boys—in particular, his autistic friend, who'd also graduated to fourth grade—was now rather obvious and became the explicit focus of some conversations with the faculty.

I happened to be observing his classroom when the children were preparing skits. They'd had a series of geology lessons and were to invent dramas on what they'd learned about rocks. The young autist at first refused to participate at all, insisting instead on criticizing what the others were planning to do. He complained to his teacher or the aide that the props the children used weren't real. For instance, the thick marker his autistic friend used to represent a microphone was "fake," or it was "cheating" to blare some songs from a tape recorder rather than really sing them. After pestering his teachers and some of the kids about this, he decided to write his own skit. His teacher let him leave the others, who were practicing on stage, to return to the classroom where he sat, writing earnestly and quickly for several minutes.

An hour or so earlier, his teacher had introduced me by name. When the autistic student returned to his classroom, I was reading some of the children's writings that were posted around the room. I didn't realize at first who had returned and busied myself with the stories and diaries I'd started reading. Suddenly, I heard a soft, low voice say, "Hi, Karen," as a student walked by, coming rather close to me. It was the shy boy I'd been observing for four years, now acknowledging me with a friendly greeting the way any child would!

At first I thought there must be some other person in the room whose name was Karen, a child maybe, but there were only the two of us. Now bent over his writing, he worked assiduously on a plot for the skit that had just occurred to him. So he *had* listened in class when he appeared to be daydreaming, else he wouldn't have known my name.

His teacher soon came to check on him. When I told her how I'd been greeted, she, too, was surprised. I marveled over the fact that, after all this time observing, all this time thinking and writing about the oft-unobserved capabilities and strengths of autistic children, I'd been caught totally off guard when one of them treated me normally. How deeply our prejudices run!

As it turned out, this boy didn't enact his skit after all. He had a conversation about it with his principal later that day in which he complained again that the skits were "fake" and that using props was "cheating." She explained, as his teacher had done earlier, that it's not cheating to use props and not fake because a skit is an imaginary enactment. To this our shy student responded incredulously, "I don't believe you!"—meaning, explained his principal, "You are not to be believed!" Perhaps he disbelieved that reality and fantasy could be combined in a single and, as it happened, social situation—a skit with players being his classmates—so accustomed was he to a bifurcation between the social world and his solitary private world. Perhaps he was also resentful that the others, even his autistic buddy, seemed easy in their integration of the social and the fantasied. "I think you are angry because you aren't joining the others in a skit," continued his principal. He glared at her for a while, then swiveled and stomped noisily back to his classroom, leaving the rest of his classmates practicing their roles. "I think he was angry," the principal told me later, "because I stood my ground that the skit was funny, didn't take his side when he called it 'stupid' or 'fake.'"

Talking it over with her later, it occurred to me that by behaving more assertively, complaining loudly and long, this boy was *feeling* normally—that is, jealously and competitively—even if he wasn't *acting* normally. He'd isolated himself from the rest of the class twice that day. To this the principal added earnestly, "Yes, and how can you behave normally unless you're having the right *feelings*?"

Indeed!

. . .

The young autist who clowned around to be "one of the boys" actually delivered a rather comical performance during his group's skit. It began with another boy's recitation of a rock's characteristics. The children had devised a "rock" concert to follow, our young autist the lead singer. At this point, the skit took a humorous turn as the actors expected and got giggles from the audience on the dual meaning of "rock." Together with another boy the young autist giddily burst forth in song, gyrating his body rhythmically as he mimicked a rock star, singing the melody's notes accurately.

Before the skit, he'd approached another boy, his prop in hand—a marker simulating a microphone—and, tapping his head with the marker, said somewhat fatuously, "This is my prop." I had to suppress a laugh as he seemed to say that his head was his main prop. Yet I couldn't be sure that he was joking, because his deadpan expression gave no indication of his intent. The other boy regarded him skeptically but with a bemused smile so, again, I couldn't be sure whether he thought the remark funny or his classmate "weird."

Everyone clapped and cheered the concert, especially the teacher, who exclaimed to the children how wonderful the skits were and how much she was enjoying herself. Soon our young autist began to clown again, saying repeatedly, "Funny, it's funny, funny, funny!" Was he showing the others, particularly his teacher, how much he understood that his skit was funny? Maybe he also wanted to prolong her appreciation of him and that of his classmates, so thrilled was he at his ability to make them laugh. He seemed to want to repeat the comical moment, even though, I thought, he'd already registered a genuine humorous moment in his gut. Perhaps he also wanted to get hold of it, like a scientist, to study it more. If so, this would be similar to an observation made by Donna Williams about processing others' speech. She became echolalic, she writes, because, in part, it gave her time to mull over the words and presumably their meaning. The autistic student may have felt compelled to repeat to himself and to everyone who would listen that the skit he'd just performed was "funny, funny" as a way of grasping the experience consciously, though I do believe he also wanted to assure himself and the others that *he* could *be* funny. Perhaps he even wanted to brag to his autistic rival, his shy friend, that he had been funny while his friend fumed over the skit being "fake" and "stupid."

One young autist resisted the idea of enactments—or that his friend had participated in a truly comical way—and the other tried palpably to grasp the skit's social meaning. This suggests that the differing reactions autists have to imaginings and to humor are likely more complex than we believe. These unusual reactions to fantasy and comedy do not mean young autists are handicapped. Their responses mean they are likely to struggle with story and humor in interesting, multiple ways. The variety in their social responses was a topic I'd wanted to speak about to the parents of the autistic boys.

Meeting with Teachers and Parents

During my first school visit, I'd invited those faculty involved in the programming for young autists as well as their parents to meet with me. A few faculty and two of the autistic boys' mothers attended. I wanted to know how the teachers and parents felt about the program for autistic youth instituted one year earlier. Since there had been much recent writing about autism's diagnosis, various methods of modifying autistic behavior, and the possible biochemical and/or neurological dysfunctions correlated with or underlying the condition, I hoped for once to be able to center this discussion on how people *feel*. How did teachers retain their composure day in and day out with these special children? How did parents cope within the family, with the public's reactions, and with their personal responses, worries, misgivings, their hopes?

I was graciously introduced to the assembled group by the first-grade teacher. She stated unequivocally that the teachers could not have met the program's expectations without the support of their principal, and somehow, she thought, I'd been of assistance. She continued by emphasizing that the results the project was producing were the direct outcome of a team approach.

I was a little taken aback to discover that, as just a visitor, I'd been part of a team effort and was tremendously flattered, but I was soon hit by familiar thoughts. It's not just the young autists who need an inordinate amount of consistent encouragement; those working with these children also need a sympathetic ear consistently. They need assurance that their work does guide autists toward a better future and that this work is going reasonably well, that one can't achieve miracles overnight, and that the best, most skilled efforts might fail temporarily or appear to flounder indefinitely; that their steady dedication every day affects young autists even when it appears otherwise—even when it seems that they are immune to kindness, refined guidance, and clever pedagogy; that while the long-term outcome might not be precisely what one wishes, the efforts expended are worth it nonetheless.

As the meeting continued, I found the mothers' caring advocacy for their autistic boys remarkable and their state-of-the-art knowledge on autism impressive. They knew, for example, that it was Leo Kanner, not Bruno Bettelheim, who originated the unfortunate appellation "emotionally cold mothers." They had read just about everything they could lay their hands on about autism and conversed straightforwardly and specifically about the "autistic spectrum" and "Asperger's syndrome." Yet they were more interested in and relieved to be talking about real children with individual needs rather than abstract diagnoses, hypothetical situations, and arcane theories. When I inquired whether they'd heard of the theory of mind studies on young autists, both mothers exclaimed heatedly that they had. We had a lively discussion about their boys' competitive feelings for one another, and one mother said of her shy son, "How could he even think about competing with his friend in school if he had no idea what his friend was all about? How could he compete if he weren't making explicit comparisons?" The mother of the young autist who'd dramatized a rock star agreed.

Both parents were enormously appreciative of every effort the school made on behalf of their children and welcomed its team efforts gladly and gratefully. Yet there was an ostensible pile-up of emotion as they spoke of their experiences securing services for their children and in supporting them emotionally, academically, and socially. One spoke of her trials in dealing with the public about her child's unusual behavior. It was as if these parents just could not get enough in the way of compassion from teachers, friends, relatives, even strangers, because each day, in some small but significant way, these remembered reserves of caring they'd received could be depleted by a single instance of tactless curiosity or one unhelpful, misguided pointer on how to deal with their children.

With these thoughts in mind, I began to speak my view on parents and autistic children. First, I commented that I found it difficult to settle on a single term to describe their boys since they were so different from one another. I wondered if in talking with the parents I should be using the word "autistic" or the even looser term "pervasive developmental disorder." The mothers assured me that "autistic spectrum" was acceptable to them since it included high-functioning autists and therefore encouraged parents to be hopeful about their children's potential.

I began to liken my experience rearing my first child with what I imagined theirs had been with their autistic infants. Although not autistic, my firstborn had been colicky, and I knew firsthand how a pediatrician could react to a worried mother with a distressed infant. I had gotten the impression that the baby doctor thought my infant's colic was due to my being a nervous mother. Well, I thought what was making me nervous was my baby's colicky misery! My analogy was inexact, but everyone seemed to get my point—in the heat of the moment vulnerable mothers may be persuaded by professionals that, indeed, their parenting is somehow the cause of their infant's troubles.

The discussion shifted to what the parents could do here and now about their children's difficulties. We discussed some practical problems facing one of the mothers who was at a loss as to what to do about her shy boy's summer schedule. She'd planned some activities for him, but worried that he'd isolate himself during the unscheduled times. I suggested that he might need some quiet time to read or think during the summer just as he did during the busy school months. I hoped to get across that parents need not feel unduly anxious about permitting a solitary time for their autistic child. His being alone at times does not necessarily mean that he will retreat forever into his inner world, never to exit it again. On the contrary, the more we can comfortably allow him his solitude, preferably during predictable times of the day, the more likely the autist will be able to meet social and academic demands energetically. He'll realize that he will have time to himself and is not required to socialize and concentrate indefinitely. Though other youngsters take this for granted, autists, who are well used to being by and within themselves, may not know it; nor do they easily believe it, even if it has occurred to them or is told to them.

Shortly after I'd shared my experience being a parent, an outpouring of feeling came from one of the mothers—all the emotions she'd had about her son seemed to erupt at once. What struck me was the complexity of feeling she expressed about her son, who was actually doing quite well in school. Knowing that things were going better for her child, she perhaps felt safe enough to express herself freely.

Feeling hope for one's autistic child, though, is not without risks. Hopes can be raised by a school's successful efforts, but still it might seem perilous to harbor aspirations for your child in case something goes wrong and all the work seems for nothing. It's difficult to discern not just what's working with young autists, but also what's going to keep on working. What will it take, many parents of these children ask, to secure their children's progress permanently?

The next day the first-grade teacher told me, "The boys' parents had so much fun talking to you!" In a million years it never occurred to me that our meeting would be fun. Isn't part of the difficulty in raising autistic children that parents find so little enjoyment in it? Yet the parents of autistic kids ought to find pleasure in talking about their children, just as any parent would. How healing in itself that could be! They ought to enjoy just being with their children—and how beneficial that surely would be.

How can we help parents have a good time with their autistic kids? And wasn't it so, I asked myself, that the young autists who prospered under my care were those whose parents enjoyed them readily?

Support for the Faculty

How did the faculty at the public school I visited enable themselves to enjoy their often diffident, perplexing students? The teachers who patiently taught the autistic boys had committed themselves to advancing the children from an asocial, nonlearning stance toward an amiable demeanor and more than a semblance of academic mastery. When teachers witnessed progress, they also learned that it wasn't linear. Being self-critical, they often blamed themselves when their students seemed to backslide. So much was riding on this project. High expectations floated thick in the air as I'd wander about the school, getting glimpses of the autists who had remained as students during the principal's final year. The three young autists I knew best continued to make reasonably good progress, but much of the time some aspects of their condition had to be worked with just as energetically as before. The most implacable aspect of the teacher's job, I thought, since I'd had the same experience, was in recognizing and in reconciling oneself to the intractability of the condition, however many gains may have accrued to the individual child. The touch-and-go part of the rehabilitation process is unnerving. If you couldn't visualize the proverbial light at tunnel's end, you'd likely conclude, as one teacher did, that "sometimes I think nothing can be done with these kids."

Yet the teachers did maintain their equanimity by talking among themselves, delighting in an autist's progress, or bemoaning a plateau in socializing or in learning. They would descend upon their principal's office, sometimes thoroughly exhilarated by a small gain or unexpected breakthrough, at other times distraught by a seemingly impassable barrier to befriending or to learning, erected, of course, by the recalcitrant, often deliberately stubborn autistic student who, feeling his oats, decided to test, for the millionth time, just how genuine the respect for and commitment to him was. The principal would make herself available for these often "mea culpa" encounters, and would tell these heroic teachers that it was no surprise to her that they were discouraged and that they weren't sure what to do about their autistic charges. "I'd remind them that it's perfectly okay to say of the autist, 'This kid is driving me crazy!' They'd say it about the other kids so I'd tell them it's okay to say that about the autistic students, that it's *normal* to feel this way about them! They're *supposed* to be feeling what they're feeling!" she concluded vehemently.

I asked her whether the teachers ever brought their autistic students directly to her for counsel. She explained, "It was good for the teachers to see me interacting with the autists. It meant I was supporting the teachers' efforts in the classroom. I'd talk to the student about what it was that he did and try to help him figure out what he could do differently next time. This is exactly what the teachers do when they haven't had it up to here," she added, gesturing upward from her chin.

"Afterwards I tell them this is just what they do. They show the kid how to behave better next time.

"Actually the teachers are as good as or better than I am about convincing the child. Precisely because they have more at stake, have a stronger relationship to the autist, they can be more persuasive." The principal's job, she said, was to help teachers help the kids, and it required from her a fair amount of confirming and validating, even identifying her teachers' efforts as intuitively ingenious.

I asked her how she felt when her teachers would tear their hair in dismay about their days with their autistic students. How did she manage to support them when they were so distraught? Was it a double whammy, because she'd ultimately be responsible for both the autists' well-being and her teachers' receptivity to working with these difficult students?

"Not at all," she declared. "I thought it was my job to help them. I was enough outside the classroom so I wasn't tired of it or frustrated by it. And I was often able to see the students' progress better than the teachers could. I didn't see the kids every day straight for six hours. I didn't have to observe the behavior that appalled or disheartened the teachers, but I *did* notice what the kids did that was terrific!"

"I think I was interested in the progress of the autists because of your work," she told me thoughtfully, "but I was especially captivated by those classrooms integrating autists because the structure was different. It matched a belief system I have about how schools ought to be run." She was referring to the team effort with the autistic children and the enthusiasm it engendered as the teachers and aides and specialists all worked together to bring about important pedagogic events: sensitively informing the autistic students of their potential for an educated, rewarding life; freely enjoying the autists' genuine academic and social successes; encouraging and uplifting the parents of these boys; and, as it turned out, informing the public about autistic possibilities as she inspired portions of this book.

Later Developments

As I got to know the autistic boys during the four years I visited their school and acquainted myself more thoroughly with their teachers' didactic purposes, I could discern that the teachers' efforts were influencing these kids. The effect was not always expected and sometimes, I thought, the teachers would misinterpret an actual step forward as a step backward. They were less prone to do so in the earlier grades, probably because everyone's hopes were high during the project's inception and because teachers in the lower grades may feel that they have more leeway to adapt and flex the program to meet students' needs. In grades three and four, accountability rears its unwelcome head. A teacher's discontent with some students could, in part, be a function of the greater expectations meted out to many students, not just to the autists.

Autistic children—and this is important for teachers of these children to recognize—don't always welcome the changes in themselves. When they are encouraged to reach out to others and do earnestly turn their attention toward learning, their lives become more complicated in ways not always congenial to them. Then it may appear that they are not responding to the program when they are actually feeling its effects. Their increased moodiness, their intensely felt jealousies and irritations, their arguments and oppositions—these and many other reactions to being in our world seem to portend failure when they actually signal success. The combined struggle of teachers and autistic kids brings them to a shared world, one with vexations as well as victories.

Sometimes, the young autist's trials center primarily on how he feels about others. Socializing more freely now, he may find himself captivated by his teacher more than he ever expected to be. The two young autists I've described as being rivals eventually formed an ongoing association in which they'd sometimes jockey with each other for attention or affection from their main teacher. Our shy autist would, for example, interrupt his teacher when she was working concentratedly with his autistic friend, softly repeating several times that he had to use the bathroom. Then he'd eye what teacher and student were doing and, suddenly turning around, determine whether they noticed that he was leaving the room. Likewise, he'd glance curiously at their table when he returned, making sure his teacher knew he was heading back to his seat as he peered at his friend's work.

If anything, these two boys seemed more sensitive than the others to their teacher's feelings. Quite possibly this had evolved as they both enjoyed their one-to-one learning times with her, while the other children had developed an easier rapport with children in addition to their teacher. Yet our bashful autist did raise his hand to be called on when another student was chairing a meeting. He had previously stared into space as his teacher led a vocabulary lesson, but when she appointed another child to call on students, acting as if he wasn't doing much of anything, he laconically raised his hand, lazily propping his forearm upward from his elbow that rested casually on his desk. Then he frowned when his classmate called on someone else.

His teacher, quiet and composed, often amused by and affectionate toward her students, worried that her shy student was not engaging as well as he might with the lessons and with the other children. I could understand her apprehension, because his efforts to participate seemed lackadaisical and disinterested. Yet his efforts were real and indicated a greater desire than I'd seen in previous years to join the others and not relate solely to his teacher, his partner, or his autistic buddy. Supporting my impression that he *was* socializing more, his principal told me he'd begun to greet her in the halls and on the playground. At first, he addressed her formally, but once he used her name jauntily after she'd called out to him playfully, just as she would with another kid.

In fact, I'd gotten the impression that this boy lived in two worlds:

"me all by myself" and "me with other people." The world in which he engaged with people, however lethargically, was, I felt, the direct result of his teachers having connected with him, having aroused his curiosity about the world of learning and the world of schoolchildren, so much so that he might have felt torn between the two seemingly competing personal and social realms. If so, this would be a sign of progress, I told his teacher, and the result of the very diligent work it takes to get through to these youngsters. This made it all the more important to build a bridge between his two worlds. Young autists need to feel that they need not choose one world over the other, that they need not deprive themselves of their cherished thoughts, or need give up on the world of people just because they don't share the autists' private world. For who among us does not enjoy socializing mitigated, at times, by a retreat into an agreeable, comforting solitude?

Toward the end of the school year, the autist who'd become jovial to attract the others also appeared to regress. He'd gotten increasingly agitated because his family was planning a trip two weeks before the end of the school year. His teacher became alarmed by his apparent regression and began to confer with the principal who, in turn, called me. We talked about how the boy's teacher could prepare him for his reentry to school just days before school let out for summer. These disruptions are particularly hard on autistic children, especially if they've gone to the trouble to form friendships, as this boy had. A routine leave-taking at summer break was to follow an unusual one, a family trip out of town, which perhaps overwhelmed him and threatened his hold on sociability more than he could comfortably withstand.

It turned out that his teacher had already devised a brilliant plan to help her student. The boy was to take a toy from the classroom on his trip. He was to keep it in his pocket so that whenever he touched it or removed it to play with, he'd be reminded of his classmates and his teacher. The toy was also to remind him that he'd be returning before school was out and that the people at school were thinking of him.

When consulted, I suggested that the boy be invited to choose the toy as his traveling "companion." But by the time I arrived for my annual visit to the school, the plan had already been put into effect, his teacher had already thought of inviting her student to choose his toy, and so no one needed my advice after all.

I was ecstatic when the boy's teacher told me how she'd instructed him about his chosen toy, a little orange troll. "Keep it in your pocket. It's your *job* to keep it in your pocket. Every time you find it there, you'll know that we're thinking about you. And it's your job to return the troll to your classroom." Ecstatic because, should he have any doubts about returning to school, he'd happily remember that he "must" in order to fulfill his obligation to return the toy to its proper place. Ecstatic, as well, to realize that a compassionate teacher, beleaguered as she was by her job of reaching unpredictable young autists, had thought of such a perfect solution.

I learned from the principal that upon rejoining his classmates our young autist acted as though he hadn't a care in the world. When it was announced at graduation that he'd won an award, he stood tall and waved both arms in the air, two fingers of each hand forming victory signs. He even approached his principal for a hug on the last day of school and, referring to summer break, said, "I will miss you." How pleased he could be with his success and how freely he could express himself!

Follow-Up

Sometime later, I learned that three of the autistic boys had been promoted to fifth grade. As noted before, one young autist had moved away and one had been transferred to another school. One of the three remaining would continue to be served by ancillary teachers. When our shy autist heard of his principal's retirement, he soon took a sudden interest in the vice-principal, as though to secure his future in the school by making a new friend of someone who'd worked closely with his principal. The teachers were also interested in collaborating with the vice-principal because they believed she would continue supporting them in their efforts with the young autists.

In the fifth grade, the shy student kept track of his fourth-grade teacher. He approached her one day and said, "Hi, Liz!"

"Hi!" she replied, glad to see him and impressed by his friendly greeting.

Looking straight at her, he asked, "How's your class this year?"

"Pretty good. How's your fifth grade going?"

"Pretty good."

Surely he felt gladdened to realize he had friends among the school's faculty, who continued to care about him even if they were no longer part of his daily life. His teacher told me it was easier to see the progress of her unusual students when she wasn't with them every day. When she wasn't their teacher, she more easily noticed their growth, just as the principal had when she'd make the rounds and witness new and promising behaviors in the autistic boys.

Upon hearing that the principal would be leaving the school, the boy who'd won an award at graduation the previous year told her forthrightly, "I don't want you to leave." They had formed a strong bond when she explained to him that kids don't get kicked out of school because they make mistakes.

"Everybody in school makes mistakes," she had clarified. "That's how you learn."

"I don't want you to leave," he now repeated.

"Most of the kids want to know who their new principal will be," she replied.

"Well, who is it?" the boy inquired.

"Someone who likes kids."

"Great!" he called out as he went on his way.

CHAPTER TEN

What to Do

[E]ach time a child moves to a new developmental stage, the way
she takes on each new challenge—walking, talking, achieving
autonomy—will give her an internal history, a set of experiences
which will shape the way she approaches the world later.
—T. BERRY BRAZELTON

I'm usually face-to-face with parents when I offer advice. As we sit in
my office brainstorming together, we talk about what to do about a
child's strengths and weaknesses, successes and failures. Thus far, I've
met with some one hundred parents of autistic children, parents who
are unusually receptive to talking things over and who seem pleased
and relieved when I speak with them about their children as I would
with other parents. As I sift through voluminous notes on parent meetings, I imagine myself talking to you in person as I muse about the
concerns you might have about your autistic child. I know my words
of advice will not apply to every parent or every child, but I hope that
some of the ideas presented here will apply to a good many situations
in which you find yourself with your young autist.

In this chapter, I make specific suggestions about how to help your autistic child learn and use language, play more freely, and above all, socialize more congenially. First, I will cover ways in which you can prepare
for and interpret the diagnostic evaluation of your child. Next, I will
discuss the importance of nonverbal communication, language aids,
play, games (board games, pretend games, thinking games), everyday
concerns, sibs and peers, and how to secure and utilize helping hands.

Your Child's Evaluation

At this writing no physical marker *unique* to autism has been identified. There are attributes associated with the condition, but not every autistic child has them all. Moreover, children who are not autistic share some of these traits. However, there *are* behavioral markers typical of autism.

To help you decide whether your child needs an evaluation for autism and to further your understanding of the condition, I'll recommend a number of books you might find useful. Bryna Siegel's *The World of the Autistic Child* is a good place to start. Many parent testimonials on their autistic kids are also helpful: Clara Claiborne Park's *The Siege* and *Exiting Nirvana*, Beth Kephart's *A Slant of Sun*, Jane Taylor McDonnell's *News from the Border*, Catherine Maurice's *Let Me Hear Your Voice*, and Russell Martin's *Out of Silence*. Read the autobiographical accounts by Temple Grandin and Donna Williams. Both authors describe their autistic childhoods, their difficulties adjusting to family and friends, their troubles in school. Read the chapters on autistic giftedness in Oliver Sacks's *An Anthropologist on Mars*.

You'll want to talk to your child's pediatrician if you suspect that he is not developing normally and if he is exhibiting autistic behaviors. It is important to act *soon*. The younger a child is identified as autistic, the sooner treatment can begin. It is important for the pediatrician or other diagnosticians to differentiate your child's developmental delays or aberrations from other, nonautistic conditions. Not all developmental disorders are due to autism. Young children can fail to speak or to meet important milestones for other reasons.

- In preparation for the evaluation it is important to keep a journal. Write down all you can remember about your child's infancy: ages of smiling, cooing, gurgling, blowing bubbles, rolling over, reaching to be picked up, sitting, crawling, standing with and without support, walking, babbling, jabbering, first words. Note not just the age at which these milestones were met but also the *ways* in which he met them. When moving about, did his body seem all of a piece? Were his first words solely about objects ("bottle," "cookie," "top") or also about people ("dada," "mama," made-up names for sibs)? When did your child begin to point? Did he point at objects only or did he include people as well? Did he expect you to follow his pointing arm and did he follow yours when you pointed at something? Write to Bernard Rimland's Autism Research Institute (4182 Adams Avenue, San Diego, CA 92116) for a checklist of autistic behaviors and fill it out. Be sure to include your checklist of what you think are your child's *adaptive* behaviors when you visit the doctor. If you think his behavior is reasonable in some way, it probably is.

• Note any unusual sensitivities your child may have had in infancy and early childhood. How does he protect himself from loud, sudden noises; unexpected physical contact; bright, boldly colored objects; strong odors; offensive tastes? Does he cover his ears, shut his eyes, turn away, scream frantically, cover his face, spit food, leave the room?

• How does he react to painful stimuli? Does he recoil from touch? Does he seem more sensitive to certain kinds of irritants, yet ignore others? Does he seem particularly sensitive to people, their speech, their approach? Does he avoid eye contact by dropping his eyes, turning his face to the side, staring into space, looking through you or toward one side of you?

• What stimuli seem to captivate him, to hold his attention, to transfix him? Perhaps the noise from fire engines, whirring motors, thunder? Is he drawn to rotating toys, shiny objects, electric lights, doors opening and closing, soft blankets, clocks ticking? Does he engage in repetitive, rapid finger, hand, or arm movements that seem to block unwanted stimuli from his view or hearing, including the very people who take care of him? Keeping such records will help professionals profile your child more accurately.

- Does your child play? Note situations in which he does play—with what kinds of toys and with whom. Note any common or repetitive play themes, and describe some typical play sequences.

- Keep a record of his developing language. List additions to his vocabulary as you go along. Note, as well, if and when he ceases talking. If your child speaks in phrases or sentences, note his syntax. Are some words regularly omitted, particularly the pronouns "I," "me," "myself"? Does he avoid the word "yes"? Does he say "no" easily, loudly, energetically? Include some sample phrases and sentences.

- Describe a typical weekday and weekend. Include any routines that your child insists upon. If he attends school, ask his teacher to describe a typical school day, specifying both troubling and adaptive behaviors. Ask the teacher to keep track of your child's self-comforting behaviors, such as rocking, rubbing the face, or other repetitive movements; stroking a soft object; holding a stuffed animal; thumb-sucking or other mouthing behaviors; talking to himself; shadowing the teacher. Include self-comforting behaviors in your report, too. These activities are adaptive and a sign of "ego strength." Include them with other adjustments, even if they seem bizarre.

- Be prepared for the evaluation. Bring your observations, your list of your child's symptoms, his developmental history, Rimland's checklist, and most important, your list of your child's adaptive behaviors. If your pediatrician appears ill-informed about autism, ask him or her to refer you to a specialist, either a child neurologist or a child psychologist. If your doctor, despite indications to the contrary, says something like, "He'll grow out of it," get a second opinion. Autistic children do not grow out of autism.

Remember: The sooner you get help, the better your child's chances of coping with autism.

It is important to stress to the diagnostician that you want an evaluation of your "whole child." She will need her strengths to combat her weaknesses. You have a right to hear from a professional what those strengths might be. While she may not be easily engaged or testable, insist, nonetheless, on an estimate of her capabilities and intelligence from observations of spontaneous behavior and from the doctor's attempt to talk to or interact with her.

If the diagnostic report does not address your child's personality fully, including her strong points, write a counterreport, and make it available to all who work with her. If you seek a second opinion, be sure to include your report in the documents you give to other physicians. Explain why you are seeking a second opinion.

Ask the diagnosing professional whether there will be an opportunity to observe your child in a playroom or an office equipped with toys so that the doctor may observe his spontaneous activity. This will be invaluable to the overall assessment and will provide a context in which to understand more formal examinations.

If the doctor or examiner suggests that you be "realistic" about your child's condition and his future, see that he or she understands that your child will need his abilities to overcome his vulnerabilities. It is the professional's *job* to identify these and to corroborate or clarify what you already know.

If you are told that you cannot be "objective" about your child, keep in mind that everyone, professionals included, has preconceived notions. This is human. Your opinions are no less valuable or valid because you are the child's parent. Quite likely, this is your first personal experience with autism. You haven't diagnosed or tested hundreds of autistic kids. The doctor has presumably had many experiences with atypical children, including young autists and, based on this experience, has undoubtedly formed personal opinions about autism's prognosis. Objectivity obtains only when doctors distinguish their personal views from facts and seek to temporarily set their opinions aside while taking a fresh look at your child and his unique personality. When the professional is candid in distinguishing his opinion from other sources of information—the latest neurological or biochemical findings; written reports of others' experience with autistic kids, including parent descriptions of procedures that work; formal test or research results—you are in a better position to evaluate his findings and opinions.

Remember: The evaluation, no less than the treatment plan, should be a team effort.

If your child is to be tested, find out from the examiner how he or she plans to gain your child's attention. If a child refuses to listen or to answer test questions, the test results may be meaningless. If the test report says that the examiner believes the test findings to be "reliable" or "valid," find out how the examiner tried to engage your child.

Your child will quite likely be upset by being tested. He won't like being talked to by a stranger. He will dislike the initial chitchat designed to make him more comfortable. He will resent having his thoughts interrupted by what he considers irrelevant or offensive questions, and he most assuredly will become angry or withdrawn if and when he realizes that the test items are getting progressively more difficult. Because you know him best, you can tell him afterward that the testing experience and the test results in no way equate to his real and full personality. You can remind him that this is doubtless true because, in all likelihood, he has refused to show his real self to the examiner. Your support will not necessarily increase his recalcitrance or diffidence. On the contrary, he will realize that you understand him and that you are advocating for him. When he perceives you as his ally, he will open up to you more eagerly. If he asks, as superhero Dirk did, why he had to answer test questions, tell him, truthfully, that you wanted to know what his strengths were. Emphasize that he will need his strong points to overcome his difficulties.

If you think your child may have responded to test items in subtle ways, request to go over the test protocols with the examiner. See if you can discern a pattern in the responses. To what questions did he react genuinely? From what items did he turn away? Did he respond by remaining silent? Maybe this information will jibe with your observations of his spontaneous behavior. The examiner needs to include your observations in the final report. Most important would be an estimate of what your child has taught himself, not just the topics or items to which he's aversive.

Remember: The lived-with and worked-with child is often quite different from the tested and theorized child.

Nonverbal Bridges to Conversation

Mute or barely speaking autistic children will sometimes warm to conversation when they discover or sense that communicating nonverbally is safe. If your child has no language or has lost the use of it, try communicating through gesture, facial expressions, childhood games, music, drawing, or writing. Sometimes it is best just to be with him, engaging in a favorite pastime, your young autist pursuing his own interests. He will feel the comfort arising from calm, silent companionship, so important to the basics of actual conversation.

There are many nonverbal cues you can use to communicate with him—for example, shrugging when you aren't sure of something, beckoning with your arm when you wish him to precede or accompany you, motioning for him to stop what he's doing or where he's going by holding your hand flat out in front of you. If he puts his hands over his ears to block loud or offensive noises, do the same, nodding agreement that the noise is intrusive. Join him when he shakes his head no or nods yes. These gestures often help him feel that body movements can substitute for words.

Keep in mind that gestural language is not an end in itself, but a way station to more developed communication. Your enthusiastic nod, signifying yes, is, likewise, a communication to him that you are pleased with him or that you intend to honor his gestural request, such as his pointing to his favorite food and drink.

Don't try to inhibit your natural facial expressions, but don't exaggerate them, either. If you do, your child may feel that you aren't being sincere or that you are trying to fool him. Smiles, frowns, serious looks, downcast sad eyes are all cues to how you are feeling and will sensitize him to the *idea* of feeling. This is important when he's not ready to hear words. Later you can play games with him, perhaps drawing cartoonish faces with different emotional expressions.

Hands-on-hips to indicate good humor when he has done something silly, mischievous, or against family rules expresses your feelings in a safe way. Also, you may playfully use vocal exclamations as a bridge to language, such as "huh?" "aha!" "oh," "oops," or "wow." He'll be able to attend to one-word communications more than he will to whole sentences. Again, you are alerting him, safely, to your emotional state.

Games that don't require words teach autistic kids to relate to others. When your child is small, you can engage her in peekaboo, pat-a-cake, or variations on these childhood diversions. Try introducing her to "joint attention" games, like "*I'm* pointing to the cookie; now *you* point to a cookie" or "Can *you* find the cookie?" If your toddler merely looks at it, praise her, and ask her to pick it up or to show you where it is with her hand or finger.

Invent hugging games to play with her. Although, as Donna Williams tells us, the child herself ought to initiate physical contact, you can prime the pump. Try telling her softly, "It's time for a little hug now," or create a song inviting her to hug you or alerting her that you are about to hug her. Give her time to reach out to you and then reciprocate by hugging her gently, never too close or too hard. Let your child cue you about how she wants to be hugged or touched, how physically close she wants to be. Some autistic children, like Marcia, enjoy hugging people who sit or stand passively by. As she becomes more comfortable with physical contact, you can initiate closeness more regularly, perhaps with a pat or walking arm-in-arm or a brief, gentle rubdown.

You might try variations on hide-and-seek with your little one. Hide an object, not yourself at first, and not something to which she is particular attached, lest she become frustrated and refuse to play. If she's munching on a cookie or other snack, cover a second cookie with a towel or hide it ostentatiously behind your back. Sometimes leave a portion of the hidden object showing so that the game proceeds easily. Then hide the whole object. Always praise her for her efforts to complete these tasks successfully. Tell her how much you liked the way she played pat-a-cake or the way she hugged you or the way she pointed to the cookie or the way she found the snack or toy.

When she's a little older, perhaps five or six, you can introduce chase games and regular hide-and-seek. Estimate whether she wants to be caught, and if not, approach her without touching her. At first she probably won't want to chase you but you can ask her to, moving away slowly and invitingly, just to see if she will pursue you. In the hide-and-seek game, start by hiding yourself, but always leave part of you showing to entice her to find you. When it's her turn to hide, cover your eyes, saying, "It's your turn now; *you* find a place to hide"—watching, though, through your fingers in case she wanders away. If she catches you peeking, tell her how smart she is. If she hides in plain view, "find" her anyway! Play these games during a set, predictable time of day so that she expects them.

By all means, indulge yourself and your child in what can be the beginnings of verbal communication during these games. He might voice playful sounds, like "eee" or "ooo" in his excitement. He might invent words for the fun of it. Take advantage of these golden proto-language opportunities, first by imitating him softly, watching, as always, for his reaction. If he tolerates this, add your own sounds or made-up words, perhaps a sound or word that rhymes with his. If his sounds approximate a real word, say it. Later, say it in a sentence, but don't comment that it is a real word. He probably knows that, but if not, he will figure it out for himself.

Some autistic children become fascinated with homonyms. To them it's an interesting puzzle that the same sounds have different meanings. I've seen this most frequently in young autists who haven't yet learned to read or spell. For example, they might interpret the word "see" as identical to "sea," as Stacy did. Even those who can read and spell will sometimes play homonym word games. To interest your child in playing with language, you might, in addition to inventing rhyming games, introduce some homonyms, such as "hair" and "hare," "pail" and "pale," with the goal of interesting her in even more word play. You can talk with her about the meanings of each pair to foster her sense of word meaning.

The same can be done with synonyms and antonyms. I've listened to autistic kids who were particularly absorbed by opposites, including one teenager who'd chant for hours, "The opposite of light is dark; the opposite of blond is black; the opposite of yes is no," soon to be followed, mischievously, by, "What's the opposite of opposite?"

Sound and word games are not so much to free an inhibited oral apparatus as they are to encourage your child to participate in and maintain a conversational stance, which foretells actual two-way talk. *Remember: A parent is the child's first teacher.* For quite a while, a parent may be an autistic child's only teacher.

Language Development

Fostering language development in your child is enormously important and, for some autists, enormously difficult. It is, of course, easier to make contact with an autistic child when she speaks to us. We then understand more precisely what her needs and wishes are. But interpreting her gestures, facial expressions, and expressive noises as if they are an attempt to communicate encourages her to attend to us more regularly.

To achieve this, one must become a close, vigilant observer. It often helps to keep a journal of the patterns in an autist's gestural or other attempts to communicate and the regularities in her truncated speech. Do grimaces and groans follow what might be, for her, an overbearing series of stimuli? Does her turning away or staring into space follow something you've reiterated a thousand times? Or does it follow an event that's totally new to her? In what situations does she repeat you? In what situations does she genuinely try to answer your questions?

All this is predicated on the assumption that her communications, verbal or not, are meaningful. If we hold firmly to the opinion, despite evidence to the contrary, that autistic children are inherently incapable of sharing meaning, then why should they talk to us? Would you talk to others if you realized they thought you were incapable of conversing meaningfully?

Your ultimate aim will be to get a discussion going in which you *share ideas* with your child. Sharing is the stuff of dialogue. To assume that an autistic child will never be able to participate in this higher-order linguistic process unnecessarily limits her progress.

As she readies herself for communication, the young autist might find it easier to attend to your words if you slow down and speak quietly. Avoid speaking condescendingly. Though she may display linguistic aberrations, her mind likely functions well. Clear, quiet, measured speech will catch her attention more than rapid-fire, boisterous, emotional talk-noise, which is just too unpleasantly distracting for her to hear and to attend to. Try to talk calmly to her when no one else is around and when the setting is peaceful, with few sudden unnerving sounds or other unexpected intrusions.

Marcia taught me how to speak with her during our early days together. She'd invariably plug her ears or turn away when I used my sometimes emotional, rapid manner of speaking or when her dorm was unbearably noisy. When I spoke more tranquilly, when the other children were engaged in quiet activity or when were alone together, she began to listen more regularly and would respond with one-word sentences or short phrases, though, even then, I had to pause between phrases to give her more time to grasp the complexities of normal speech.

I've known autists who have concluded that people speak to rattle their nerves. These kids are sometimes so convinced that their environment is a dangerous, intrusive place that whatever you do or say appears to confirm their worst expectations. Because they were not as withdrawn as some other autists I'd known, Stacy and Dirk would react more quickly, urgently, and sometimes violently to overstimulating conversation.

Stacy often feared what I was about to tell her. She anticipated me in this way because so often I had talked to her about scary events—thunderstorms, for example. Rainstorms became potently associated in her mind with talking-to-Karen. If I had some inkling of what she did not want to hear, I'd quietly explain what I did not intend to discuss. I'd say that I did not, at the moment, wish to talk with her about thunderstorms but about what she had learned in school. If she persisted in panicking about storms, I'd ask her whether her teacher showed her how to predict the weather for the rest of the day. Then she would become more responsive to what I did want to discuss with her. Again, my tone had to be soft and gentle, the pace of speaking a little slower than normal, rather rhythmical, soothing.

If your child has a good grasp of language, he might focus on one or two topics to the exclusion of everything else. You may be told by teachers, friends, neighbors, relatives, or experts to discourage him from indulging his favorite topics or diversions. This is misguided. Though his teacher will doubtless ask him to leave his private world to attend to learning, you, as his parent, can allow him his world. What's more, he won't attend to you and what you have to say if you don't attend to him. True, he may wish to ignore his immediate environment, concentrating only on his special, sometimes arcane, interests. Listen to him with the aim of finding something, anything, that interests *you* in what he says. Then respond to what *you* are interested in. When he joins you in the beginnings of conversational give-and-take, continue with this plan, but do not overtax your child. At first, spend just a few minutes each day talking with him reciprocally. Gradually increase the times spent talking together as he, also gradually, accustoms himself to this new form of interacting.

If he resists such a plan, realizing that you are trying to lead him into a shared world and away, briefly, from his solitude, assure him that you are truly interested in his thoughts and ideas, but that sometimes it's *his turn* to listen to you for a few minutes, or that it's time, now, to *talk together*. Then he will get the feeling that you do not expect him to be with you forever, talking indefinitely. Invite him to choose a topic to share, and once again, find something in what he says that interests you. In this way you'll start a cycle, not just of conversing but also of relating, that mitigates the effect of his solipsistic world. Eventually he might find these talks fun, more pleasurable than talking to himself or thinking alone.

Behavioral methods can sometimes enhance this process, but they can't substitute for it. A behavioral therapist might attempt, by direct instruction, to turn your child's talk away from his own interests toward something shared: "Remember? We are talking about school now, not superheroes." Or, in the case of a child "perseverating" on one topic, "Now it's time for you to let go of the superhero talk and answer my questions about school." Such a therapist might offer tangible, material rewards if your child complies. What you want to accomplish, though, is to impress upon him the *inherent* value of relating to *you*, not the value of receiving candy or other treats, or tokens for these treats. While you may want to turn your child's face gently toward you, or ask him outright to pay attention, and look at you while you're talking together—let *him* decide if he wants to focus on your eyes—your goal is to elicit a natural flow of language from him to you, from you back to him. The behavioral methods are adjuncts to the basic interpersonal process you are striving for.

The more you get to know about your child's special interests, the more he will want to tell you about them. He might repeat words that belong to a single category, as Greg did when he spelled animal names in the game of Hangman. This is an important cognitive achievement. It means a child has begun to classify objects spontaneously. Create word lists to see if your child will add some words to yours or if he will identify your category. If he responds with his own list, ignoring yours, tell him how much you like his list, but now it's time to listen to yours. When he is comfortable with your participation in his sorting activities, choose several words, playfully, that fit a different category. If he is listing animals, you can list plants. If he doesn't add anything to your list, tell him there are many objects in the world that can be grouped together and invite him to join you in a search for other sorting schemes.

You can begin to add connectives among the words you are gathering together. If his category is animals and he's listed alligator, elephant, robin, and whale, connect these by saying, outright, "Alligators, elephants, robins, and whales are all animals." If he appears to understand, tell him you now realize that he knows the difference between animals and plants. He'll benefit from knowing that you appreciate what he has taught himself. Continue to explore different categories and subcategories with him. This encourages variation in his listing behavior. Any variation in his customary behavior that you are able to develop is a big plus. You might begin with, "Cookies are a kind of . . . ," waiting for him to finish the thought. If he says cookies are snacks instead of food, praise him and up the ante: "Yes, cookies are a kind of snack, and snacks are a kind of . . ."

The possibilities are endless. If your child states that cookies are "things," you can respond, "Yes, cookies are things; they are not people. Tell me some other things; name some people." If he chooses to talk only about things: "Tell me some things you can eat and things you can't."

If your child struggles with pronouns and refers to both herself and to you as "you," or avoids saying "I," "me," and "mine," try interpreting her literally. If she says, "You want cookie," answer her truthfully: "Yes, I do want a cookie now," or "No, I just had lunch."

If she says, simply, "Want cookie," try asking her, "You mean, *you* want a cookie?"

If she becomes frustrated, angry, apprehensive, withdrawn, or frightened, explain that you need to know when she is talking about herself and when she's talking about you. It's best in these situations to refer to her by name: "I need to know when you're talking about Susie or talking about Mom." You may find that, in the effort to clarify things, she will begin to use her name and eventually the pronoun, "I," as Stacy did when she started to refer to herself as "you" or by her name, but then burst forth with, "I mean, *I* don't want to go to dinner." Your child may refer to herself as "me," as in, "Me want cookie." Accept this for the moment without correcting. She's getting the idea, or becoming comfortable with the important idea that different pronouns refer to people differentially.

Autistic kids often struggle with sentences because they are mystified by syntax. They sometimes become near-mute when they get discouraged by their verbal clumsiness or when they need time to process all the separate elements of a sentence. One language aid is to begin a sentence and wait for your child to finish it. Kids who find talking painful are often relieved at having to supply only one word or just a few. If you want to know what your child wants for supper, you could begin with, "Jimmy wants to eat . . ." If you wish to know what he would like to play with, "Jimmy wants to play with . . ." Later you can ask with whom he'd like to play: "Jimmy wants to play with toys and . . ." You hope, of course, that he will specify Mommy or Daddy. Letting him finish sentences encourages your child to add more words as he feels hopeful about completing them.

Be advised that kids with better developed language might resent this strategy. Try to assess how much receptive, silent language your child possesses. A child with good receptive skills might interpret a "fill-in-the-blanks" scheme as condescending. It might interrupt his special, private thoughts. Other strategies, like the classifying games described previously, are more likely to work with these children.

As he becomes more fluent, try to distinguish your child's self-talk from his attempts to talk to you. There may be more of the latter than you expect. Keep a record of the themes he typically uses to communicate. These will be the ones you'll want to expand upon in your attempts to get him to speak more reciprocally.

Musical Activities

Your child may be talented in some way, but even if he is not, a good way to approach him is through the arts and reading. If he's drawn to music, try to join him in song or other musical activities. Even if he isn't particularly gifted, singing about human emotions allows him to explore how people feel without attributing to himself or to you the feelings expressed by the song's lyrics.

First, listen attentively to his singing, to the particular songs he chooses to warble. Then begin by humming along with him. Equip him with musical toys to expand his repertoire. When he's accustomed to your presence during musical moments, try singing "conversationally" with him. Let him choose his favorite songs; next select a verse or several lines that you particularly like or that you think fits his experience. For example, if he chooses a pop song, you can vary the words so that it catches his interest. If he protests the lyrical changes, tell him that he can sing the way he wants to and so can you. If his lyrical choices are particularly apt, as Marcia's were when she sang the song about Michael coming ashore in a music boat, you could sing your child's own name if the lyrics apply to him. Or if he sings nursery rhymes, as Stacy did, and bursts forth with, "And everywhere that Mary went, the lamb was sure to go," respond by singing something like, "And everywhere that Mary went she surely had a friend." So what if it doesn't rhyme? Maybe your child will sing something that does!

Drawing

Drawing, likewise, enables an autistic child to communicate. At first she may want to exclude you from this activity. Ask her permission to draw your picture as she is drawing hers. If she says or shakes her head no, don't push it, but stay with her. If she draws something recognizable, draw something in response, but let the drawing sit on the table until she's ready to notice it. As she gets used to your presence, try guessing out loud what she's depicting. If she becomes angry at wrong guesses, encourage her to tell you what she's drawn: "Oops, I was wrong. So tell me, please, what it is."

You'll want your shared drawing activity to lead to communication. Start drawing people engaged in human poses, but slowly and deliberately. Watch for your child's reactions. If he tolerates what you're doing, try writing cartoon captions to accompany the people you've drawn. Write short messages in bold, large letters. Then read the messages to him, softly and slowly. Or if he can read, remain silent so that he may decipher your messages himself.

Storytelling

When he's a little older—say, six, seven, or eight—ask whether he'd like you to tell him a story. Follow up by writing or typing the story for him to look at and possibly to read. Then read it with him, and if he will permit it, discuss it. Ask if he'd like to tell or write a story for you. If he's old enough, encourage him to use the typewriter or a computer to tell his tales. When you write to him, begin with short phrases, and always choose something that interests him. If he follows your lead and writes a message to you, respond with another short message, as if you were answering him in conversation.

To activate beginning reading in your child, or to enhance beginning reading already in progress, you might want to try the "organic" method, so termed because its originator, Sylvia Ashton-Warner, wished to preserve the natural connection between a child's experience and his first written words. If she's in school, be sure to check with her teacher so your reading exercises aren't at odds with hers. You may ask your child to dictate her favorite words, which you write on separate pieces of paper, or she may wish to do this herself. Print the words in large, bold letters, the way a teacher would. If she doesn't recognize the words, draw a picture on the paper or have her draw one as a visual cue for the word. Then read the words with her, pointing to each one as you read. Ask her if she'd like to read some of the words. After she's mastered a small vocabulary of nouns and verbs— introduce nouns first, then verbs—ask her to arrange the words as she wishes. Accept, of course, any words she volunteers. Forget, for the moment, the linguistic connectives and let her play at arranging her words any way she wants.

When she's mastered a small written vocabulary, tell her that there are certain words we need for a complete sentence, such as "the" and "and." Write them yourself. If she doesn't use these spontaneously, interpolate them in phrases, if she will let you. Take turns reading the phrases or sentences. Again, these lessons should be short at first so that she doesn't get tired or discouraged. Gradually increase the reading time.

Be sure to notice your child's ability to tolerate increasingly longer times spent with you. Don't give up on her if she rejects you after an apparent breakthrough. She's still getting accustomed to one-to-oneness. Or she's asserting her right to choose what you do together. You can say, "Okay, this is enough for today; but tomorrow's another day, and I want you to try with me again." This prepares her for a forthcoming social event which may help soothe her fears of, or insecurities about, being with people. Make sure that she understands that you require from her a limited, predictable togetherness; otherwise, she will conclude that she must be with you, and others, endlessly.

Chat Time

It is important that you take note of your child's reaction to the social exercises described previously, including his facial expressions, gestures, expressive noises, conversation, limited though it may be. Explore his nonverbal and barely verbal behavior as best you can. Respond to his communications as if he were speaking to you normally.

When you sense that he feels safe and comfortable being with you, use more of your time together just to chat. It's probably best to begin chat times when you are alone together, without distractions that could interfere with the rapport you've established. Speak uncomplicatedly, but as normally as you can, about his favorite topics, his preferred toys and activities, the day's schedule, what he did yesterday, what he might do tomorrow. If his other parent is at work and his sibs at school, imagine with him what he thinks they are doing. Ask him to guess their favorite pastimes. Ask him to imagine what you are doing when you are at work, what you do when you are having fun.

Lastly, begin to talk to him directly about thoughts and feelings. If he's interested in animals, imagine with him whether animals have thoughts; do they have feelings as people do? If he's interested in mechanical devices, ask him, do motors really run themselves? Or do they have to be started and stopped by us? How does he feel about animals? About objects? Does he like animals or objects better? How about people and animals? People and objects? Does he think you like people or animals better? People or objects better? On a scale of one to ten, where would he put his affection for people, animals, objects?

Remember: Getting a conversation going with your autistic child in much the way you'd talk to any child is a great boon to his ego and to his language development. The two of you speaking freely together will make him feel like a regular kid.

Play

One of the most valuable lessons an autistic child, even a very young one, can learn is the long-term utility of variation both in what she says and does. I remember watching a film of an autistic eighteen-month-old when I had just begun to work with Marcia. I was startled to witness that this little girl, who had learned to walk some months before, would consent to do so only in circles and in only one direction. What an uncommonly dedicated pursuit of sameness in such a little person!

Her therapist, a Dutch psychiatrist, first approached her by walking in circles with her. I was amazed by the simple efficacy of the intervention he later chose to encourage variation in her locomotion. He took her by the hand and gently circled her little body in the opposite direction. After some weeks of this, the little girl began to perambulate in both directions, albeit still in circles. Her small face seemed to light up just a bit as she began to gaze more openly at her doctor.

Playing with your child offers you many opportunities to vary her behavior by introducing new toys or objects when the time is right and by encouraging new and different play themes. Observing her reactions closely will teach you when it's time to introduce something fresh and novel.

Before you begin to enter your child's play or to initiate play sequences with him, note any objects, toys, equipment, or sensory stimuli to which he seems especially drawn. These will form the basis for shared play activities.

If your child doesn't play yet, select one or two toys or objects that you think might interest him. Play with and explore them yourself, talking to your small child gently, slowly, about what you're doing, but don't say too much. If he turns away or makes angry noises, respect his wish that you stop this activity, and after a few minutes of silence, tell him that you'll try again tomorrow. Stay with the same toys or objects for several days or a week, even if he ignores you or pushes you away. At least your behavior will be predictable, which eventually will create a context in which he might tolerate what you're doing and saying.

If he shows some minimal, passing interest in a toy or an object, begin to play with him. If you're exploring the roundness of a ball, rolling it, cradling it, tossing it, roll it to him to see whether he will pick it up to hold it, explore its shape, or toss it. Then ask him to roll it away; maybe he'll even roll it to you. Start a game by saying, "Go away ball; come back, ball."

If he seems interested in your twirling a top, see if you can make it twirl toward him. If he stares at sunlight streaming through a window, show him how you can create different effects by partially closing the blinds or drawing the curtains. If he protests your dimming the lights, say, "I *closed* the blinds [curtains]; now I'm *opening* them." Or get some colored cellophane and hold it up to the light, thus inviting him to join in shared explorations. If he's interested in machines whirring, let him turn them on and off, with your supervision, of course. Supply him with battery-operated toys that he can manipulate in this way. Talk to him as he plays: "Now you're turning it *off*; now you're turning it *on*." If he's interested in electric lights, play little games with him by telling him he can be the "boss" of the lights when it's time for dinner, or when it's time for bed. He can turn them on for dinner, off for bed.

All the while, be responsive to his nonverbal cues and to his words or statements. Your aim is to give him the feeling that playing is fun, and that if a ball, a top, a machine, sunlight, and electric lights are fun, other objects will be, too. Gradually add other items to the pile to which he's already responded favorably. If he rejects any or all of these, ask him to select which new items he likes and which he doesn't. Honor his choices. Make a game of rejecting some toys and accepting others. Encourage him to say *no* and *yes* to the toys.

If your child does play, sit with her as she explores favorite objects or toys, or as she engages in what seems like repetitive play, like shaking a rattle or sifting sand through her fingers. Insist that you be together for a short time each day while she plays. Do this without requiring, at first, that she join you or requiring that she let you join her. If she takes the toy you've got, don't protest; rather, ask her to give you something in return. Tell her that you need the toy so the two of you can play together. Then offer to give it back. Say, "Now I'm *taking* the toy; now I'm *giving* it back." If she turns away or stares straight ahead, tell her that you will ask to play with her again tomorrow.

Don't be afraid to use a "trial-and-error" approach with your child. This is the only way you will hit upon something that works. Be careful, though, not to give up on an activity too soon. She may be testing the effects of her nonresponsive behavior on you. If after a couple of weeks of concentrated, regular, consistent effort on your part with apparently little response from her, switch to something else, explaining briefly that you think she wasn't interested in what you were doing or playing with before, which is why you're trying something new. Ask her to point to something she'd like to play with or to fetch something from her room that interests her. Be overjoyed if she does so, and of course, respect her choice.

If she still rejects you, tell her outright what your goals are. If she protests this, listen. You've started a dialogue, which is one of your aims.

Pretend Games

Your child might want you to join him in his pretend play or in his imaginary conversations with imaginary playmates. Join him on his terms first. If his imaginary play scares him, suggest simple resolutions of the play. For example, if he sets up an imaginary situation in which a doll or a pretend person becomes frightened and wants to discontinue the play because he, himself, is frightened, introduce another doll to reassure his doll, or talk to the imaginary character in a reassuring voice.

Gradually vary these imaginary scenarios, if he will let you, to promote variation in his overall behavior. Add a toy, an idea, or a theme one at a time to avoid overwhelming him.

It is important not to get too emotionally involved in your child's pretend dramas lest you be unable to help her with the feelings they arouse. Showing interest in them and providing resolutions if the play is too scary, too repetitive, or gets out of hand, is important, but don't take over completely. After all, the dramas are the result of her imagination, not yours. You don't want to become so involved that you can't find an easy exit. If the scenes seem preposterous, add a touch of reality, but not condescendingly. If she imagines something that can't possibly happen and seems so wrapped up in it that she attends to little else, don't correct her, or say, "That's not real." Say instead, "Tell me how this all began," or "How's it going to turn out?" If the pretend person is always getting into trouble or into dangerous situations, ask, "Why is that person always in trouble or always scared? How can we help?"

You may want to ask how she feels about her imaginary characters. Does she like them or hate them? Of a threatening character's outrageous instigations, you can suggest, "It's time for your imaginary person to behave, to be nicer to you." Depending on your tone of voice and the rapport you've established, you may find that she listens to you more than you anticipated. As always, take note of any reactions, nonverbal as well as spoken. These will help you fine-tune your interventions in the future.

Board Games

Board games help your child learn how his mind works both similarly to and differently from yours. If he enjoys games, let him choose which ones to play. At first, do not attempt to change his special rules and procedures. Tolerate his cheating, even if it's relentless. Teaching him different ways of playing games can wait until later. It's better to familiarize yourself with his ways of playing his favorite games and to inquire, from time to time, how he happened to think of playing this way. As he becomes accustomed to playing games with you, you can begin to play by the rules. Narrate why you are doing what you are doing, that you think this is what the game's rule is, that you and he can check the rules together, or that you think one might gain an advantage by moving a game piece a certain way.

Note any patterns in his game-playing. For example, if you are playing checkers, note whether he advances carelessly to your side of the board without concern for his back men or the overall game strategy. Narrate why you keep your back men in place. Note whether he plays offensively, defensively, or whether he tries to combine aspects of both. Explain the advantages of attending not just to what he's doing but also to what you're doing. Gently introduce new strategies to him, giving him a chance to try them in a "practice" game. If he resists, suggest that he watch what happens when you make a few "practice" moves. A collaborative spirit as you introduce new game ideas will work better than an adversarial one.

You might differentiate between "luck" games and "thinking" games. Does he prefer luck games like Candy Land or Chutes and Ladders, or is he willing to try chess, checkers, Othello, Monopoly, and the like? While playing thinking games, he'll require a good deal of benign teaching and patience, a lot of practice with you as his collaborator and not so much as his opponent.

Thinking

Your child may be interested in exploring how the world works. Experiments with water can help him plan, infer, and predict. Join him in these explorations as a quiet observer at first. Make available an array of differently sized and shaped containers, and let your child explore how the water looks in the different vessels. Does he notice that the water level rises or recedes depending on size and shape? If so, ask him to explain, if he will. If he won't discuss it, tell him what you think. You can use sand, marbles, beads, or other small solid items in the same way as he plays with different containers.

If he's interested in aspects of nature, ask him to help you care for a houseplant or something growing in the garden. Help him keep a weekly record of the plant's growth, how much water it needed, whether it seems to be turning toward the light. Suggest that he predict from week to week how the plant will fare.

If you have pets, get him to help you take care of them. Try to interest him in their behavior—why a dog barks when it does, why a cat meows, why animals approach us, and why they wander away. Help him keep records of what interests pets as they roam the house or run around the yard. You'll be sensitizing him to animal motivation and reactions that may attune him to human behavior.

Always supply your child with the information he needs or asks for; help him get it himself by joining you in looking for information in the dictionary or the encyclopedia. Refer him to *The Guinness Book of World Records*, a world atlas, or any source of information that's likely to provide grist for the workings of his young mind. Don't be afraid that you'll turn him into a "little professor." Becoming knowledgeable about the world is his way of coming to terms with his immediate surroundings. Enjoy his bragging; he will feel good knowing something that others don't yet know.

While talking with your child about his thoughts, you may notice that he becomes fatigued by the intensity of your discussion. He may be overstimulated, not just by conversing but also by his own mental processes. If so, he will need to rest. He will need a time-out from discussions that inundate him with more thoughts than he can comfortably manage. You can help him comfort himself by providing a calming, soothing activity or a special place to which he can retire. Then he'll be better able to process what has gone on between you and to engage in solitary, dependable, familiar activity. Don't worry if this seems unduly isolating. More than regular kids, autistic kids need scheduled peaceful times to recuperate from the stresses of interacting, thinking, learning, *trying*.

Intelligent autists can be encouraged and aided in their theory of mind facility. Be open-minded yourself about your child's ability to think.

She may show no interest in her mind or yours, but that's different from not being able to understand the mind concept. Clarifying what your child says by asking her what she means or guessing her meaning are good ways to sensitize her to the mind's functions—yours and hers.

She may at first display what psychologists call "prelogical" or "preconceptual" thinking. She may confuse causal associations with haphazard associations. She may believe a causal connection can be reversed, as Stacy did when she believed that being outside would stop the rain and thunder. To her, going in when it rains suggested going out to stop the rain.

Or he may believe, as Dirk did, that sharing an attribute with someone else or with a fictional someone automatically, even necessarily, means he is in all ways like the real or fictional person. Dirk firmly believed that he would be able to fly just because he wore a Superman costume.

Your child may believe that actions upon two such different categories of entities as people and objects will have the same effect. Stacy believed that because she could break objects, she could break feelings.

Immature thought, which is present in all young children, is a way station to more advanced systematic thought. It is important to listen carefully to what your child believes to be true. Don't correct her at first; try instead to understand what she believes, and then ask her how she knows. This may happily link what she believes to something she's actually observed.

Or, if a child believes that because A causes B, then B causes A— as when a child believes that because the rain can have an effect on us, we can have an effect on the rain, you can say, "Do you think that the rain makes us come inside?" Next step: "Do you think because the rain 'makes' us come inside, we can 'make' the rain stop by going out?" You'll have to adapt your questions to the specifics of your child's beliefs to make your meaning clear. His thoughts may be complex, but your language must be plain.

If you correct your child prematurely, he may become inhibited in revealing more of his thoughts. Your aim will be to keep a discussion going. If he confirms your guesses, feel free to thank him for letting you know what he thinks. When he seems comfortable talking about his thoughts, you can begin to introduce "counterevidence"; that is, you can talk to him about a causal event that doesn't reverse itself, as in, "We don't think, do we, that because we've pushed the ball, the ball will push us." It's important to encourage him to keep on exploring, because only with continued investigations of how the world works will he be able to sort out and make sense of his observations.

If your child confuses the properties of people with those of objects, as Stacy did when she told me she could break my feelings, invent exploratory games so he can test whether this is true. If he behaves as though he can turn you off the way we can turn off an electric light or a running motor, play this out with him. Ask him the whereabouts of the switch that makes you do something.

If she thinks that she can make you disappear by shutting her eyes or plugging her ears, remind her that she can still hear you when her eyes are closed and she can still see you when her ears are plugged. Then it may become clearer to her that her behavior reveals a belief or a wish.

Sometimes, "preconceptual" thinking can be taken by the child to the realm of metaphor. It's important, even if difficult, to differentiate immature thought from metaphorical thought. The latter bespeaks advanced cognition. When Stacy told me, as she flung objects across the floor, that she was *trying* to break my feelings, she alerted me to the fact that she now likened one thing to another: she *wished* feelings could be broken, like objects, but deep down she knew otherwise. Try though she might, she knew she couldn't break them.

Your child will eventually, perhaps spontaneously, differentiate people from objects. She will learn not to concretize that which is better symbolized. Stacy realized she could not actually see feelings being broken the way she could observe a toy being broken. So she invented an expressive metaphor to signal how she felt, a manner of speaking with me about her intensity of feeling toward me. I thought she meant to say something like, "I wish I could break your loving feelings, because they make me feel too close to you; but I know I can't rid myself of feeling the way I rid myself of toys."

Toys and equipment that I like to call "cognitive" can assist your child's theory of mind aptitude. These are toys that naturally invite the child to manipulate and learn. They help children plan ahead, test outcomes, predict events, and, ultimately, feel proud as a child "explorer" or a child "scientist."

Nesting toys and graduated blocks help very young autists learn about size and shape and invite them to compare objects. Puzzles of all kinds are also valuable for learning about size and shape, and they teach children how to fit one thing with another. All of this helps your child feel that certain aspects of his experience are sensible and reliable, a benefit to his view of himself in the world.

If your local science museum has a gift shop, find out about its science toys. One great science toy, called the "swinging wonder," illustrates Newton's second law of motion—changes in motion are equal to the applied force and in the direction of the applied force. Don't explain this at first. Let your child explore how the toy's five metal balls swing back and forth. Only later ask him to predict what will happen if he swings one, two, or three balls. Be sure you supervise this play because the balls, which are suspended by strings from a wooden frame, easily become tangled, which might frustrate your child. Explain to him that your job is to keep them untangled; his is to figure out how the toy works by playing with it carefully.

A child of six or seven may figure out how the swinging wonder works. A child of ten or older may be able to articulate the physical principle this toy demonstrates. Be sure to praise your child's every insight. Let him discover how this and other science toys work, and note the development in his thinking as he explains what he's doing and why.

Like the swinging wonder, magnets invite your child to explore the physical world. Let him experience the feeling in his hands when two magnets are attracting and repelling. Discuss with him what he thinks is happening as he plays with them. Encourage him to ask questions about what he's observing.

Magnet marbles fascinate young children. When they are able to pry open the marble's plastic covering, they soon discover that the object inside is a magnet. As they try to string magnet marbles together, even young children learn fairly quickly how to connect a marble being repelled at one end of the string; they'll readily attach the marble at the other end. They've learned that at one end of the string the marble attaches, and at the other end it repels.

Let your child explore the marbles before asking him to explain his actions. Accept his explanations, even if they seem wrong. Eventually you can ask pointed questions, encouraging him to think out problems more maturely. If he says he switched the marble to the other end of the string "just because," you can tell him that, indeed, he caused something to happen. If he says he switched the marble because it "likes" the other end better, ask him whether objects have feelings. Your aim is to get him thinking, whether or not he comes up with a fully correct answer.

Magic tricks also invite children to explore. Try showing your child how simple magic tricks work. He may feel "tricked" himself, as Greg did when we played with the rope-in-bottle trick, so let him invent his own magic and be appropriately impressed. Later, discuss with him that the trick's effect is an illusion; an event appears to happen in one way when in reality it happens in another. For example, the "magic money changer" appears to make a coin disappear when, in fact, the "magician" merely removes it from view.

The money changer consists of a hollow wooden rectangle into which a smaller rectangle can be inserted. The latter has a sliding internal piece with two coin-sized slots, only one of which is visible at a time. When a coin is placed in the visible circle, it appears to vanish as the "magician" pushes the insert against a tiny, hidden wire resting inside the larger wooden holder. This moves the slot containing the coin out of sight. All that can be seen is the empty slot.

Most children will remove the insert to look inside the wooden holder. Some kids actually notice the tiny wire at one end of it. Praise your child if he happens to discover the wire. Otherwise, ask him where he thinks the coin is, especially if he shakes the insert and can hear the coin rattling. Give him some clues to make correct guesses more likely, and tell him, when he's discovered or understood the trick, how well he can think out problems, how well his brain is working.

Building with blocks aids spatial organization in your child and also fine-motor and gross-motor coordination. He will have to think ahead to build a tower, a house, a garage for his cars. You can invent games with blocks, like taking turns building high towers to see which one topples first. See if he will build with the SOMA cube, seven differently shaped blocks that form a cube or such other objects as a tower, a dog, a castle. This is an advanced toy, appropriate for a child of nine or ten, unless your child is especially drawn to fitting shapes together or is spatially talented.

Cuisenaire Rods help with math understanding, but your child should just play with them first. The set comes with a poster for teachers and parents that will guide you in discussing these brightly colored, differently sized blocks with your child. He may discover on his own that rods of the same color are the same length. If not, you can show him that, say, the light green rods are shorter than the dark green ones. Then he may discover on his own that two light green rods equal one dark green.

Help him seriate the rods by length. After he's become accustomed to manipulating the rods, you may begin to teach him basic mathematical operations, which are illustrated by the poster. Ask your child's teacher how to use Cuisenaire Rods, or write to the Cuisenaire Company of America (New Rochelle, NY 10805). Or get John Holt's *How Children Fail* (revised edition, Perseus Publishing, 1995), and read the chapter demonstrating Dr. Caleb Gattegno's math teaching.

Shared storytelling, riddles, and jokes, inventing comparisons and analogies are all aids to developing theory of mind and social processes. Begin with storytelling, and discuss simple story themes to accustom your child to narrative and metaphor. Read stories to her and try to get her to talk about story meaning. Encourage her to discuss why a storybook girl or boy behaved as she or he did. This invites your child to ponder what the author meant to say. Above all, tell personal stories to your child about herself, her day, her past, her family, her future. Urge her to add details. Ask her to tell a story about what happened to her or to someone she knows. If she resists the story format—the fiction of it—encourage her to tell it as fact. Explain the difference between fictional and documentary accounts.

Then branch out into riddles; a good source for these is *The Six-Million Dollar Cucumber*, compiled by E. Richard Churchill (Dell, 1976). Riddles encourage linguistic fluency in your child as he plays with the idea that words change meaning in different contexts or that humor derives from extending a fact to its absurdity. For example, he might learn to appreciate the humor in: "What animal has the poorest manners? The goat. It is always butting in." Or to appreciate the ridiculous in: "Why did the mother buy her six children a dachshund? She wanted a dog they could all pet at once." Many autistic children attend to such specific details as the length and contour of animals. Their natural predilection for observing keenly would allow them to appreciate the amusing idea of a long animal being necessary for six children to pet simultaneously.

Similarly, easy-to-understand jokes help your child understand humor. If he has no perceptible reaction to riddles or jokes, tell him why you think they are funny. Ask him to make up some riddles or jokes, and even if they aren't funny, try to guess why he might think so. Always begin with the simple and progress gradually to the complex.

Simple comparisons can pave the way for more complex analogies. Begin with something like this: "Cats and dogs are both animals." Then ask your child to finish this thought: "Trees and flowers are both . . ." Move on to something more complicated, as in "A leaf is to a tree as a petal is to a . . ." If he seems interested in these exercises, or actually enjoys them, encourage him to search for comparisons and analogies himself. Ask him to explain his choices. Appreciate them even if they seem unusual or not quite right. As you continue to play with him in this way, he'll become more adept at comparing and analogizing in ways that make sense. If he protests these exercises, tell him that you require a bit of "thinking homework" each day.

Remember: Happily playing, learning, and thinking with your child will convince him that socializing is worth the effort.

Everyday Concerns

Parents can't always behave optimally toward their kids. When you feel frustrated or angry at an apparently endless impasse, the best thing to do is to go on to something else—a book, a household chore, time alone in your room, a cup of tea in the kitchen—before your feelings

overwhelm you. Doubtless you have learned to read your child's behavior and anticipate when he will act in ways that have frustrated or
annoyed you before. It's best to act on this knowledge sooner rather
than later, before your feelings pile up and become unmanageable for
you both. You can always try again later when you've calmed down
or feel more hopeful about him. It's best, especially if your child goes
ballistic with little warning, to arrange a system with your spouse, a
nearby relative, baby-sitter, or trusted neighbor, to take over while
you remove yourself, temporarily, from your child. Knowing you have
this backup will lessen your anxiety and enable you to survive the
worst in his behavior.

*Remember: Your child probably picks up on how you feel about
him even if he acts as if he couldn't care less.* Autistic kids care about
their parents' upsets just as ordinary kids do.

Even if your child is progressing, his development will not be linear.
No child's is. Young autists, especially, experience gaps in development, because they've been out of touch with the social world for a
while. Don't be alarmed if he seems to progress faster in some areas
than in others. Every positive gain is encouraging. Autistic kids may
advance more quickly in the cognitive sphere, their emotional understanding lagging behind. Praise his new understanding and new
knowledge, and comfort yourself that with your guidance his emotions
will catch up.

*Remember: All children sometimes experience a gap between their
level of thinking and their ability to handle their emotions reasonably.*

Read child-development books, many of which appear in the references, to familiarize yourself with typical behaviors at various ages.
Such books will give you some notion of what to expect when your
child leaves his solitary world to relate to you, to talk, to play, to

learn. He needs your support for every step forward even though he remains behind in some areas. The actual age at which he meets a developmental milestone is not as important as the fact that he's met it.

He also needs to be comforted when he's yet to become accustomed to a new way of looking at things, to a new way of being. This is often frightening to autistic kids, who resist any and all changes, even if they are for the better. Reassure him that all children have mixed feelings about growing up. Discrepancies in development may even out by adolescence or early adulthood. Your concrete, reasonable hopes for him will foster his own, which, in turn, will motivate him to keep trying and to feel okay about his future.

Your child's wish for control over everyday events has likely been your concern. As he leaves his private solitary world for the people world, he may try to exercise more control over you and other family members than he did before. *This is a propitious development.* It means the people world has become attractive to him. Respond by telling him the ways in which he can control his environment and by assuring him you will help him to do so. Help him predict the day's events. Invite him to participate as you schedule the day. He might like to write his own schedule. If he schedules something weird, let it go, and check with him at the end of the day to see if what he anticipated actually happened. You might develop this into a game in which you schedule something preposterous and ask him if it really happened.

Talk with him about the fact that he can choose, within limits, what to wear to school, which toys to play with, what he wants for gifts, and the like. About things he can't control, explain that these are group choices. Assure him that he will have a vote just as the others do. Don't be discouraged if he tests you on this, or gets angry and threatens to have a tantrum. Stick to your guns that there are some events he can control and some he can't. Respond to his temper matter-of-factly. Go about your business if he threatens to get out of control, telling him that you'd like to talk to him when he calms down. You'll have to teach him how to handle times away from you. Give him a specific time when you'll rejoin him. If he's amenable to using a timer, set it for, say, ten minutes, and tell him you'll check in with him then. If he hasn't calmed down, reset it, explaining to him what he has to do to get your attention again. Suggest a favorite activity for him while he's waiting for you or guide him to one of his favorite places in the house so he'll learn to comfort himself while he's regaining control.

As your child becomes more aware of himself in a social world and begins to compare himself to others, he may conclude that he is hopelessly odd, weird, unlikable, or incompetent, all because he's autistic. Tell him: *everyone has something in his life that is unfair.* Explain that life can be plagued by unexpected adversities that no one can predict and that we all must overcome as best we can.

As always, start the discussion on a positive note. Remind him that because he's accomplished in certain areas—say, at recognizing tunes, remembering facts, classifying natural phenomena, acing board games—in essence, "doing hard stuff well"—he has it in him to become proficient in other ways. If he mopes about not being very intelligent, tell him he must be, or he would not know as much as he does, wouldn't be able to read or to draw as well as he does, wouldn't have made as much progress as he has.

When he seems easy with your reassurances, you can branch out into the more difficult topic of his insecurities. Repeat to him: *we all have areas in which we feel less competent.* If he brings his social problems to you, ask him how *he* feels about *others.* If he responds that it is *they* who don't like *him,* tell him you'll help him cope. Try to find out as much as you can about the situations that make your child most uneasy. Discuss concrete strategies he may use with kids who tease and taunt him, like ignoring them, separating himself from them, reminding himself that *they* are the ones being unfriendly, not he. Suggest that he find someone who shares some of his interests so that he may more easily ignore the unfriendly behavior of the others. If your child attends school, ask his teacher for suggestions to help with social impasses.

Tell him about the memoirs of Temple Grandin, Donna Williams, and the autobiographical account by Paul McDonnell (in Jane Taylor McDonnell's *News from the Border*). Tell him these people wrote about their social problems in ways he might find interesting, inspiring, and liberating.

If his social problems continue and his self-esteem seems to plummet, consult a professional to help with self-image problems. In some locales, there are social-skills groups that can help your autistic child. Getting together with other parents of autistic kids provides support for you during these trying times and may lead to friendships for your child. Psychotherapists interested in young autists can provide guidelines for raising your child's self-esteem.

Sibs and Peers

Other children's reactions to your autistic child will be influenced by your responses to her. In a supportive, nurturing, tolerant environment that intimates hope for all, young children will not necessarily pick up on autistic oddities. Both sibs and peers will appear "naive" about autism unless someone communicates to them that something's wrong with your child or unless she behaves in a relentlessly bizarre, withdrawn, or hostile fashion. At some point in her development you may want to discuss with your other children that your autistic child is different from them in certain easily observable ways. If you add that everyone is different—that is, unique—and that your autistic child shares some traits with her sibs, your other children will have a generally benign context in which to understand autistic behaviors. As always, stress with all your children their skills and traits that are especially promising. In this way, they'll learn that human differences are to be respected and enjoyed.

When your young autist is interacting with his sibs, you can be a little less guarded than you would with a child from another family. Your other children quite likely will approach your autist naturally, intuiting what is likely to interest him. You must, of course, protect your children from mishap, undue stress, and disappointment, but as long as things are going reasonably smoothly, stay on the sidelines and make note of developing friendly scenarios among your children. Intervene quickly when things threaten to get out of hand. Advocate for all your children by saying something like, "It's okay for you to get tired of one another," and, "Now it's time for each of you to be by yourself doing something quietly."

Remember: The more your autistic child interacts with his sibs, the more naturally and realistically he'll interact with other children.

If an older relative or neighborhood child is more likely to be patient with your young autist than his agemates, enlist his or her help in getting your child engaged in playing and learning. Sometimes older kids invent clever games and learning activities. You can always discuss with your young aides the kinds of exercises you have developed for your child. Perhaps a babysitter would like to join you in your effort to draw your child out of his solitary world.

Prepare him in advance for a visit from a prospective friend from school or from the neighborhood. Remind him what his companion's interests are and discuss the schedule of events, including what he'd like to do and what you both think his companion would like to do.

Discuss the schedule with him the day before, with a warm-up reminder an hour or so before the visit.

Play dates should be brief at first. Get your child to participate in the planning and scheduling of these. Be ready to offer snacks, TV, or some other calming, diverting activity if he becomes frustrated, angry, or withdrawn. If conflicts arise, intervene immediately rather than hope things will straighten themselves out. Though your child and his sibs might be able to work things out on their own, a child outside the family will doubtless intimidate your autistic child more than his sibs do. Your child and his guest will need your firm hand sooner.

It's easier to calm things down when you troubleshoot potentially explosive situations early. Make sure that the parent of your child's companion is ready to pick him up after a short visit. You can gradually increase the length of your child's play dates, depending on how able and willing he is to tolerate social discourse. You'll need the cooperation of other parents, who may have to be on call initially, so that the prospective friend isn't turned off by too much autistic bluster.

Try to have the visit end on a happy note. This is what the children will remember, not the length of time they spent together.

You can coach your child in maintaining himself in structured activities with his sibs or peers. When you play with him, try to imagine how your other children or a child outside the family would react to your autist's social clumsiness, his arguments and oppositions, his daydreaming. You'll need to accustom him to the structured format of sports or board games before he'll be able to brave these activities with his sibs or companions. After he's got the hang of a game's rules and procedures, playfully introduce the behaviors you think characteristic of other children when he resists adjusting to the game's requirements. Try coaching him directly on how a companion might feel about his reluctance to join social activities. Teach the value to *him* of following rules, the predictive power of surmising what another person would do in a structured situation. All this gives him the opportunity to practice being with others.

After some social successes, you might see your child develop conflicts over excelling versus befriending. His comparisons with other kids may intensify, and he may exaggerate both his ineptness and the others' social facility. Moderate his exaggerations by talking to him matter-of-factly. Most children experience a dilemma over excelling and befriending as they attempt to achieve well and to be loyal to their friends all at once. Tell him this is a normal childhood problem. Tell him, as well, that it's a sign of progress that he wants to achieve and to make friends. Have him weigh the pros and cons of always winning at games versus attending to his friend's feelings. You're not aiming for a specific outcome. You want him to think and to implement his own social resolutions. As he does so, he will feel more competent, which in itself encourages more coping attempts.

The more he interacts with others, the more your child will react to taunts and gibes from his peers. He may expect that they'll treat him as gently and respectfully as you and your other children do. Yet he may no longer be content to ignore his peers or to turn away from them. Try teaching your child the difference between being laughed at and laughing with someone. Your goal is to sensitize him to those moments when he could share a joke or some fun with another kid. Teaching him the difference between being mocked and sharing comic moments could help enormously when he's dealing with painful social situations. You can prompt your child by telling jokes with the explicit instruction that if the kids make fun of him, he can also make fun, by joking. Don't get discouraged if he can't manage this immediately, consistently, or adroitly. Just one experience of deflecting his peers' mocking attitude will act as a powerful incentive to maintain his newly laid-back demeanor.

If, on the contrary, your child seeks revenge, as Greg did, for the taunts and gibes he's suffered at the hands of his peers, explain, first, that he has every right to be angry. Then warn him of the dangers of retaliation: that it's not safe for him to start fights or in any way seek revenge. Explore with him what he can do with his anger, for example playing out scenes with dolls or action figures, writing in a journal about how unfair it is that he gets teased, or talking it through with you or his sibs. The latter will convince him that his family is behind him, backing him up in his attempts to deal with his peers. The other main point to get across is your young autist's safety. Hearing that his safety is his family's primary concern will convince him of your sincerity in protecting him and will enable him to listen to your suggestions on how to cope with his feelings.

Helping Hands

A team approach is best whether your child is in a regular school or a special school. Public schools are mandated to educate your child. If classroom staffing is inadequate, write to the Autism Society of America (7910 Woodmont Avenue, Suite 300, Bethesda, MD 20814-3015) for advice on increasing educational services in your child's school. Or join a parent group so as to combine your efforts with others to secure the kind of school setting autistic children need. The Autism Society has chapters in every state and can help you find a parent group in your area.

Whether your child is in a regular or a special class, it might be staffed, in addition to the main teacher, with a student teacher and/or an aide and such ancillary teachers as a language specialist. The main teacher, who usually coordinates the faculty administering the program to special-needs students, will doubtless welcome support from you. Offer to help her coordinate everyone's efforts on behalf of your child. You can help by regularly attending parent–teacher conferences or meeting other routine requirements; you can volunteer for classroom activities and outings.

Review your child's program with his teacher so that you may support it at home in your discussions with him about school. It's very important for you to be in regular touch with his teacher, to hear about his progress not just in learning but also in socializing. The teacher will have different goals from the ones you've set at home. But this need not be confusing. It can be a learning experience for your child, because he will learn to respond differently to different situations. As he realizes something like "I read in school; I play at home," he will also respond differently to different people. It's just as important for his teacher to know what he's doing at home as it is for you to know what's going on in school. Explain to him that these talks will help you and his teacher plan for him. Discuss with him that family and school, while different, are similar in their aims to provide the best they can for him.

Autistic children who are ready for school learning can usually understand and learn to accept classroom rules. Rules can actually be reassuring to these kids because they make classroom life more predictable. Yet some kids, once they've understood the implications for them of classroom rules, may argue with their teacher or their parents, insisting that the rules aren't "fair" or are "stupid." They may assert that *they* should be the ones making the rules. Parents and teachers should realize that despite their unreasonable protests, the kids have, nonetheless, acknowledged the rules and allowed that there are social constraints.

Engage your child in a pros–cons discussion of the rules. Tell him it's not sufficient to flatly reject them. He must propose a more just or intelligent rule. A matter-of-fact attitude works best in these situations. Get him to see that his stubborn social intransigence won't get him very far, but reasonable talk will. Remind him of the value of group decisions. Just as everyone in your household has a say in some of the family rules, his teacher may lead a discussion in which the students voice their opinions about classroom rules.

You can help your child anticipate the school day by making a weekly calendar of school events. Ask his teacher whether you should supplement her teaching at home and, if so, how. Your aim is to clarify what is expected of your child and to help him see that you and his teacher are working together. Make sure he understands that homework times with you will be shorter than schoolwork times with his teacher, that he will have more time to play and to pursue his favorite diversions at home.

Share with his teacher the observations you've made on how he learns best. Discuss with her his special interests and any particular talents he may have. She can use this information in class to build on his strengths. Don't be reticent about suggesting ways to approach him. Make sure to ask your child's teacher about classmates who've made overtures to him or have been patient with him. If she hasn't thought of it already, suggest to the teacher that she pair him with another, willing student to share such classroom tasks as caring for a classroom pet, gathering up student papers, cleaning erasers and the chalkboard. Get the teacher's advice on how to go about arranging play dates for him, including whether she thinks the classmates' parents would support your efforts to get the kids together. Advance planning could save you and your child the disappointment of having a child or parent hesitate to socialize with your young autist.

If his school has no art, music, or gym program, try to introduce one or all of these into the curriculum. If you meet with resistance or such programs are slow in developing, provide your child with art and music materials and the exercise he needs. Join him in using crayons or markers and paper, in playing toy musical instruments or the piano, or in playing ball. As he becomes interested and more proficient, invite his sibs or some neighborhood kids to join you, gradually increasing the time he engages in these social activities.

Don't be discouraged or alarmed if your child shows increased moodiness or agitation about school. This is quite likely the result of his becoming more responsive to his teacher, to learning tasks, to his classmates, to classroom events. The teacher and the curriculum are having an impact on him, which is what you want. Discuss with his teacher ways in which you and the school personnel can support your child during troubling times to help him maintain his gains.

If he has adapted to classroom learning, he's probably bonded with his teacher in some way. His trust in her will help him overcome his resistance to learning and to making friends. Talk these issues over with him and his teacher. You may want to schedule a meeting with the two of them to review ways to help him feel comfortable with the school's expectations. He may need specific guidance on how to keep plugging away at learning and socializing despite apparent setbacks in his progress. He will doubtless have to be reminded *many times* that other students resist learning on occasion or become confused about certain learning tasks.

Remember: Your child will not suddenly become "normal" by virtue of being in a regular classroom or by adapting reasonably well to a curriculum designed for autistic kids. But with adequate support, he'll cope as best he can, reward enough, hopefully, for parents and teachers alike.

Parents and teachers do not have to be the autistic child's therapist, nor should they expect themselves to be. If your child seems stuck and the methods you and the teacher have tried to help her don't seem to be working, you may want to consult a psychotherapist. There may be psychological aspects to her rejection of learning, to her turning away from other students; there may be aspects to her pessimistic attitude that you or her teacher haven't thought of. Sometimes a fresh perspective on a knotty problem reveals unnoticed factors and suggests new tactics. She might welcome the opportunity to talk with someone about how she feels about being autistic. These talks may enable her to imagine a more viable future, one that includes more consistent learning and socializing attempts.

If your child is in therapy, insist on keeping the communication channels open between you and her therapist. To accomplish this, the therapist doesn't have to divulge every confidence she shares with him or her. It's the therapist's *job* to work out with your child how and when to discuss with you what's going on in therapy. The therapist also needs to hear from your child's teacher how things are progressing in school. Quite likely the teacher will want guidance from the therapist on better ways to approach her autistic student. Everyone concerned with these often difficult-to-reach kids—parents, teachers, therapists, language specialists—should be in regular contact regarding how she is processing the curriculum, dealing with social overtures, reacting to classroom events and happenings at home.

First rule of thumb on finding professionals for your child: they should like kids! You can assess this by visiting a classroom to observe whether the teacher enjoys her job and likes *being* with kids. You can ask prospective tutors, language specialists, or psychotherapists what they especially enjoy about their work. Since the work with autistic children is arduous, try to determine whether they like being with these kids enough to sustain themselves in the educational or therapeutic endeavor enthusiastically. Experience with autistic kids can be helpful but an inventive, energetic, yet less experienced person can be just as good. What you want is a forward-looking professional who can envision positive effects of the work he or she is doing with your child.

I hope these imagined talks I've had with you about your young autist's needs and troubles, his abilities and his prospects, have started you thinking about ways to promote his development. I hope "talking things over" with you has also inspired you to find ways of reaching your child that closely fit his or her unique experience, ways that, not knowing your child personally, I have doubtless missed.

Remember: An autistic child's parents and a community of helpers dedicated to him are his best hope for the future.

CHAPTER ELEVEN

Hopes for Autistic Children

We still are dreamers.

—PARENT OF A YOUNG AUTIST

While I was writing this book, I happened to turn on the radio during a panel discussion on autism that included several teachers of autistic children and a psychologist specializing in the condition.[1] The call-in forum encouraged parents to speak their views. They could not get enough of talking enthusiastically and affectionately about their children, very like many of the parents I'd known.

A mother of a nine-year-old girl was especially articulate. She recounted her autistic daughter's school successes, telling the radio audience how well her child was doing in a regular classroom. She gave an impassioned speech about her daughter's special qualities, her musicality, her poetic language, her sense of humor.

One of the participants interceded, "I think autism is a terrible disease, and we ought to get rid of it."

Undaunted, the girl's mother responded, "I'm not at all sure that if there was a pill to cure autism—and I don't think there will be—that I'd want my daughter to take it. It would be a loss of some sort," she concluded, referring to the qualities she'd listed so tenderly. Gracefully, she resisted succumbing to the expert's unwarranted pessimism about her daughter's condition.

. . .

Autism, as lived out, is not so much a disease as it is a social condition. It is more promising and accurate to think of autism as a set of social predicaments aided and abetted by specific neurological impediments that challenge autistic people over the course of their lives as they stretch for or forbear socializing.

The medical model allows us to test for and attempt to remediate the neurological, biochemical dysfunctions, but often it does not acknowledge what the young autist himself can do to ameliorate the effects of his condition. If we understand his problems as biological only, we deny such a child the mastery that flows from making human choices. Anthropologist T. M. Luhrman, who makes a similar point, writes of the hazards in viewing psychiatric disorders as primarily medical. This, she says, discourages those diagnosed from recognizing that they are thinking and feeling, albeit sometimes differently from other people. "They become lesser persons, lesser agents, lesser moral beings."[2]

As I've stressed throughout this book, our respect for the autist's perspective, our understanding of and empathy with his condition, is what lays the groundwork for luring him away from his private world and into the "people world." Showing him that he makes a difference to us, that we care about what he does, thinks, and feels, that we care about him as a person, helps prepare him for the idea that he is capable of participating in his own recovery.

Unless he is attracted to the people world, though, he will not wish to join us. Showing him that he matters to humankind and that there are those who wish to assist him with his troubles socializing and conversing, with his problems approaching others despite his autistic ways, engenders the hope that he *can* improve his lot in life. He becomes more optimistic about his future day by day, as any child would, as he perceives more clearly that each small gain, each hesitant but significant step, leads him ever closer to being the happier person he wishes to be, at ease with himself, at ease with others.

Demoralizing those parents who are dedicated to tackling autism's quandaries is not the answer. It is the *team approach* that works best in assisting autistic youngsters. Parents, more than experts, are aware of the intractable realities of living with these children. Those of us interested in them and in their condition ought to help parents *enjoy* their kids. We ought to *applaud* a parent who rejoices in her child's achievements. We who would instruct, guide, and enlighten parents' efforts need not dwell on the obvious social perils besieging young autists and their families. We ought to recognize each autist's actual weaknesses *and* strengths, noticing the veritable child without eliminating from our vision the hoped-for child. He will need to use his strengths to combat his weaknesses. Helping a child resolve some of his social dilemmas has its own merits and ought to be honored.

As they cope with a withdrawn or wild young autist, parents and teachers may believe that it's impossible for them to alter their attitudes or feelings toward these notoriously challenging kids. But feeling the "right" feelings goes a long way toward easing autistic indifference. Although we cannot accomplish a change of heart by fiat, we ought to consider that our emotions and attitudes affect the young autist from the outset. This encourages in us the realization that the baby's or toddler's reactions to his parents, his sibs, his teacher—*his* behavior toward *you*—makes sense. While it may not make sense when your baby refuses your loving arms, his tearful upsets do make sense when you remember his sensitivities, his feelings of inadequacy, his worry that something's terribly wrong, his agitation when those around him become frustrated at not being able to relate to him.

Your feeling that his behavior makes sense, in turn, contradicts the young autist's inveterate pessimism, because he perceives that important people in his life have become more selective in their guardedness about his future. They may recognize, for example, that his actions are clumsy but that he nonetheless displays a phenomenal memory for weather facts, show tunes, baseball statistics, animal lore, or chess moves. Though he may test just how sincere you are in granting him his skills, interests, and predilections, the notion that people appreciate what he has accomplished tempts him to acquaint himself with his place in society.

Psychotherapy and Team Efforts

Much of this book describes conversations between an autistic youngster and me as we talk or play together in the consulting room. It has been my aim throughout to demonstrate how three important settings—the therapy hour, the home, and the classroom—can structure situations to increase the likelihood that a young autist will emerge from his isolation to speak with us, to relate better generally, in essence, to *be among us* more companionably. But how better to identify the specific circumstances that challenge autistic indifference and engage young autists in their own recovery? How to know which of our attitudes will enlist their participation in a social world?

The psychotherapy setting is a special sort of social milieu, permitting the child and me to be comfortably together without the world's distractions. In important ways, it is not unlike the mother–infant communion, when mother and baby are pleasurably and safely connected to one another. Yet the social benefits of the mother–baby duo are often missing in the early life of an autistic child. As a baby, he is often wildly overstimulated, literally pushing himself away from his mother's cuddling or languishing limply in her arms.

The child who tolerates attentive empathy in individual therapy—who learns to do it—experiences or reexperiences an attunement that ordinarily reverberates between parent and small child. This is not to say that the psychotherapist functions as a mother to such a child. Nor should a therapist baby him, return him to infantile pleasures. This is the last thing a young autist needs. Infantilizing him would create a false sense of security and would debilitate his struggling ego. Rather, he needs to develop the social and intellectual skills more or less appropriate to his chronological age.

Yet the one-to-oneness in the therapeutic encounter restores and fortifies a fundamental sense of *us*. The child is then enabled to respond to his parents at home, primed as he is for "us-ness." Over time, he likely connects more closely with his family than he did before. The feeling of *being understood*—feeling tuned in to—helps the young autist adapt to society.

Being protected in the company of a trusted person convinces the autistic child of the worth of the "people world." The interpersonal therapy setting has in common with the parent–child duo the hugely gratifying communion with a sympathetic other that many young autists lack or have lost, until someone dedicated to them restores it. With this restoration, the child not only experiences hope for himself in a social world, often for the first time, but he also reveals more of himself to his parents, sometimes in subtle ways, confiding more of his feelings and thoughts. His parents, in turn, realize they have found something new, originated by their child, to which they can relate.

This is what psychotherapy can offer young autists that behavioral therapies cannot. A behavioral program focuses on substituting new behaviors for maladaptive behaviors but, ordinarily, without any input from the child, the one who is asked to change. Though many autists need social training by behavioral methods and specific, direct linguistic assistance, these interventions can be productively supplemented for children and families who are receptive to the "talking cure." In this more open-ended context, the autist who learns to take charge of his own therapy begins to understand and to help himself in the presence of a responsive, encouraging other.

Not all autistic kids need psychotherapy. Some regroup with people by reacquainting themselves with their parents spontaneously. Or they reconnect by way of an important attachment to their teacher. But some need therapy to help with their insecure and often angry feelings at being autistic. Others need it when the efforts of parents, teachers, and specialists run aground because of the child's resistance to change. Young autists, like other children, sometimes reject even well-intentioned efforts on their behalf.

Psychotherapists to autistic kids must remember that they are often most at ease within their solitary worlds. We must not aim to deprive a child of his world, even if we could. He has likely lived in his private realm for many years, a protected sphere that interests, even fascinates him, one that often gives him great pleasure. He enjoys the control he exerts over it, because it is not subject to the vagaries of interacting with people. In this world he can imagine acting more freely, while in the people world he feels constrained by his extrasensitivities, by the unexpected that arises from relating to others, and by the demands, real or imagined, that they place on him. We should not cavalierly deny, nor even dilute, what he reaps from his world.

Yet, many autists with whom I worked responded well to the opportunity to reflect upon themselves. Introspection didn't seem alien to them. When they began to trust that I wouldn't intrude haphazardly into their thoughts, they engaged in this basic psychotherapeutic process rather easily, sometimes ardently. They explained themselves to me with the same earnest fervor they had displayed before, when they delved into conversations about dinosaurs, the weather, chess, superheroes, stories and histories, the "good" and "bad" in people.

There are hazards intrinsic to the therapeutic process for autist and therapist alike. When an autistic child begins to share her thoughts with another person and to perceive the benefits of doing so, she begins to experience herself in a new way. She must adapt to aspects of a developing self. Adapting to the new is not generally part of an autist's repertoire, even if a new thing or experience appears to be fun or gratifying. It is important for everyone involved, her parents, her therapist, above all the young autist herself, to realize that doubts about and retreats from the therapeutic process are to be expected. They are normal. If we get unduly discouraged or worried, we may dishearten or confuse the child, whose grasp of the new is tenuous at best. Too many times she's seen the world retreat at her clumsiness and her eccentricities. She's altogether too likely to conclude that contending with the people world is just not worth it.

Often a therapeutic benefit accrues to the young autist simply because he begins to relate well to someone outside the family. Taxonomist Greg and superhero Dirk could conceive of having friends because they thought of me as a friend. Greg's befriending attempts succeeded more than Dirk's, probably because Greg's family sought to blunt the impact of the rejections he suffered at the hands of his peers, while Dirk's parents reproached Dirk for his social failures. Scribe Wendy was also well integrated into her family, but she had had few successes engaging with her teachers, and before therapy her peer relationships had been chronically unsteady.

All three children became visibly relaxed when they were with me, realizing that they had a friend who would not vanish for some perplexing reason, for some autistic impropriety they hadn't even registered.

The fact that a friendship could have such favorable effects on these young people encouraged me. I had known since my work with singing Marcia, dramatizing Stacy, and mute Paulie that the unexpected that arose from human interaction threatened them, had many a time interrupted their attempts to be close, had, in Paulie's case, inhibited him to such an extent that he wouldn't even venture a human approach. Paulie's parents were gladdened, as was I, when their reclusive son, who had never seemed to notice anyone outside his immediate family, appeared to react to me in some mysteriously promising, outgoing fashion. He soon sensed, his parents told me, their burgeoning hopes for him, especially when they dropped him off for our meetings, which eventually seemed to excite Paulie enough for me to detect a certain anticipation in his gaze as he watched dreamily for my next action or coyly listened to my next few words.

Young James coped better in social situations the more he negotiated with me. Since his declamations often abrogated the rights of others as this "little professor" attempted to control and predict their every action, it was essential for his success in the people world for him to admit and honor the fact that others had their own plans, interests, minds, and feelings. He behaved as if he were a young prince, centered squarely in his solitary universe, into which he'd invite others now and then, but only on condition that he dictate their actions, thoughts, and feelings.

Yet James found an honorable way to resist my misguided efforts to help—actually to admonish my behavior—by holding to his view, albeit passively, of the taking-turns rule. His apparent disinterest in me and in the board game we were playing masked his wish that I acknowledge his understanding of, and need to abide by, the rule he'd learned in school. He didn't protest my talkative behavior openly as other children do. He ignored my habitual invitation to him to choose a shared activity, wishing silently that I'd take my turn selecting something. He simply declined to respond until it occurred to me that his inaction signified his belief that I ought to behave differently. It wasn't that he wished to remain estranged from me. On the contrary, he was bewildered when I seemed to avoid taking my turn, violating a social norm.

As James became bolder in arguing with me about the proper way to conduct a therapy session, I realized that he challenged me on my own turf and in my modality as a therapist. This was the very development I'd been working toward. I hoped that he would stand up for himself when with other people, that he'd express his opinions forthrightly and persuasively. Even though he seemed a little pugnacious when he practiced being himself, I loved it when he did so. Who was I to dispute his new assertiveness, especially when it arose from our conversations and thus was a personal reaction to me and my life's work? Together, James and I created the conditions in which he could affirm himself, much like Wendy, who zealously defied me as she refused to let me see the stories she'd written.

By his inaction or by his occasional mystifying silence, James was able to create in me the need to reevaluate continuously, not just what I wished to see in him, but also where I, personally, was coming from.[3] Although I didn't tell James outright that his behavior made me feel a certain way, my actions seemed to speak to him. When I got up from our game to do something on my own, as he, apparently ignoring me, was flipping through a book, James behaved as if I'd said that my behavior toward him had been so off the mark that it had caused him to withdraw, as if I'd remarked, "Hey, before I was wrong about you when I said, 'Maybe you don't feel like playing with me right now. You wish, perhaps, that you and I could be together, but still do our own thing.'"

Although he didn't acknowledge my changed attitude openly, he did rejoin me in our game and confided in me again. He told me he was once more worried about emergencies. This admission led to our discussion of life situations that felt like emergencies and those that didn't.

Therapeutic Dilemmas

Therapeutic dilemmas occur in work with autistic children as the result of two factors. One derives from the autistic personality, which creates a catch-22 as the child engages with you at the same time that he seeks to protect himself from this commitment. Just when he ventures toward you, he feels he must withdraw his overtures. The very act of relating mobilizes his desire to remain apart. Beth Kephart describes this phenomenon in her young son when she writes beguilingly: "He escapes into a room in his head like a ship to sea, even as the gulls fly above, imploring: land, land."[4] The other factor is an unreflective interpretation of the child's behavior that does not take into account his immediate, anguished ambivalence over intimacy. James had become consciously aware of the intensity of our relationship when he withdrew from shared activities, returning to them only after I followed his lead and began, like him, to do something on my own.

A similar impasse occurred when ten-year-old Stacy understood how close she and I had become. She had left her pretend world for good. She became acutely involved, if ambivalently, in our special times together. She'd ask for her favorite snacks during our individual meetings, only to reject noisily the very drink she said was her favorite. She would, impishly at first, request cherry soda, then boisterously refuse to drink it, fiercely teasing me as she ceaselessly pushed it—and me—away. Why, I asked myself, did she not enjoy my bringing her favorite drink to our special meetings?

Initially, I thought Stacy playacted an early childhood drama about being fed. What she meant to express, I realized later, was her reaction to closeness *per se*. Being with me *and* drinking her favorite soda was simply too much. My suppositions startled her, much like the sudden noise of a vacuum cleaner or the unbearable screech of a fingernail on the blackboard. In fact, as I spoke with Stacy about her cherry drink, she grabbed and split in half a tiny dollhouse vacuum cleaner as though to alert me to my misunderstandings of her. When I tried to articulate her conflict by saying, for example, "Maybe you're not sure you like me, so you don't feel like drinking your snack," she threatened to break yet more toys.

It wasn't at all that she didn't like me, although she *was* angry that I didn't understand her. Indeed, her affection for me contributed to the overstimulation she experienced when she was presented with her favorite drink by her favorite person. Since my theses seemed so wrong, there was no way she could clarify them by rephrasing them and asking me afterward, "Do you mean . . . ?"

Giving Stacy her favorite drink confronted her with the dilemma that were she to accept it, she risked feeling closer to me than was safe. Yet refusing the drink meant forgoing something she dearly loved, which hardly felt pleasurable *or* safe. Her conflict was often so excruciatingly painful that she dissolved into desperate, angry tears or started flinging toys around, intending to break them. Then she was trying to break my feelings. She wished to crush the affection she felt toward me and I toward her lest she be hurt by being loved too much. When push came to shove, she, like many an autist, chose the thing over the person.

Did I feel insulted as Stacy withdrew from me to slurp her soda, wide eyes pinned to the cherry red bubbles? Probably. That is why I tried to analyze her behavior—in effect, to get closer to her, no matter what. I had forgotten that being less withdrawn than a kid like Marcia did not mean that Stacy wasn't feeling inundated, intimidated actually, by intimacy.

Perhaps if I'd distanced myself a bit, rather than talking to her in an intense voice, or accepted her wish to remain distant from me, quietly straightening up the session room or reading a book so she could consume her snack in peace, she would have found my presence less overbearing, as James had when faced with a similar conflict. Then Stacy might have enjoyed her cherry drink and begun, a few minutes later, to chat happily with me again.

The Threat of Separation

Just as autistic kids find forming and maintaining social bonds troubling, they have difficulty coping with separations from people who have become important to them. Both Stacy and Marcia tried valiantly to adjust to my absences when I worked and lived with them at the

Orthogenic School. After Marcia began to relate to me, my yearly vacations loomed large as she wept for hours upon my return. Even maddeningly taciturn Marcia seemed to feel the loss of her favorite people when they were away. My fancy psychological explanation for her weeping upon my return is that I was safe as a loved person only when I was actually present. She could not risk weeping for me in my absence, so she waited until she was sure my vacation was over and done with.

Stacy knew that she'd suffer not just temporary losses—when I was ill with the flu or away temporarily—but that I would eventually leave her once and for all. She concluded that this must be so, because she saw that other staffers left the School and the kids they cared for.

During the years I worked there, we felt that the most important aspect of our work with our troubled charges was the quality of our personal relationships with them. For autistic students, a most important aspect was the inception of a relationship. This may explain why those working with these children were particularly prone to imagining that only they were strongly attached to them. The autistic kids were so hard to understand, to relate to, to *be* with, that once the hurdle of forming an attachment had been cleared, the ensuing interactions took on an urgent, precious quality.

The kids also felt the urgent devotion. All too often Stacy imagined what would happen to her hard-won friendship with me, wondered what would happen to her if it were permanently interrupted as, inevitably, it would be. That is why, as I was leaving Chicago, she responded so quickly and earnestly, so poignantly, with her request that I take her with me to Boston.

I was to discover, years later, that even those autists who live at home withdraw or become anxious at the threat of a rift from their favorite tutors or teachers. This stems partly from their having had to struggle so hard to trust others outside the family. When the autistic kids move ahead a grade, or when a teacher or tutor moves away, or when they finish their therapeutic work and have to say good-bye to their therapist, the intimidation attending this loss affects them more than it does a regular kid. Autistic children doubt their ability to interest others, so any interpersonal loss discourages them from trying again. Their view that the next person to come along might not appreciate or understand them inhibits them from reaching out freely to an unfamiliar someone.

Eleven-year-old Nate, who'd escape into the world of books, anticipated that we'd eventually part. But he enjoyed his supportive, congenial family. When a separation surfaced, either from a favorite teacher as he graduated to the next grade or from me, he could approach it with greater equanimity than did Stacy or Marcia. He knew he would never lose the family who saw to his needs so reliably.

Yet it was important for Nate to assure himself and me that our relationship, or perhaps, the *idea* of our relationship, would survive therapy's end. He dramatized his wish by declaring that the chessmen he called "commanders" would withstand their final battle. In doing so, he revealed his view of relationships. He feared they might become undone because he'd always dreaded feeling and remaining close to people. The only reason he could think of to explain our separation was that something must have gone wrong; he must not, he thought, have been attentive enough to our interactions.

This time, he did not want to return to a friendless existence. Rather than finishing his last therapy hour by having one of the commanders—that is, one of us—perish, he playacted that they—we—endured. At this turning point, he felt he must reassure himself through play that the affectionate bond between us would live on despite our parting. In this way he tried to overcome his social insecurities.

Nate's ability to adapt rested largely on his parents' resolute efforts to ease the impact of his condition. This convinced me, as did the progress of other autists who relied on their responsive families, that the best hope for an autistic child is his family. As long as the family is reasonably cohesive and the child is normally intelligent and shows a linguistic aptitude or other natural skills, home life is best for fostering his development. And if the child's autism is diagnosed early, professional assistance can be magnified many times over by a supportive family.

Placing him in an institutional setting will likely increase an autist's isolation. Relationships that live on are key to helping autistic kids endure, not just emotionally and socially, but also physically.[5] Even at their best, institutions cannot provide a permanent, viable, social experience for young children. The emphasis here is on "permanent." The Orthogenic School was a viable social milieu, but it lacked a sense of permanence for many of its students. Even if the institution allows family visits or brings the family in for treatment, the child, besieged by anxiety at the apparent loss of his family and home in an environment that seems strange and forbidding, will find it difficult to remember that his family still cares about him. As noted previously, autistic youngsters who suffer the loss of their families are thereafter unlikely to respond propitiously to people if they understand that their habitat is subject to personnel changes. The family is the autist's best hope for a return to the social world—a family, nurtured and encouraged, to be sure, by the community of helpers ready to assist in this momentous yet rewarding task.

Sensitive, reticent, and skeptical though he may be, if the child has already experienced interpersonal triumphs, our judicious hopes for him will mitigate against his assumption that the loss of an important person is an irreversible tragedy. Such a child needs the conviction of all who remain with him that separations can be coped with, that his feelings about them make sense, and that new people in his life offer different, but equally valuable, social opportunities.

Parents are Part of the Team

Psychotherapists to autistic kids are well positioned to help their parents. A therapist who connects with a young autist and promotes his social development can also offer guidelines to his parents on how to encourage similar developments at home. Therapy with such a child ought to be focused on overcoming his social reclusivity and not on, say, the angry feelings he may have toward the important people to whom he is nonetheless unsteadily attached. A therapist simply does not have the luxury of speaking with an autistic kid about mixed feelings toward family members if he has spent much of his life remote from them. Only after he has left his solitary world, and only if he brings his mixed feelings spontaneously to the therapeutic hour, may the therapist help him sort out his ambivalence toward those close to him with any degree of success.

By early adolescence Gregory had combined the animal world with the people world. But I had to keep from saying too much. I'd learned that he would not respond if I asked him about the negative feelings that might be fueling his metaphorical dramas. Talking with him about his mixed feelings toward the people who had taken such good care of him would undermine the progress he'd made in relating to them. Even a mild suggestion about how he might possibly resent his sibs evoked loyal statements from him as he attempted to show me how important his family had become. Much better were my comments that he appreciated his parents' kindness and that he enjoyed the company of his brother and sister. Then he could hear me ask, "Why not make friends?"

Greg had become particularly responsive to his mother, who usually brought him to his therapy appointments. She told me that Greg eagerly anticipated his visits with me. He may have thought something like, "My mom takes me to this nice person, who has interesting things to play with. She's a grown-up who likes me, just as my mom does."

I doubt that Greg's alliance of me with his mother went much beyond this. And I didn't encourage it to develop in an adversarial way by remarking that he may have harbored negative feelings toward her—or me. Greg's major problem, notwithstanding his inner struggle over the "good" and "bad" in him and the "good" and "bad" in others, was in approaching and negotiating within the people world. As I encouraged him to feel good and hopeful about himself, the intensity of the inner struggles seemed to abate, as if by magic. He brought his feeling of "good me" to new and different situations that, naturally, promoted more interesting relationships within his family and more lasting friendships with his peers. As we worked together toward his social adaptation, for which he repeatedly sought help as he dramatized his difficulties with his classmates, Greg and I were able to envision social vistas for him never before imagined possible.

As he came to feel more relaxed in my company, Greg seemed to behave more sensitively toward his mother. It might have also worked the other way around: pleasing his mother by being more sensitive to her perhaps allowed him to relax with me. They'd leaf through library books together, discussing the text informally and amiably. He began to tolerate my conversations with her, sometimes joining in. Before, he'd tense up, fretting that his mother would divulge something he didn't want me to know, or he'd protest that we were interfering with his solitary agenda.

He helped his mother more often, just as he had helped me pick up marbles. He'd even try to comfort her when she was upset by trying to reason with her that her upsets were unnecessary. He soon volunteered to take care of a household pet. His teacher reported that he was volunteering in class, both to assist others with school assignments or to help with a classroom chore, like gathering up student papers. When I heard of these new developments, I wondered whether Greg's newly resilient sense of self in therapy had affected his relationship with his mother and his teacher or, on the contrary, whether these improved relationships had increased Greg's ability to use his therapy visits.

When I supported his sense of himself by saying of the jackal, "He wrote who he was!," I encouraged Greg to drop his reclusive stance. This worked because he felt strong in the presence of another person, one to whom he'd opened up many times through metaphorical dramas. He was then able to take chances with others, notably his mother, who had always enjoyed Greg's company, but who now felt easier being with him more flexibly. She realized, she told me, that he wasn't keeping his feelings from her as he had before, which inspired her to behave differently toward him, to act rather like she did with her other children.

Therapists of autistic kids must sensitize themselves to the child's greater openness, both with his parents and with his therapist. This greater receptivity to social situations reverberates from one setting to another, from home to therapy, back and forth. Such resonances can also occur between the child, his teacher, and his parents. Then parents and teachers alike will find ways to use their parenting styles and teaching skills more freely and effectively in devising strategies to help young autists that work.

If psychotherapy benefits autistic children, it's because empathy and intimacy become associated with good things happening. Being with the therapeutic other becomes unassociated from such scary or perilous events as being subject to unbearable stimulation or to feelings of inadequacy in significant, earthshaking ways. Practicing being himself in therapy aids the young autist in buffering his senses from interpersonal stimuli, because he has the feeling that his strong self can find ways to ameliorate their effects. This strong self, in turn, is more likely to hone interpersonal skills within the family, to risk contact with an increasingly larger social group, to perfect talents in the arts or in science.

• • •

Wendy began to feel closer to her mother, and her mother to Wendy, when she began to open up to me in therapy. She always had a viable relationship with her mother, yet she would vehemently object when her mother asked to see her writing, especially if she sensed her mother was more than casually interested in it. Her mother worried that Wendy was trying to shut her out; she also became apprehensive when her daughter would withdraw from her peers or behave diffidently toward her teacher. Wendy's mother was most disturbed when Wendy would recoil from intimacy just when her mother most needed it.

My goal was to draw mother and daughter even closer, and more safely. Soon Wendy's mother became relieved by the single fact that she saw her daughter begin to interact with me, reciprocating my overtures. This reassured her, helped convince her that something could be done about her daughter's tendency to withdraw into her own world, that she could be gently coaxed by someone outside the family to be with people more cordially.

A decisive moment in Wendy's therapy came when she realized that imitating someone is not the same as being inspired by her. Earlier she thought if she "copied" her mother too assiduously, she might "copy" her mother's emotions, feel them exactly as her mother did. Now she understood that when she wanted to model herself on her mother's qualities, especially her artistic gift, she need not fret about being inundated by the stimulation emanating from her mother or by the understandable excitement her mother displayed at viewing Wendy's art. She could retain the feeling of being inspired without risking her emotional safety.

After acknowledging Wendy's progress, her parents began to up the ante, to wonder whether their daughter was capable of developing skills in areas in which she'd shown little interest before. Could she tackle tasks that she'd never attempted to master?

I assured her parents that Wendy was capable of developing her natural gifts and interests but warned them that if they pressured their daughter too much, she might refuse to listen to them and might withdraw from areas in which she'd excelled. I spoke with them about how all children, not just autistic kids, need support in their chosen realms, especially when they have experienced success. The fact that I advised them about Wendy as I would any parents tempered their apprehensions and expectations. "I guess if she *wants* to learn how to play softball, she *will!*," they concluded. A few months later, Wendy's mother told me that Wendy had not only agreed to try out for the softball team, but had actually paid attention to the game, learned the rules, how to bat, how to be a team player, how to be "one of the girls"!

I've already commented on how hopes soar among some parents of autistic kids as the result of the dedication of their teachers or other professionals and the perception that help has been forthcoming in tangible, welcome ways. It's as though the years of dismay and despair must be balanced by aspirations and accomplishments that would be unrealistic for any child in a short time.

I've had to suggest to the parents of these children that the remarkable achievements of, say, Temple Grandin or Donna Williams are not attainable by all young autists, just as regular kids cannot be expected to be young Albert Einsteins or Mary Cassatts. The hope that a child will achieve what Grandin and Williams have attained is particularly prominent among parents whose children are gifted or who react auspiciously to a therapeutic encounter. Hopes mount beyond what the autist, intelligent or gifted though he may be, can comfortably manage. The hazard of this situation is that the autistic child will withdraw from the people world, concluding that his early successes weren't numerous or significant enough.

The remedy for the hopeful parent of a responsive young autist is for those of us who work with the family to support both child *and* parent in the child's efforts to learn, to communicate, to socialize. It is more important to develop these three areas in his repertoire than any single skill or achievement. Psychotherapy can help because the therapist, more than parents or teachers, has the luxury of following the child's interests. Teachers impart knowledge; parents help kids adapt socially. The therapist follows the child's own thoughts and balances the team's efforts. A child like Wendy, then, can learn in therapy, just as she does at home, to communicate and to socialize while writing and drawing. A child like Greg can learn in therapy, just as he does in school, to communicate, even socialize, while lecturing on his chosen topic, animal taxonomy. He had to develop memory and classification skills in order to acquire this knowledge. As I listened to him, tracking his evolving mastery, he felt that I was truly interested in him, which had a ripple effect on his behavior elsewhere.

I am convinced that perhaps *the* most important benefit of psychotherapy—one that can also be realized at home and in school—is the child's coming to know his own mind as he explains it to another person. Feeling more secure in knowing what he is all about, he is more likely to become curious about the minds of others. Why do they come to the conclusions they arrive at, rather than those the autist has deduced? How to make sense of the sometimes wondrous disparity between two different perspectives when both suddenly seem relevant? An ability and a willingness to appraise the other's mind motivate the young autist to measure his performance, successes, and conclusions against those of other people. This not only promotes the acquisition of knowledge and the refinement of skills, it also enhances communication and, above all, social learning.

How They Fared

How did the autists I've portrayed fare after my work with them ended? Marcia returned home a year after I left Chicago. I had no contact with her after that.

Stacy also returned to her family several years after I left the Orthogenic School. Before she left, she wrote to me occasionally. Her letters told of what she was learning and of such daily events as class field trips. I was heartened to see that she'd learned to write. Since she sometimes mentioned other staffers, I assumed she had formed new relationships. Her spelling was accurate, but her handwriting was erratic, the letters often huge. She exaggerated her letters just as she had elongated a word's vowels or had spoken precisely to insure that I caught her meaning. Perhaps she imagined getting my attention with her boldly and massively written messages.

I later discovered that Stacy tried resolutely to form new relationships but, alas, she was not strong enough to bear the many staff changes. Much of what she had gained from her teacher seemed to vanish if she was moved to a different classroom. She had to begin anew with each new teacher.

The same was true of her reaction to my leaving. She became disconsolate at the mere mention of my name. She lost many of the fundamentals of relating along with the person who left her. Perhaps Stacy hoped I would return to take care of her if she wrote to me in dark, bold letters.

Burt continued to make slow gains in a hospital's special program for autistic youth. Paulie and Dirk moved away while I was working with them, so I have no recent information on how they got on in life.

The others at this writing are doing remarkably well. Greg is about to finish high school, excelling in biology and computer science. James is flourishing. His parents told me that he's expanded his social circle and spends most evenings on the telephone, arranging dates with his friends. Now preadolescent, Jamie excels in all school subjects.

Wendy's parents revel in her successes, both academic and creative. They are relieved that she enjoys a busy social life. Though quite shy, Wendy has formed meaningful friendships within a small group of her peers. Nathan has several close friends. He attends high school, where he excels in the humanities but balks at math. He resisted math, he once told me, because he realized that mathematical procedures, such as the rules of "borrowing" and "carrying," gave him no leeway to make up his own.

What to make of these successes? All four children had the consistent support of their parents, despite the trying setbacks they experienced helping their kids, and despite the discouraging reactions of those who believe autism to be a terrible disease to be gotten rid of as soon as possible. The parents had all sought help early. Greg's and James's parents brought them to see me when their boys were quite young—Greg was five; James was two and a half. Though Wendy and Nate were older when their parents sought my help, all along they had chosen the most compatible teachers they could find for their children, had arranged play dates for them when their kids seemed unduly isolated, had marshaled the help of relatives when fatigued by their children's demands and unsettled by their quirks. Finally, all four children had developed language before the age of five.

The conclusion? Identify autistic youngsters during their early years to provide them with the tutorial and therapeutic assistance they need to continue to grow and thrive emotionally, linguistically, socially, and cognitively. Provide parents with the helping hands they require.

Teachers and Team Efforts

I referred earlier to the fact that our feeling the "right" feelings helps autists transcend their condition. This applies both to school and to home. "Helping autistic kids is really a matter of liking them," said the principal of the public school I visited. Liking autistic kids is feeling one of the right feelings. To search for something likable about them may seem a daunting assignment but when, much to your surprise, they begin to talk to you or to a peer, or shyly join a group activity, you'll find, henceforth, that liking them becomes easier.

Appreciating autistic children is not the only "right" feeling. The frustration that ensues when teachers' efforts do not go well is entirely natural. Honoring your covenant to them is taxing and arduous, sometimes without a reward in sight. During these times, it's critical to have the support of those with whom you work—other faculty, administrators, the child's parents. Parents, too, need the continual support of their families, friends, and neighbors, in addition to encouragement from professionals who work with their children.

"You're supposed to be feeling what you're feeling. You say about a regular kid, 'This kid is driving me crazy.' You can say that about your autistic students, too," said the principal of the teachers I observed, cheerleading her faculty by supporting their personal responses to their students. "It's time we went beyond coddling the fragile feelings of the autistic kids," said one of the teachers, validated by the faculty in her heroic efforts to reach these special children. "It's time we expected them to learn, just as we do the others." She liked them, so she could comfortably question overcoddling them. She could give them much more than affection. She knew love was not enough.

My observations at the public school suggested that its pedagogy, effective for the regular students, was remarkably effective in reaching the young autists. The slogan "No child left behind" applies to all children, autists included. Polly Morrice, the mother of an eleven-year-old autistic boy, writes that better remedies are needed for families with such a child: "[P]ublic schools should not be acting as emergency rooms for autistic children. . . . [Schools] need partners in the challenge of helping students with the disorder."[6] Morrice wants the federal government to reimburse schools for the costs of educating any child who is disabled, noting that currently only 17 percent of the cost is paid by the federal government, rather than the 40 percent required by law.

The public school I observed had devised an innovative curriculum implemented by competent teachers. It was funded generously enough to allow for ample space in which to teach and for ancillary teachers. Its principal had the luxury of speaking directly to her autistic students about, for example, what they'd done wrong and how they could behave differently next time. She did this with all the students in the school, as did the teachers with their students. And the autists knew it. They knew they were being treated like regular kids.

It's true that teachers don't routinely rub down students' backs nor do they help kids hold their pencils. But good teachers do attend to individual student needs to introduce them more effectively to the curriculum. They create a psychological space in which all students are likely to learn. This ambience extended to the autistic group, as teachers, aides, and specialists noted what seemed to work with their shy, often factious, intriguing but unconventional kids. The all-school policy embedded in the three *R*s posted in the principal's office and around the school—respect for self, for others, and for property— roused teachers and students, autists included, to maintain a classroom climate of learning and socializing.

The nature of the student–teacher conversations, the myriad contexts that offered a well-rounded education, the ease with which the teachers expressed their feelings about teaching and learning—these inspired the students as they struggled to learn.

The communications to autists in the classrooms I observed were clear and simple without being condescending or unnatural. Speaking with young autists is probably one of the most difficult tasks in helping them progress. For autists to learn how to use language more productively, what they hear us say must catch their attention and not appear labored. Yet, our words must be chosen with care, our language must be respectful and not too different from what we would say to any child.

When one of the teachers noticed her shy student's reluctance to take his place for a group lesson, she spoke softly and cogently to him as she said, "You're only thinking of where you should sit, not the lesson." This statement reminded me of the many times I had seemed to speak truisms to the autistic kids with whom I worked. For example, as I spoke with Gregory about his acting up in school, I found myself saying, "Your suspension upset your parents." Yet I knew my words had to appeal to him in order to assure his cooperation in a plan to reduce his antisocial behavior. And Greg seemed reminded of how much his parents cared about him, how often they'd gone to great lengths to help him. Likewise, the shy student who hesitated to take his seat could attend to his teacher's remark, because he evidently perceived little criticism in a statement that captured his predicament precisely. His teacher may have implied, "You can think about where to sit or you can think about the lesson." Then it was up to him to decide which came first.

Or, reconsider the teacher who helped her autistic student with a separation from school and classmates, when he was scheduled to take a trip just before school let out. Referring to the little troll he'd chosen as his traveling companion, she said to him, earnestly and carefully, "Every time you find it . . . you'll know that we are thinking of you," and "[I]t's your job to return it to your classroom." He could readily hear that his classmates cared about him and that his teacher entrusted him with the care of a classroom toy, an assignment that surely made him feel important and proud to fulfill.

However essential it is for young autists to receive special instruction in speech and communication, basic academic skills, drill in handwriting, and other subjects, it is also important for them to have access to a varied curriculum. Since many intelligent autists are gifted in the arts, a well-balanced program that offers art instruction, or just the opportunity for these kids to exercise their artistic skills and aesthetic urges, often softens the blow to their egos that derives from being behind academically or handicapped in some way. Similarly, the opportunity to write original stories about their experiences or to dictate them to their teachers and parents not only helps with language skills but gives them a forum in which to communicate meaningfully with another person. Music programs assist the musically gifted in expressing emotions connected to song and dance and also, according to experts who have used music therapy with autistic children, bond them with other musically competent people. Even those not musically inclined would benefit from music class as they learn to express their emotions through singing and to move their bodies in rhythm.

In the school I observed, the special gym program was also beneficial to the young autists, achieving its aims to improve their coordination and build muscle strength, and easing them into a freer kind of socializing. The gym exercises and games also freed their bodies, to create an atmosphere of relaxed enjoyment, which in turn encouraged the autistic boys to express their emotions to one another as they, for example, began to cheer and whoop excitedly when one of them hit a home run. These curricular successes came with minimal alterations in the program. The autistic boys met in the same room as the regular students and used the same equipment. The gym teacher's aim was the same: to help build and strengthen the bodies of the students, to help them refine their sports understanding, to become team players, to help them develop their ability to catch, bat, jump, and run.

If a teacher discusses her students' reactions to the learning materials, it helps them sort out their feelings about being taught. The autistic kids, too, are encouraged to sort their feelings as they listen to their peers' comments during a teacher-led discussion. In the school I observed, teachers went a step further. They would comment on their own feelings of elation or frustration, to be sure, within limits and when appropriate. They shared the students' excitement about a class skit, or they commiserated with kids about the hot weather or pages missing from a workbook. In essence, they would comment publicly on their own state of mind. Talking about one's mind helps kids learn over and over, again and again, about minds and the mind's theories. The view that autists cannot theorize depresses the mind's incentive to engage its own thoughts. It deprives autistic kids of the social stimulation that develops higher-order thinking.

The developmental orientation of the teachers in the school I observed helped particularly the young autists. Conversant with typical developmental gains at different ages, the teachers were able to track when these kids progressed, either spontaneously or through instruction. The ability to spot gains in understanding their peers or in academics enabled these teachers to adjust the curriculum to fit their students' conceptual level. In other words, they were primed to mark not just the failures of the students but also their developmental successes.

The teachers' orientation permitted me to discuss with them the consequences of any child becoming more aware of himself as a person, aware of himself in the company of others. While ordinary kids, for example, experience conflict over their affiliative and academic needs, often perceiving their simultaneous expression as incompatible, the same can be said of young autists, except that, unlike the regular kids, autists tend to give up much sooner when confronted with social dilemmas. They may prefer to stay the academic course without any regard whatsoever for the feelings of their companions.

As they become more aware of themselves and their predicaments, autistic kids will react to their greater self-understanding, sometimes auspiciously. They may try to help their classmates, as Gregory did when he coached them about biology. More important, though, is their clear understanding that they are different from their classmates, as well as their realization that, realistically, there are ways in which they can never match some of the achievements of their peers. They will recognize their social handicaps and that they must work extra hard to overcome them.

So far, so good. Being sensitive, they are nonetheless at risk for becoming unduly discouraged and despairing; they then sometimes resort to their customary autistic ways, concluding prematurely that if one is not the top student or the center of the social scene, one's very real achievements have little true value. It's important for teachers (and parents, friends, and neighbors) not to share this despondency but to realize that it's part of development to encounter new problems with new insights.

It's important to avoid viewing a temporary impasse as a permanent setback. If a young autist of nine or ten perceives more fully what his personality is like and the probable struggles he will encounter with schoolwork and befriending others, he may seem to roam two worlds simultaneously in an effort to maintain his inner, private world, lest the world of people fail him. This represents a realistic assessment of his condition and its uncertainties and should be acknowledged as such. For only with an accurate appraisal of his condition can he move beyond it. Our getting dispirited only strengthens his grasp on the private world he is so loathe to relinquish. Undue pessimism may convince him that he is, indeed, subject to a Sisyphean fate in which he is forever doomed to shove that monumental rock up the infinitely stretching mountain path, only to watch it tumble down carelessly, only to conclude that he must begin the meaningless, impossible task yet again.

Hopes for the autistic boys did surge among the faculty of the public school I visited, just as they did for the boys' parents. The teacher of the shy, reticent fourth-grader realized that her student had become more aware of his condition and his peers' personal reactions to him.

She was pleased by this development, just as she was by his friendly greeting after he'd moved on to the next grade.

A year later, on Valentine's Day, our bashful student was sitting off a little to the side, yet eyeing the festivities closely. His eyes began to mist, and he quietly excused himself to get a drink at a nearby water fountain. There he was able to compose himself sufficiently to return to his classmates, eyes clear and demeanor pleasant. He took his seat and waited patiently as the others talked excitedly among themselves.

No doubt he was wondering whether the other kids would give him valentines. He may even have guessed, accurately, that he wouldn't get many. But why would he estimate at all if he had no interest in, nor any idea of, his classmates' intentions? If he hadn't cared about the kids and their opinions, he would not have felt like crying.

Need I add that being nervous about the number of valentines received on this special day is a normal reaction? I believe it was, in part, the caring atmosphere of the school, its students, and faculty that prompted him, in return, to care about them. Not so incidentally, he had the foresight to divert attention from his upset by going to the water fountain to compose himself. His was not an autistic isolating behavior. It was a typical diversionary ruse that helped him cope with the events of a holiday, the theme of which specifically engages children's feelings about one another.

No matter how skillful and responsive we are to the autistic child's needs—and this school's faculty was remarkably sensitive to the shy boy's feelings—sometimes he seems, willy-nilly, to feel most protected when his world revolves solely around his own behavior. This is why it is so important to get across to him that he need not give up his world in which he is king. He need only try to be a more willing participant in our world.

Help Me

Autism is one of those human dilemmas that forces upon us a vigilant openmindedness to comprehend its ambiguities. When we try to uncover autism's enigmas, all too often we fail to probe its mysteries respectfully. Rather, we conclude that autistic individuals should be acting differently. The little "autist artist," the girl who reached for my arm to be led into the art room, should learn not to talk in opposites but to give her energies to taking turns. She should ask directly for her turn to paint rather than declare impassively, "No painting." Kanner's young patient, Donald, should speak as expected to his doctor, because language is what separates us from animals. He should shed his mysterious ellipsis and forthrightly answer the question, "What's ten minus four?" He should say, "Six," not "I'll draw a hexagon."

Autistic people are continually and not so subtly pressured to do or to be . . . what? Many are kind, intelligent, and earnest—even caring. After all, Temple Grandin did save Oliver Sacks's life! But this is not enough. They should join us more. They should *want* to join us more.

In our quantifying society, where we grasp ever more assiduously for the mythical norm, we have forgotten how to enjoy human differences. Measuring, labeling, and evaluating others have led us either to eschew human variation or to become alarmed by it. What could the twelve-year-old possibly have meant by typing SCBBCXZZZCBNJGHELP-MECZDFF? Couldn't he have just asked for help? Actually, no. By surrounding his plea with seemingly irrelevant random letters, he showed me just how difficult it was for him to communicate. The sibilants in his message intended to create in me the buzz of the noisy world he experienced, the very auditory stimulation that inhibited him from getting close to people. Although we haven't yet charted or graphed the inimitable human dimension typical of autistic people, it is very much there, attested to by parents, poets, artists, musicians, educators, and yes, even by psychotherapists. If only we would focus as much on the worked-with and lived-with child as we do on the theorized and tested child!

Being put off by the impertinence of indifferent autistic individuals, we perhaps exact an eye for an eye by proclaiming that neither can they be helped nor lived with. If so, we foreclose the opportunity to ask the vital question. In what special way are autistic people expressing their legitimate take on humanity? Helping young autists requires us to consider the lengths we can and must travel to honor their status as fellow humans. It requires that we make inner peace with undertaking such a challenge in the wake of theories that rob autistic people of their sensibilities. To disavow their human response is a revisitation of the original autistic experience in which little children slip away from us into their own venerated worlds. By objectifying them with labels, tests, experiments, and theories that state or imply that they lack human mentality, the world of people deserts them. Without this world, what chance do they have of bridging their world and ours?

Acknowledgments

I could not have written this book had I not learned to observe children's behavior. I owe a substantial debt to two renowned psychologists, one whom I knew well, the other whom I know through avidly reading his many works. Bruno Bettelheim taught me the importance of a child's every action, every word. Jean Piaget's meticulous accounts of children's behavior strengthened the covenant I made to note the minutest detail in what children do and say. The respect these two scholars showed young people impressed me as a student and even as I write: Bettelheim's for children's feelings and motives, and Piaget's for children's reasons, even as they differ from our own.

I am deeply grateful to Inge Fowlie, Mauri Formigoni, Lou Harper, and Shelton Key for our colloquies during my Orthogenic School days, for their direct help with my autistic charges, and for their emotional support as I tried to get through to these challenging children.

Many people read parts of this book during its various lives. I was lucky to have their hearty support, especially when my mind threatened to go blank. Special thanks to Mike McCone for reading early drafts and for recognizing their potential during the arduous process of bringing the book to completion. For their enthusiastic responses to the themes contained herein, I also thank Betty Lou Bradshaw, Ted Bradshaw, Elizabeth Colt, Mike Curtis, Addie DiIorio, Madeline Feingold, Elio Frattaroli, Dawn Prince-Hughes, Margot Griffin Kenney, Peg McKinlay, Dick McKinlay, Louise Rosenkrantz, Sharada Thompson, Karen Waltuck, and Bob Weiss.

Stan Berman, Gail Donovan, Bruce Feingold, J. J. Hanley, Tom Horton, Diana Grossman Kahn, Kathy Lubin, Dorothy Miller, Andrea Farkas Patenaude, Tsipa Peskin, Harvey Peskin, Jacqui Sanders, Richard Sens, Alice Shabecoff, Philip Shabecoff, Michael Thompson, and Fae Tyroler, each in his or her own way, hastened this book's progress. Thanks also to my agent, Theron Raines, for advocating the book over many years, for making valuable substantive suggestions, and for introducing me to the wonderful people at St. Martin's Press.

Myriad thanks to Diane Reverand, my editor at St. Martin's, whose infectious enthusiasm about the book kept me going during the hours I spent revising. Her simpatico editing and substantive commentary alerted me to better ways of writing and focused me more clearly on the themes I tried to illuminate.

Melissa Contreras of St. Martin's was graciously available to answer my every question and efficiently managed many important details up until the very last minute!

Thanks to Wah-Ming Chang, St. Martin's Press's production editor, for deciphering my handwriting and coordinating the many changes to the book, both editorial and substantive. Heartfelt thanks to Shea Kornblum, who designed the elegantly aesthetic book jacket that captures the profile of an autistic child perfectly.

Linda Witnov saved me from my awkward computer self by preparing countless drafts, leaving me free to think rather than wrestle with that machine. Thanks to Joe Zelan for getting the revisions on the computer (that machine, again!).

Special thanks to Kathy Carlson for brainstorming with me about the book's title and for suggesting one so apt.

Many loving thanks to Saul Zelan for setting me straight about the pediatrician's perspective on patients big and small, normal and troubled.

Many loving thanks to Jeana Zelan for her solicitous reading of portions of this book and for our many lively discussions on the pleasures of writing.

Muchas gracias con cariño to Liliana Ramirez-Cortes for cheering me on during the book's later stages.

I am enormously grateful to Kris Field for the vigorous and compassionate help she gave to this book. I am in her debt for listening to me rant and rave endlessly about writing impasses, for sharing my excitement when the ideas flowed and the writing took off, for reading drafts of the entire book, for convincing me that regular schools can serve autistic children resourcefully, and last, but decidedly not least, for introducing me to marvelously talented and dedicated teachers.

I will be forever indebted to my collaborator in mind and spirit, Joe Zelan, who appreciatively listened to me spin ideas on autism for over a decade, who encouraged me to "check up on the children" when I worked at the Orthogenic School, who attended to every detail and nuance in my writing, critiquing the good and the bad, winnowing the words and keeping the cadence. And for just being there.

Notes

Prologue

1. See Bettelheim's *Love Is Not Enough* (Free Press, 1950) and *The Empty Fortress* (Free Press, 1967) for a description of the staff's work with troubled youth. Bettelheim's *A Home for the Heart* (Knopf, 1974) details the Orthogenic School's structure and functioning.
2. Kanner, Leo. "Autistic Disturbances of Affective Contact," *Nervous Child* 2: 217–50.
3. Ozonoff, Sally, Geraldine Dawson, and James McPartland. *A Parent's Guide to Asperger Syndrome and High-Functioning Autism.* New York: Guilford, 2002.
4. Ibid., p. 64.
5. See Uta Frith's *Autism: Explaining the Enigma* (Cambridge, Massachusetts: Blackwell, 1989) and Bryna Siegel's *The World of the Autistic Child: Understanding and Treating Autistic Spectrum Disorders* (New York: Oxford University Press, 1996).
6. NPR's *All Things Considered*, March 2001.
7. "Panel Finds Earlier Autism Tests Will Lead to Better Treatment," *New York Times*, June 15, 2001.

Chapter One: The Diagnosis Is Not the Person

1. Siegel, Bryna. *The World of the Autistic Child: Understanding and Treating Autistic Spectrum Disorders.* New York: Oxford University Press, 1996, p. 9.
2. Misguided psychological and psychoanalytic attempts to help parents of autistic children are described in Catherine Maurice's *Let Me Hear Your Voice: A Fam-*

ily's Triumph over Autism (New York: Ballantine, 1993). Positive results for autists of behavioral training are reported by O. Ivar Lovaas ("Behavioral Treatment and Normal Educational and Intellectual Functioning in Young Autistic Children," *Journal of Consulting and Clinical Psychology* 55: 3–9, 1987; "Long-Term Outcome for Children with Autism Who Received Early Intensive Behavioral Treatment," *American Journal on Mental Retardation* 97: 359–384, 1993). Bernard Rimland reports on the effects of vitamin supplements in the quarterly publication of the *Autism Research Review International.* Additional information on the effects of vitamins on the autistic condition is provided by Eric Schopler and Gary B. Mesibov in *Neurobiological Issues in Autism* (New York: Plenum, 1987). The effect of psychotropic medication on her autistic son is described by Jane Taylor McDonnell in *News from the Border* (New York: Ticknor and Fields, 1993). The treatment of "hyperaudition" in her autistic daughter is recounted by Annabel Stehli in *The Sound of a Miracle* (New York: Avon, 1991). Theory of mind studies are described in Uta Frith, *Autism: Explaining the Enigma* (Cambridge, Massachusetts: Blackwell, 1989), and Simon Baron-Cohen, Helen Tager-Flusberg, and Donald J. Cohen (eds.), *Understanding Other Minds* (New York: Oxford, 1995).

3. Astington, Janet Wilde. *The Child's Discovery of the Mind.* Cambridge, Massachusetts: Harvard University Press, 1993.

4. Spurling, Hilary. *The Unknown Matisse: A Life of Henri Matisse, The Early Years, 1869–1908.* New York: Knopf, 1998, p. 46.

5. Bettelheim, Bruno. *The Empty Fortress.* New York: Free Press, 1967, p. 63.

6. Bohr, Niels. *Volume III: Essays 1958–1962 on Atomic Physics and Human Knowledge.* New York: Wiley, 1958. Bohr's relevance for psychology is discussed in Elio Frattaroli's *Healing the Soul in the Age of the Brain: Why Medication Isn't Enough* (New York: Penguin, 2002). Therein Frattaroli asserts Bohr's principle of complementarity—the necessary interaction between the observer and the observed—to be the "single most important [scientific] idea of the twentieth century" (p. 182).

7. Phillips, Adam. *Terrors and Experts.* Cambridge, Massachusetts: Harvard University Press, 1996, p. 90.

8. Asperger, Hans. "'Autistic Psychopathy' in Childhood." In Uta Frith (ed.), *Autism and Asperger Syndrome.* Cambridge, England: Cambridge University Press, 1991, p. 37.

9. The November 1998 *APA Monitor* cites additional studies in the search for the causes—or correlates—of autism. Scientists in recent years have identified "candidate genes" that might affect neurotransmitters or compromise the immune system to increase the risk of autism from viral infection. Moreover, research is under way to identify malfunctioning regions of the brain that could compromise language development in young autists.

10. Asperger, "Autistic Psychopathy," p. 90.

11. Kanner, Leo. "Autistic Disturbances of Affective Contact," *Nervous Child* 2: 217–250. Also Kanner's "Early Infantile Autism," *Journal of Pediatrics* 25: 211–217.

12. Park, Clara Claiborne. "Exiting Nirvana," *American Scholar* 67(2):28–42, p. 33.

13. TEACCH is a division of the School of Medicine at the University of North Carolina at Chapel Hill. The TEACCH program has developed structured teaching approaches that benefit students with autism (see Eric Schopler and Gary B. Mesibov, *Learning and Cognition in Autism*, New York: Plenum, 1995).

14. Lord, Catherine. "The Complexity of Social Behaviour in Autism." In Simon Baron-Cohen et al., *Understanding Other Minds*, p. 292.

15. Trevarthen, Colwyn, Kenneth Aitken, Despina Papoudi, and Jacqueline Robarts. *Children with Autism: Diagnosis and Interventions to Meet Their Needs*. Bristol, London: Jessica Kingsley, 1996, p. 169.

16. Siegel, Bryna. *The World of the Autistic Child*. New York: Oxford University Press, 1996, p. 86.

17. Deacon, Terence. *The Symbolic Species: The Co-evolution of Language and the Brain*. New York: Norton, 1997, p. 274.

18. For example, a British physician suggested in 1998 that the increase in reported cases of autism and the use of an updated MMR (measles, mumps, rubella) vaccine might be linked. Parents of autistic kids pressed researchers to determine whether there was an association. But a California study (reported in the *Journal of the American Medical Association*, March 7, 2001) found no correlation between the common childhood vaccine and rising cases of autism. Yet the parents' outcry for continuing investigation into the environmental triggers of autism could well result in some answers to questions that have vexed us for decades. In fact, a vocal group of parents of autistic children did continue to question the effects of the MMR vaccine. This led pediatrician Neal Halsey in 1999 to urge that vaccine manufacturers remove thimerosal from vaccinations given to children. An article, "The Not-So-Crackpot Autism Theory," in *The New York Times Magazine* (November 10, 2002, p. 69) concludes, "If the autism trend begins to recede now that thimerosal [a mercury-containing preservative] has been removed, it could certainly suggest a cause. If it does decline, we might have Neal Halsey to thank."

19. Frith, Uta (ed.). *Autism and Asperger Syndrome*. Cambridge, England: Cambridge University Press, 1991, p. 15.

20. Trevarthen et al., *Children with Autism*, p. 169.

21. Rimland, Bernard, "On Autism: An Interview," 1994, the Autism Research

Institute (pamphlet); the Autism Society of America, personal communication, 1997; Oliver Sacks, *An Anthropologist on Mars* (New York: Knopf, 1995), p. 247; "Understanding Autism," *Newsweek*, July 31, 2000.

22. The study was conducted by epidemiologist and pediatrician Robert S. Byrd of the University of California, Davis, and was reported in *The New York Times* ("Increase in Autism Baffles Scientists," October 18, 2002).

23. Ozonoff, Sally, Geraldine Dawson, and James McPartland. *A Parent's Guide to Asperger Syndrome and High-Functioning Autism.* New York: Guilford, 2002.

24. Siegel, *World of the Autistic Child*, p. 12.

25. Sacks, *Anthropologist on Mars*, p. 241.

26. We are told repeatedly that a large number of autistic individuals are mentally retarded. We must ask, though, by what means these individuals were so identified. If standard IQ tests were used to evaluate them, we'd do well to question the linkage of autism to mental retardation. A large number of autistic children are simply untestable by ordinary means. In fact, Oliver Sacks tells us that the talented autist Stephen Wiltshire earned a verbal IQ score of only 52 (ibid., p. 202). And it's entirely possible that some of the mentally retarded individuals showing autistic behaviors are not autistic at all. The overall mental deficiency of many mentally retarded individuals may be the cause of their autistic-like behavior, just as blind individuals often engage in seemingly autistic mannerisms because of their visual handicaps.

27. Dolnick, Edward. *Madness on the Couch: Blaming the Victim in the Heyday of Psychoanalysis.* New York: Simon & Schuster, 1998, p. 227.

28. Teitelbaum, Philip, Osnat Teitelbaum, Jennifer Nye, Joshua Fryman, and Ralph G. Maurer. "Movement Analysis in Infancy May Be Useful for Early Diagnosis of Autism." *Proceedings of the National Academy of Sciences* 95(23):13982–13987.

29. Lord, "Complexity of Social Behaviour."

30. Valenstein, Elliot S. *Blaming the Brain: The Truth about Drugs and Mental Health.* New York: Free Press, 1998, p. 134.

31. Gould, Stephen Jay. *The Mismeasure of Man.* New York: Norton, 1996, p. 186.

32. Grandin, Temple, and Margaret H. Scariano. *Emergence Labeled Autistic.* Novato, California: Arena, 1986, p. 25.

33. Bettelheim, *Empty Fortress*, p. 402.

34. Williams, Donna. *Nobody Nowhere.* New York: Times Books, 1992.

35. Williams, Donna. *Like Color to the Blind.* New York: Times Books, 1996.

36. Williams, Donna. *Somebody Somewhere.* New York: Times Books, 1996, p. 76.

37. McDonnell, Paul. *News from the Border*, pp. 367 and 376.
38. Sacks, Oliver. *Anthropologist on Mars*, p. 295.
39. Ibid.

Chapter Two: Gregory's Journey

1. In her interesting book on mothers and infants, *Mother Nature: A History of Mothers, Infants, and Natural Selection* (New York: Pantheon, 1999), primatologist Sarah Blaffer Hrdy discusses avoidant behavior in young children. She notes (quoting researcher Mary Main) that avoidance might be adaptive for infants in certain situations. So that their parents will continue to care for them, angry young children may employ "avoidance in the service of attachment" as they inhibit gazing at their caretakers (p. 523). Young autists, too, may use avoidant behavior adaptively when they are angry at not being understood or when they feel rejected. These withdrawn children may sense that they will have a better chance of avoiding parental displeasure if they prevent their parents from perceiving their anger or other negative emotions.

2. Grandin, Temple. *Thinking in Pictures: And Other Reports from My Life with Autism*. New York: Doubleday, 1995, p. 100.

Chapter Three: A Meeting of Minds

1. Frattaroli, Elio. *Healing the Soul in the Age of the Brain*, p. 146.

2. Coles, Robert. *The Mind's Fate: A Psychiatrist Looks at His Profession*. Boston: Little, Brown, 1995, p. 183.

3. Jarrold, Christopher, "Pretend Play in Autism: Executive Explanations," in James Russell (ed.), *Autism As an Executive Disorder*. Oxford, England: Oxford University Press, 1997.

4. In some instructions to parents filling out a family questionnaire, a behavioral pediatrician informs them, "Children do not have much insight into their own behavior, so the majority of the information is obtained from the parent and teacher inputs." Yet it is the *child* who is asked to change.

5. Trevarthen et al., *Children with Autism*, p. 136.

6. McDonnell, Jane Taylor, *News from the Border*; Catherine Maurice, *Let Me Hear Your Voice*; Russell Martin, *Out of Silence: A Journey into Language*. New York: Henry Holt, 1994.

7. In *Toward a Theory of Instruction* (Cambridge, Massachusetts: Harvard University Press, 1966), Jerome Bruner differentiates two learning styles, coping and defending. He contrasts a child's active attempt to learn school assignments with a child's need to defend himself against the feelings (panic, for example) that certain schoolwork may arouse in him. I am suggesting that, similarly, there may be two playing styles. Autistic children, who are confronted by their

own feelings while playing, may seek to defend themselves by disrupting their play or by avoiding playful activity entirely.

8. Bettelheim adapted psychoanalytic theory to shape the treatment milieu in which the Orthogenic School students lived.

9. McDonnell, Paul, Afterword to *News from the Border*.

10. Martin, *Out of Silence*, p. 236.

11. Kephart, Beth. *A Slant of Sun: One Child's Courage*. New York: Norton, 1998, p. 10.

12. Dirk had been given the Peabody Picture Vocabulary Test.

13. Williams, *Nobody Nowhere*, p. 4.

14. Ibid., pp. 20–21.

15. The idea that an autist might feel merged with another arose from a now out-dated view that the autistic condition is a form of childhood psychosis. This idea is discussed in Bruno Bettelheim's *The Empty Fortress* and in Margaret Mahler's "On Child Psychosis and Schizophrenia: Autistic and Symbiotic Infantile Psychoses," in *Psychoanalytic Study of the Child* 7:286–305. (New York: International Universities Press, 1952).

Chapter Four: I Can See Me in Your Eyes

1. Bettelheim, *Empty Fortress*, p. 17.

2. Williams, *Like Color to the Blind*, p. 10.

3. "Life in a Parallel World," *Newsweek*, May 13, 1996, p. 70.

4. Stacy may have avoided the personal pronoun "I" because of its association in her mind with the word "eye." In describing her relationship to her friend Ian, Donna Williams writes, "I looked deeply into his eyes with no 'I' within me with which to know me in relation to him" (*Like Color to the Blind*, p. 15). Likewise, in talking with Stacy I often felt that there was no "I" there, but even more often I felt this way with Marcia. One day I asked her, "What is so terrible about saying 'I'?" Marcia reacted by flushing and, pointing to her eyes, said irritably, "Eye, eye, eye." It was as though the homonymous linkage between "I" and "eye" should be obvious to anyone who wondered about her "I" evasion. She, like the little girl described in *Newsweek*, may have avoided saying "I"—to her mind, the same as saying "eye"—because she was afraid it signified looking at people, looking deeply into their eyes.

5. Stacy may have listened to the words of the song "Beyond the Sea" ("Somewhere, beyond the sea/She's there watching for me") and may have understood that it was about a person imagining a loved one waiting for him "beyond the sea." Initially she reacted overtly only to her homonymous association to the word "see" as she checked other people's eyes, as described on pp. 96–99.

6. Donna Williams opens her book *Nobody Nowhere* with accounts of her mother's impatience with and rage at young Donna.

7. Furth, Hans G. "Research with the Deaf: Implications for Language and Cognition." *Psychological Bulletin* 62:145–164, 1964.

Chapter Five: From Solitude to Sociability

1. Bettelheim, *Empty Fortress*, p. 17.
2. Park, *Siege*, p. 51.
3. Parents who brought their children to the Orthogenic School were asked to give an account of their child's early and recent history. Marcia's mother's report was given to a staffer other than me.
4. In his many books, David Elkind describes the adolescent's self-conscious comparisons between himself and others. See *Children and Adolescents: Interpretive Essays on Jean Piaget* (New York: Oxford University Press, 1981); *The Hurried Child: Growing Up Too Fast Too Soon* (Reading, Massachusetts: Addison-Wesley, 1981); *All Grown Up and No Place to Go: Teenagers in Crisis* (Reading, Massachusetts: Addison-Wesley, 1984).
5. Rimland, Bernard. "Treatments to Be Avoided." *Autism Research Institute Newsletter*, ARI publication, July 1993.

Chapter Six: Theory of Mind Problems

1. Frith, Uta. *Autism: Explaining the Enigma*. Cambridge, Massachusetts: Blackwell, 1989.
2. Williams, *Like Color to the Blind*, p. 15.
3. Frith, *Autism*, and Bruner, Jerome, and Carol Feldman, "Theories of Mind and the Problem of Autism," in Simon Baron-Cohen, Helen Tager-Flusberg, and Donald J. Cohen, *Understanding Other Minds: Perspectives from Autism* (New York: Oxford University Press, 1995.
4. Bruner and Feldman, ibid., pp. 282–283.
5. "A Gallery of Human Oddities Who Are, After All, Human," *New York Times*, 8/23/98, pp. 29–33.
6. "Blind to Other Minds," *Newsweek*, August 14, 1995, p. 67. The Sally–Anne test is described yet again in a later *Newsweek* article, this time in a feature story, "Understanding Autism" (July 31, 2000, p. 49).
7. Lord, Catherine. "The Complexity of Social Behavior in Autism," in Baron-Cohen et al., ibid.
8. Russell et al., ibid., pp. 296–297.
9. Ibid., p. 295.
10. Frith, *Autism*.
11. Sacks, *An Anthropologist on Mars*, p. 246.
12. Frith, *Autism*, p. 118.
13. Ibid.
14. Ibid., p. 175.

15. The *Oxford English Dictionary* (2d ed.), S.V. "telepathy."

16. Dunbar, Robin. *Grooming, Gossip, and the Evolution of Language.* Cambridge, Massachusetts: Harvard University Press, 1996, p. 88.

17. McDonnell, Paul. *News from the Border*, p. 331.

18. Ibid., p. 372.

19. Dunbar, *Grooming, Gossip*, p. 90.

20. Gardner, Howard. *Extraordinary Minds*. New York: Basic Books, 1997, p. 134.

21. Astington, Janet Wilde. *The Child's Discovery of the Mind*. Cambridge, Massachusetts: Harvard University Press, 1993, p. 2.

22. Sigman, Marian, and Lisa Capps. *Children with Autism*, p. 2.

23. Bruner, Jerome. *The Culture of Education*. Cambridge, Massachusetts: Harvard University Press, 1996, p. 100.

24. Ibid., p. 178.

25. Ibid., p. 177.

26. Bruner and Feldman, "Theories of Mind," p. 285.

27. Ibid., p. 285.

28. Dunbar, *Grooming, Gossip*, p. 99.

29. Bruner, *Culture of Education*, p. 179.

30. Deacon, Terence. *The Symbolic Species: The Co-Evolution of Language and the Brain*. New York: Norton, 1997, p. 274.

31. Bruner, *Culture of Education*, p. 179.

32. Grandin, *Thinking in Pictures*, p. 136.

33. Sacks, *Anthropologist on Mars*, p. 280.

34. Ibid., p. 287.

35. Dyson, Freeman. "The Scientist As Rebel," in *New York Review of Books*, May 1995, p. 33.

36. Ibid., p. 33.

37. Williams, *Nobody Nowhere*, p. 217.

Chapter Seven: Self-Revelations

1. Stern, Daniel. *The Interpersonal World of the Infant*. New York: Basic Books, 1985, p. 277.

2. Wendy agreed to let me write down her poem, which she had arranged with poetry-kit words. "You can have my poem," she said, "it's your poetry kit." I supplied the punctuation for the poem as the kit has none.

3. Bettelheim, *Empty Fortress*, p. 3.

4. Ibid. Bettelheim links self-knowledge to our knowledge of others: "If we wish to understand the human being in all his intricacy, we must fall back on the earliest method for comprehending man: to know oneself so that one may also

know the other. This is why a deficiency in self-knowledge means a deficiency in knowing the other."

5. Stern, *Interpersonal World*, p. 124.
6. Ibid., p. 140.
7. Maurice, *Let Me Hear Your Voice*.
8. McDonnell, *News from the Border*.
9. Kephart, *Slant of Sun*.
10. Maurice, *Let Me Hear Your Voice*, p. 185.
11. Ibid., p. 195.
12. Bettelheim, *Empty Fortress*, p. 179.
13. Grandin, *Thinking in Pictures*, p. 104.
14. Bettelheim interprets Marcia's statement on p. 201 of *The Empty Fortress*.
15. Bettelheim's view that Marcia wished to possess me is discussed on p. 207.
16. Stern, *Interpersonal World*, pp. 69–123.
17. Stacy learned the word "abominable" in conversation with me about her pretend people. When they were treating Stacy badly, I'd playfully say their behavior was abominable and tell them to stop bothering her. Then I'd hear my own voice as Stacy repeated my words and intonation, much like a little girl imitating her parents as she talks to her dolls.
18. Williams, *Nobody Nowhere*, pp. 10–11.
19. Ibid., p. 17.
20. Williams, *Somebody Somewhere*, p. 10.
21. Williams, *Nobody Nowhere* (author's note), p. xiv.
22. Bruner, *Culture of Education*, p. 177.
23. Freud, Sigmund. "Civilization and Its Discontents," in Peter Gay, *The Freud Reader*. New York: Norton, 1989, pp. 732–733.
24. Sendak, Maurice. *One Was Johnny*. New York: Harper & Row, 1962.
25. Russell, *Autism As an Executive Disorder*, p. 265.

Chapter Eight: Risking Friendships

1. Grandin, *Thinking in Pictures*, p. 132.
2. In many of his works Bettelheim remarked that those working with emotionally disturbed children could learn about their own suppressed desires by understanding the behavior and motives of their patients. Similarly, the Orthogenic School children learned about how people think by observing the behavior of others, autists included.
3. McDonnell, Paul, in Jane Taylor McDonnell, *News from the Border*, p. 363.
4. Grandin, Temple *Thinking in Pictures*, pp. 132, 133.
5. Eliot, George. *Adam Bede*. London: Penguin Books, 1859/1989, p. 313.
6. The dissociation of autistic individuals appears to arise from a generalized re-

sponse to the overstimulation they experience in the presence of other people. This is different from the dissociation that occurs as a result of specific traumatic experiences.

7. Psychoanalysts Donald Winnicott and Heinz Kohut have observed independently that the developing child actually benefits from the benign "mistakes" a parent makes. If the parents were always kind, always right, omniscient, and omnipresent, the child would never learn on his own, never become independent. Winnicott calls mothers "good enough" when they genuinely care for their children yet have their own lives ("Ego Distortion in Terms of True and False Self," in *The Maturational Processes and the Facilitating Environment.* New York: International Universities Press, 1965, pp. 37–55). Kohut refers to the ordinary, expected mistakes made by parents as "optimal failures" (*The Restoration of the Self.* New York: International Universities Press, 1977). These theories apply to relationships other than parent–child, notably intimate friendships, in which both partners gain from defining themselves in a supportive context that does not, however, always perfectly meet the partners' needs.

8. Grandin, *Thinking in Pictures*, p. 132.

9. Gopnik, Alison, Andrew N. Meltzoff, and Patricia K. Kuhl. *The Scientist in the Crib.* New York: William Morrow, 1999, p. 57. The three-year-olds Gopnik studied were shown a candy box, only to find that it held pencils. When asked about what they believed was in the box, they steadfastly insisted that they had always thought pencils were in the box, not candy. When one of Gopnik's students told the children, firmly, that they hadn't initially said pencils, that they had said the box held candy, the children changed their minds about what they believed. Could it be that the children were responding to an authority view, a knowing adult who could teach them about things, beliefs included? In the hide-and-seek game, Stacy learned from an older child, an authority of sorts. These events seem to reflect the impact of the teaching environment upon very young, normal children and upon an autistic child as well.

It should be noted that those in the autistic group described by Gopnik did not appear to possess a theory of mind. Yet it's difficult to evaluate this impression, since Gopnik asserts that "most people with autism are also mentally retarded" (p. 54). Unless we control for intelligence within the autistic group, we don't know whether the inability to understand false beliefs results from impoverished cognitive ability or from the autistic condition. Marian Sigman and Lisa Capps, authors of *Children with Autism: A Developmental Perspective*, state that the strongest predictors for the future of autistic children are their intellectual abilities and their language skills (Cambridge, Massachusetts: Harvard University Press, 1997, p. 144).

10. Ashton-Warner, Sylvia. *Teacher.* New York: Bantam, 1963. Ashton-Warner writes that she selects words from children's conversations to teach them in

reading lessons. She also uses a key vocabulary "common to any child in any race, a set of words . . . organically associated with the inner world," such as "Mommy," "Daddy," "kiss," and "scared." Eventually she helps them write sentences about themselves and their lives. It was this step that disconcerted Marcia and often made her angry. When I would suggest that she sequence the words meaningfully, she would avert her face, I thought at the time, to avoid revealing herself. But she may have wanted to write—that is, tell—about herself and her life not to me, but to her teacher!

11. By this time in Stacy's recovery I was able to intercept her assaults on others by standing between her and the intended victim or by firmly holding onto the object she was about to toss. This proved sufficient to defuse her anger and she'd soon back off, often retreating to repetitive activity (such as sorting like items into neat piles) until she brought her emotions under control. But when she was newly admitted to the Orthogenic School, I had to take her firmly by the hand, lead her into the hall, away from the others, and sit with her until she calmed down. At these times I often held her hands to prevent her from attacking me—or more simply, moved out of her reach so as to evade her attacks.

12. Williams, *Like Color to the Blind*, p. 8.

13. Yeats, W. B. "Per Amicus Silentia Lunae." *Mythologies*. London: Macmillan, 1959, p. 331.

14. Gardner, Howard. *The Unschooled Mind*. New York: Basic Books, 1991, p. 110.

Chapter Nine: School Days

1. In their book *Creative and Mental Growth* (New York: Macmillan, 1965) Viktor Lowenfeld and W. Lambert Brittain discuss the "schemas" in drawings of children who are about seven years old. The "human schema" appears after the child has experimented with artistic shapes, and it varies a great deal among individual children. A child's schema is often repeated across differing thematic renditions. The schema is no less than a stable "symbol" for the human figure. It is stable because it is conceptual.

2. Camus, Albert. *The Myth of Sisyphus*. New York: Vintage, 1991, p. 121.

Chapter Eleven: Hopes for Autistic Children

1. KQED radio, *Forum* with Michael Krasny, May 2000.

2. Luhrman, T. M. *Of Two Minds: The Growing Disorder in American Society*. New York: Knopf, 2000, p. 285.

3. Psychoanalyst Fred Pine has written of the benefit of therapist self-disclosure, especially during impasses with a patient (*Direction and Diversity in Psychoanalysis,* New Haven, Connecticut: Yale University Press, 1998). He notes the

uses of carefully worded and timed self-disclosing statements with troubled (but presumably nonautistic) adults.

4. Kephart, *Slant of Sun,* p. 77.

5. Many "failure to thrive" children may actually be autistic. When their caretakers attempt to feed them, autistic infants may refuse the food because of their overly sensitive reaction to a human presence.

6. Morrice, Polly. Op-Ed, *The New York Times,* December 11, 2002.

References

References with asterisks are child development books or books on children's learning.

*Ashton-Warner, Sylvia. *Teacher*. New York: Bantam, 1963.

Asperger, Hans, " 'Autistic Psychopathy' in Childhood." In Uta Frith (ed.), *Autism and Asperger Syndrome*. Cambridge, England: Cambridge University Press, 1991.

*Astington, Janet Wilde. *The Child's Discovery of the Mind*. Cambridge, Massachusetts: Harvard University Press, 1993.

Baron-Cohen, Simon, Helen Tager-Flusberg, and Donald J. Cohen. *Understanding Other Minds: Perspectives from Autism*. New York: Oxford University Press, 1993.

Bettelheim, Bruno. *Love Is Not Enough*. New York: The Free Press, 1950.

———. *The Empty Fortress*. New York: The Free Press, 1967.

———. *A Home for the Heart*. New York: Knopf, 1974.

Bohr, Niels. *Volume III: Essays 1958–1962 on Atomic Physics and Human Knowledge*. New York: John Wiley and Sons, 1958.

*Brazelton, T. Berry. *Families: Crisis and Caring*. Reading, Massachusetts: Addison-Wesley, 1989.

*Bruner, Jerome. *Toward a Theory of Instruction*. Cambridge, Massachusetts, Harvard University Press, 1966.

———. *The Culture of Education*. Cambridge, Massachusetts: Harvard University Press, 1996.

Bruner, Jerome, and Carol Feldman. "Theories of Mind and the Problem of Autism." In Simon Baron-Cohen et al., *Understanding Other Minds: Perspectives from Autism*. New York: Oxford University Press, 1993.

Camus, Albert. *The Myth of Sisyphus*. New York: Vintage, 1991.

Coles, Robert. *The Mind's Fate: A Psychiatrist Looks at His Profession*. Boston: Little, Brown and Company, 1995.

Deacon, Terence. *The Symbolic Species: The Co-evolution of Language and the Brain*. New York: Norton, 1997.

Dolnick, Edward. *Madness on the Couch: Blaming the Victim in the Heyday of Psychoanalysis*. New York: Simon & Schuster, 1998.

Dunbar, Robin. *Grooming, Gossip, and the Evolution of Language*. Cambridge, Massachusetts: Harvard University Press, 1996.

Dyson, Freeman. "The Scientist As Rebel," in *The New York Review of Books*, May 25, 1995.

Eliot, George. *Adam Bede*. London: Penguin Books, 1859/1989.

*Elkind, David. *Children and Adolescents*. New York: Oxford University Press, 1981.

———. *The Hurried Child*. Reading, Massachusetts: Addison-Wesley, 1981.

———. *All Grown Up and No Place to Go*. Reading, Massachusetts: Addison-Wesley, 1984.

Frattaroli, Elio. *Healing the Soul in the Age of the Brain: Why Medication Isn't Enough*. New York: Penguin, 2002.

Freud, Sigmund. "Civilization and Its Discontents." In Peter Gay, *The Freud Reader*. New York: Norton, 1989.

Frith, Uta. *Autism: Explaining the Enigma*. Cambridge, Massachusetts: Blackwell, 1989.

——— (ed.). *Autism and Asperger Syndrome*. Cambridge, England; Cambridge University Press, 1991.

Furth, Hans G. "Research with the Deaf: Implications for Language and Cognition." *Psychological Bulletin* 62:145–164, 1964.

*Gardner, Howard. *The Unschooled Mind*. New York: Basic Books, 1991.

———. *Extraordinary Minds*. New York: Basic Books, 1997.

*Gopnik, Alison, Andrew N. Meltzoff, and Patricia K. Kuhl. *The Scientist in the Crib: Minds, Brains, and How Children Learn*. New York: William Morrow, 1999.

Gould, Stephen Jay. *The Mismeasure of Man*. New York: Norton, 1996.

Grandin, Temple. *Thinking in Pictures: And Other Reports from My Life with Autism*. New York: Doubleday, 1995.

Grandin, Temple, and Margaret M. Scariano. *Emergence Labeled Autistic*. Novato, California: Arena, 1986.

*Holt, John. *How Children Fail*. New York: Perseus, 1995.

Hrdy, Sarah Blaffer. *Mother Nature: A History of Mothers, Infants, and Natural Selection*. New York: Pantheon, 1999.

Jarrold, Christopher. "Pretend Play in Autism: Executive Explanations." In James Russell (ed.), *Autism As an Executive Disorder*. Oxford, England: Oxford University Press, 1997.

Kanner, Leo. "Autistic Disturbances of Affective Contact." *Nervous Child*. 2:217–250, 1943.

———. "Early Infantile Autism." *Journal of Pediatrics* 25:211–217, 1944.

Kephart, Beth. *A Slant of Sun: One Child's Courage*. New York: Norton, 1998.

Kohut, Heinz. *The Restoration of the Self*. New York: International Universities Press, 1977.

Lord, Catherine. "The Complexity of Social Behavior in Autism." In Simon Baron-Cohen et al. *Understanding Other Minds: Perspectives from Autism*. New York: Oxford University Press, 1993.

Lovaas. I. Ovar. "Behavioral Treatment and Normal Educational and Intellectual Functioning in Young Autistic Children." *Journal of Consulting and Clinical Psychology* 55:3–9, 1987.

———. "Long-Term Outcome for Children with Autism Who Received Early Intensive Behavioral Treatment." *American Journal on Mental Retardation* 97:359–384, 1993.

*Lowenfeld, Viktor, and W. Lambert Brittain. *Creative and Mental Growth*. New York: Macmillan, 1965.

Mahler, Margaret. "On Child Psychosis and Schizophrenia: Autistic and Symbiotic Infantile Psychoses." In *The Psychoanalytic Study of the Child*: vol. 7, pp. 286–305. New York: International Universities Press, 1952.

Martin, Russell. *Out of Silence: A Journey into Language*. New York: Henry Holt, 1994.

Maurice, Catherine. *Let Me Hear Your Voice*. New York: Ballantine, 1993.

McDonnell, Jane Taylor. *News from the Border*. New York: Ticknor and Fields, 1993.

McDonnell, Paul. Afterword to *News from the Border*. New York: Ticknor and Fields, 1993.

Oxford English Dictionary (Second Edition, on Compact Disc).

*Ozonoff, Sally, Geraldine Dawson, and James McPartland. *A Parent's Guide to Asperger Syndrome and High Functioning Autism*. New York: Guilford, 2002.

Park, Clara Claiborne. *The Siege: The First Eight Years of an Autistic Child*. Boston: Little, Brown and Company, 1982.

Park, Clara Claiborne. "Exiting Nirvana." *The American Scholar*, Spring 1998, pp. 28–43.

———. *Exiting Nirvana*. Boston: Little, Brown and Company, 2001.

Phillips, Adam. *Terrors And Experts*. Cambridge, Massachusetts: Harvard University Press, 1996.

Pine, Fred. *Direction and Diversity in Psychoanalysis*. New Haven: Yale University Press, 1998.

Rimland, Bernard. *Autism Research Review International* (quarterly publication).

———. *Autism Research Institute Newsletter*.

Russell, James (ed.). *Autism As an Executive Disorder*. Oxford, England: Oxford University Press, 1997.

Russell, John. *Matisse: Father And Son*. New York: Abrams, 1999.

Sacks, Oliver. *An Anthropologist on Mars*. New York: Knopf, 1995.

Schopler, Eric, and Gary B. Mesibov (eds.), *Neurobiological Issues in Autism*. New York: Plenum Press, 1987.

———. *Learning and Cognition in Autism*. New York: Plenum Press, 1995.

Sendak, Maurice. *One Was Johnny*. New York: Harper & Row, 1962.

*Siegel, Bryna. *The World of the Autistic Child: Understanding and Treating Autistic Spectrum Disorders*. New York: Oxford University Press, 1996.

*Sigman, Marian, and Lisa Capps. *Children with Autism: A Developmental Perspective*. Cambridge, Massachusetts: Harvard University Press, 1997.

Spurling, Hilary. *The Unknown Matisse: A Life of Henri Matisse, The Early Years, 1869–1908*. New York: Knopf, 1999.

Stehli, Annabel. *The Sound of a Miracle*. New York: Avon, 1991.

*Stern, Daniel. *The Interpersonal World of the Infant*. New York: Basic Books, 1985.

Teitelbaum, Philip, Osnat Teitelbaum, Jennifer Nye, Joshua Fryman, and Ralph G. Maurer. "Movement Analysis in Infancy May Be Useful for Early Diagnosis of Autism." *Proceedings of the National Academy of Sciences* 23:13982–13987, 1995.

Trevarthen, Colwyn, Kenneth Aitken, Despina Papoudi, and Jacqueline Robarts. *Children with Autism: Diagnosis and Interventions to Meet Their Needs*. London: Jessica Kingsley, 1996.

Valenstein, Elliot S. *Blaming the Brain: The Truth About Drugs and Mental Health*. New York: The Free Press, 1998.

Williams, Donna. *Nobody Nowhere*. New York: Times Books, 1992.

———. *Somebody Somewhere*. New York: Times Books, 1996.

———. *Like Color to the Blind*. New York: Times Books, 1996.

Winnicott, D. W. "Ego Distortion in Terms of True and False Self." In *The Maturational Processes and the Facilitating Environment*. New York: International Universities Press, 1965.

Yeats, William Butler. "Per Amicus Silentia Lunae." *Mythologies*. London: Macmillan, 1959.

Index